T0188429

Intermittent Demand Forecasting

Intermittent Demand Forecasting

Context, Methods and Applications

John E. Boylan
Lancaster University
Lancaster, UK

Aris A. Syntetos
Cardiff University
Cardiff, UK

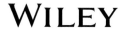

This edition first published 2021
© 2021 John Wiley & Sons Ltd

The right of John E. Boyan and Aris A. Syntetos to be identified as the authors of this work has been asserted in accordance with law.

Registered Offices
John Wiley & Sons, Inc., 111 River Street, Hoboken, NJ 07030, USA
John Wiley & Sons Ltd, The Atrium, Southern Gate, Chichester, West Sussex, PO19 8SQ, UK

Editorial Office
9600 Garsington Road, Oxford, OX4 2DQ, UK

For details of our global editorial offices, customer services, and more information about Wiley products visit us at www.wiley.com.

Wiley also publishes its books in a variety of electronic formats and by print-on-demand. Some content that appears in standard print versions of this book may not be available in other formats.

Library of Congress Cataloging-in-Publication Data applied for

ISBN 978-1-119-97608-0 (hardback); LCCN - 2021011006

Cover Design: Wiley
Cover Image: Mata Atlantica - Atlantic Forest in Brazil © FG Trade/Getty Images, Turbine © Brasil2/Getty Images

Set in 9.5/12.5pt STIXTwoText by SPi Global, Chennai, India
Printed and bound by CPI Group (UK) Ltd, Croydon, CR0 4YY

C9781119976080 _120521

For Jan and Rachel

Contents

Preface

The images on the front of this book highlight a crucial tension for all advanced economies. There is a desire to travel more and consume more, but also a growing awareness of the detrimental effects that this is having on the environment. There is a belated realisation that those of us living in countries with developed economies need to consume less and waste less.

Waste can occur at all stages of the supply chain. Consumers may buy food they never eat or clothes they never wear. Retailers and wholesalers may order goods from manufacturers that never sell. These wastages can be significantly reduced by better demand forecasting and inventory management. Some items conform to regular demand patterns and are relatively easy to forecast. Other items, with irregular and intermittent demand patterns, are much harder.

Wastage can be addressed by changes in production, moving away from built-in obsolescence and towards products that can be maintained and repaired economically. For this to be an attractive proposition, spare parts need to be readily available. Unfortunately, these items are often the most difficult to forecast because many of them are subject to the sporadic nature of intermittent demand. Although there have been significant advances in intermittent demand forecasting over recent decades, these are not all available in commercial software. In the final chapter of this book, we highlight the progress that has been made, including methods that are freely available in open source software.

The reasons for the slow adoption of new forecasting methods and approaches in commercial software are varied. We believe that one of the reasons is a lack of appreciation of the benefits that may accrue. Because intermittent demand items are so difficult to forecast, it may be thought that *highly accurate* forecasting methods can never be found. This may be true. However, it is possible to find *more accurate* methods, which can contribute towards significant improvements in inventory management.

There is also a need for greater awareness of the methods that have been developed in recent years. Information on them is scattered amongst a variety of academic journals, and some of the articles are highly technical. Therefore, we have set ourselves the challenge of synthesizing this body of knowledge. We have endeavoured to bring together the main strands of research into a coherent whole, and assuming no prior knowledge of the subject.

There are various perspectives from which demand forecasting can be addressed. One option would be to take an operations management view, with a focus on forecasting and planning processes. Another would be to take a more statistical perspective, starting with mathematical models and working through their properties. While some of our material has been influenced by these orientations, the dominant perspective of this book is that of operational research (OR). The start point of OR should always be the real-life situation that is encountered. This means that it is essential to gain an in-depth understanding of inventory systems and how forecasts inform these decisions. Such an appreciation enables a sharper focus on forecasting requirements and the appropriate criteria for a 'good forecast'.

In this book, the first three chapters focus on the inventory management context in which forecasting occurs, including the inventory policies and the service level measures that are appropriate for intermittent demand. Recognising the interconnection between inventory policies, demand distributions, and forecasting methods, the next two chapters focus on demand distributions, including evidence from studies of real-world data. The following two chapters concentrate on forecasting methods, with discussion of practical issues that must be addressed in their implementation. We then turn to the linkage between forecasts and inventory availability, and review how forecast accuracy should be measured and how its implications for inventories should be assessed. We also look at how stock keeping units should be classified for forecasting purposes, and examine methods designed specifically to address maintenance and obsolescence. The next two chapters deal with methods that can tackle more challenging demand patterns. We conclude with a review of forecasting software requirements and our views on the way forward.

We are grateful to those pioneers who inspired us to study this subject, and who have given us valuable advice over the years, especially John Croston, Roy Johnston, and Tom Willemain. We would like to express our thanks to those who commented on draft chapters of this book: Zied Babai, Stephen Disney, Robert Fildes, Thanos Goltsos, Matteo Kalchschmidt, Stephan Kolassa, Nikos Kourentzes, Mona Mohammadipour, Erica Pastore, Fotios Petropoulos, Dennis Prak, Anna-Lena Sachs, and Ivan Svetunkov; and to Nicole Ayiomamitou and Antonis Siakallis who helped with the figures.

Lancaster and Cardiff

January 2021

John E. Boylan

Aris A. Syntetos

Glossary

ADIDA	aggregate–disaggregate intermittent demand approach
AIC	Akaike information criterion
AR	autoregressive
ARIMA	autoregressive integrated moving average
ARMA	autoregressive moving average
APE	absolute percentage error
BO	backorder
BoM	bill of materials
BS	Brier score
CDF	cumulative distribution function
CFE	cumulative forecast error
CSL	cycle service level (all replenishment cycles)
CSL$^+$	cycle service level (replenishment cycles with some demand)
CV	coefficient of variation
EDF	empirical distribution function
ERP	enterprise resource planning
FMECA	failure mode, effects, and criticality analysis
FR	fill rate
FSS	forecast support system
FVA	forecast value added
HES	hyperbolic exponential smoothing
INAR	integer autoregressive
INARMA	integer autoregressive moving average
INMA	integer moving average
IP	inventory position
KS	Kolmogorov–Smirnov (test)
LTD	lead-time demand
MA	moving average
MAD	mean absolute deviation
MAE	mean absolute error
MAPE	mean absolute percentage error
MAPEFF	mean absolute percentage error from forecast
MASE	mean absolute scaled error

ME	mean error
MMSE	minimum mean square error
MPE	mean percentage error
MPS	master production schedule
MRO	maintenance, repair, and operations
MRP	material requirements planning
MSE	mean square error
MSOE	multiple source of error
MTO	make to order
MTS	make to stock
NBD	negative binomial distribution
NN	neural network
NOB	non-overlapping blocks
OB	overlapping blocks
OUT	order up to
PIS	periods in stock
PIT	probability integral transform
RMSE	root mean square error
rPIT	randomised probability integral transform
S&OP	sales and operations planning
SBA	Syntetos–Boylan Approximation (method)
SBC	Syntetos–Boylan–Croston (classification)
SCM	supply chain management
SES	single (or simple) exponential smoothing
SKU	stock keeping unit
SLA	service level agreement
SMA	simple moving average
sMAPE	symmetric mean absolute percentage error
sMSE	scaled mean square error
SOH	stock on hand
SOO	stock on order
SSOE	single source of error
TSB	Teunter–Syntetos–Babai (method)
VZ	Viswanathan–Zhou (method)
WMH	Wright Modified Holt (method)
WSS	Willemain–Smart–Schwarz (method)

About the Companion Website

This book is accompanied by a companion website.

www.wiley.com/go/boylansyntetos/intermittentdemandforecasting

This website includes:
- Datasets (with accompanying information)
- Links to R packages

1

Economic and Environmental Context

1.1 Introduction

Demand forecasting is the basis for most planning and control activities in any organisation. Unless a forecast of future demand is available, organisations cannot commit to staffing levels, production schedules, inventory replenishment orders, or transportation arrangements. It is demand forecasting that sets the entire supply chain in motion.

Demand will typically be accumulated in some pre-defined 'time buckets' (periods), such as a day, a week, or a month. The determination of the length of the time period that constitutes a time bucket is a very important decision. It is a choice that should relate to the nature of the industry and the volume of the demand itself but it may also be dictated by the IT infrastructure or software solutions in place. Regardless of the length of the time buckets, demand records eventually form a time series, which is a sequence of successive demand observations over time periods of equal length.

On many occasions, demand may be observed in every time period, resulting in what is sometimes referred to as 'non-intermittent demand'. Alternatively, demand may appear sporadically, with no demand at all in some periods, leading to an intermittent appearance of demand occurrences. Should that be the case, contribution to revenues is naturally lower than that of faster-moving demand items. Intermittent demand items do not attract much marketing attention, as they will rarely be the focus of a promotion, for example. However, they have significant cost implications for a simple reason: there are often many of them!

Service or spare parts are very frequently characterised by intermittent demand patterns. These items are essentially components or (sub-) assemblies contributing to the build-up of a final product. However, they face 'independent demand', which is demand generated directly from customers, rather than production requirements for a particular number of units of the final product. In the after-sales environment (or 'aftermarket'), we deal exclusively with 'independent demand' items. Service parts facing intermittent demand may represent a large proportion of an organisation's inventory investment. In some industries, this proportion may be as high as 60% or 70% (Syntetos 2011). The management of these items is a very important task which, when supported by intelligent inventory control mechanisms, may yield dramatic cost reductions.

Intermittent Demand Forecasting: Context, Methods and Applications, First Edition.
John E. Boylan and Aris A. Syntetos.
© 2021 John Wiley & Sons Ltd. Published 2021 by John Wiley & Sons Ltd.
Companion Website: www.wiley.com/go/boylansyntetos/intermittentdemandforecasting

Industries that rely heavily on after-sales support, including the automotive, IT, and electronics sectors, are dominated by intermittent demand items. The contributions of the after-sales services to the total revenues of organisations in these industries have been reported to be as high as 60% (Johnston et al. 2003). This signifies an opportunity not only to reduce costs but also to increase revenues through a careful balancing of keeping enough in stock to satisfy customers but not so much as to unnecessarily increase inventory investments. There are tremendous economic benefits that may be realised through the reappraisal of managing intermittent demand items.

There are also significant environmental benefits to be realised by such a reappraisal. Because of their inherent slow movement, intermittent demand items are at the greatest risk of obsolescence. The problem is exacerbated by the greatly reduced product life cycles in modern industry. This affects the planning process for all intermittent demand items (both final products and spare parts used to sustain the operation of final products). Better forecasting and inventory decisions may reduce overall scrap and waste. Furthermore, the sustained provision of spare parts may also reduce premature replacement of the original equipment.

The area of intermittent demand forecasting has been neglected by researchers and practitioners for too long. From a business perspective, this may be explained in terms of the lack of focus on intermittent demand items by the marketing function of organisations. However, the tough economic conditions experienced from around 2010 onwards have resulted in a switch of emphasis from revenue maximisation to cost minimisation. This switch repositions intermittent demand items as the focus of attention in many companies, as part of the drive to dramatically cut down costs and remain competitive. In addition, the more recent emergence of the after-sales business as a major determinant of companies' success has also led to the recognition of intermittent demand forecasting as an area of exceptional importance.

Following a seminal contribution in this area by John Croston in 1972, intermittent demand forecasting received very little attention by researchers over the next 20 years. This was in contrast to the extensive research conducted on forecasting faster-moving demand items. Research activity grew rapidly from the mid-1990s onwards, and we have now reached a stage where a comprehensive body of knowledge, both theoretical and empirical, has been developed in this area. This book aims to provide practitioners, students, and academic researchers with a single point of reference on intermittent demand forecasting. Although there are considerable openings for further advancements, the current state of knowledge offers organisations significant opportunities to improve their intermittent demand forecasting. Numerous reports, to be discussed in more detail later in this chapter, indicate that intermittent demand forecasting is one of the major problems facing modern organisations. Specialised software packages offer some forecasting support to companies but they often lag behind new developments. There are great benefits that have not yet been achieved in this area, and we hope that this book will make a contribution towards their realisation.

There are three main audiences for this book:

1. Supply chain management (SCM) practitioners, broadly defined, who wish to realise the full benefits of managing intermittent demand items.

2. Software designers wanting to incorporate new developments in forecasting into their software.
3. Students and academics wishing to learn and incorporate into their curricula, respectively, the state of the art in intermittent demand forecasting.

In summary, business pressures to reduce costs and environmental pressures to reduce scrap (often introduced in the form of prescribed policies imposed by national governments or the EU for example) render intermittent demand items, and forecasting their requirements, one of the most important areas in modern organisations.

There are great benefits associated with forecasting intermittent demand more accurately, and those benefits are far from being realised. This may be explained by the well reported innovation–adoption gap, which arises from the divergence between innovations and real-world practices. Organisational practices typically lag behind software developments, and software developments typically lag behind the state of the art in the academic literature. It is the aim of this book to bridge these gaps and show how intelligent intermittent demand forecasting may result in significant economic and environmental benefits.

In the remainder of this chapter, we first discuss in more detail the potential benefits that may be realised through improved intermittent demand forecasting. We then provide an overview of the current state of supply chain software packages and enterprise resource planning (ERP) solutions with regard to intermittent demand forecasting. This is followed by a section where we elaborate on both the structure of this book and the perspective that we take regarding the material presented here. We close with a summary of the chapter.

1.2 Economic and Environmental Benefits

Intermittent demand for products appears sporadically, with some time periods showing no demand at all. Moreover, when demand occurs, the demand size may be constant or variable, perhaps highly so, leading to what is often termed 'lumpy demand'. Later in this chapter, we discuss why forecasting sporadic and lumpy demand patterns is a very difficult task. Specific characterisations of intermittent demand series are considered in detail in Chapters 4 and 5.

1.2.1 After-sales Industry

Intermittent demand items dominate service and repair parts inventories in many industries (Boylan and Syntetos 2010). A survey by Deloitte Research (2006) benchmarked the service businesses of many of the world's largest manufacturing companies with combined revenues reaching more than $1.5 trillion; service operations accounted for an average of 25% of revenues. In addition to their contribution to revenues, these items present a distinct opportunity for cost reductions. Maintenance, repair, and operations (MRO) inventories typically account for as much as 40% of the annual procurement budget (Donnelly 2013). Increased revenues and reduced costs naturally lead to increased profits. Many organisations have repeatedly testified to the importance of after-sales services for their businesses and the profits they generate. Companies such as Beretta, Canon, DAF Trucks, Electrolux, EPTA, GE Oil & Gas, and Lavapiu have reported contributions of the after-sales services to their total profit of up to 50% (Syntetos 2011). Comparable numbers have been reported by Gaiardelli et al. (2007), Kim et al. (2007), and Glueck et al. (2007), while after-sales service has been identified as a key profit lever in the manufacturing sector (Manufacturing Management 2018).

Intermittent demand items are at the greatest risk of obsolescence. Many case studies (e.g. Molenaers et al. 2012) have documented large proportions of 'dead' (obsolete) stock in a variety of industries, with serious environmental implications. However, under-stocking situations may be as harmful, given the potentially high criticality of the items involved. In civil aviation, for example, lack of spare parts is one of the major causes of 'aircraft on ground' events (problems serious enough to prevent aircraft from flying). Badkook (2016) found that a quarter of the aircraft in an (un-named) airline's Boeing 777 fleet were affected by such aircraft on ground events over a year.

1.2.2 Defence Sector

Defence inventories, which are highly reliant on spare parts, have been repeatedly identified as a high risk area with a direct impact on a nation's economy. In the United States for example, the Department of Defense (DoD) manages around five million secondary items. These include repairable components, subsystems, assemblies, consumable repair parts, and bulk items. They reported that, as of September 2017, the value of the inventory was $93 billion (GAO 2019). Although a matter of concern, there had been no substantial reductions in inventory values over the previous decade (being, for example, $95 billion in 2013 and 2010; GAO 2012, 2015).

A major determinant of the performance of an inventory system is the forecasting method(s) being used to predict demand. Inaccurate forecasts lead to either excess inventory or shortfalls, depending on the direction of the forecast error. Over-forecasting can lead to holding stocks that are simply not needed. According to the US Government Accountability Office (GAO 2011, p. 11), 'Our recent work identified demand forecasting as the leading reason why the services and DLA [Defense Logistics Agency] accumulate excess inventory'.

Unfortunately, progress in improving forecasting and inventory management has been slow in many industries, with the defence industry being a case in point. The GAO of the United States reported, 'Since 1990, we have identified DoD [Department of Defense] supply chain management as a high-risk area due in part to ineffective and inefficient inventory management practices and procedures, weaknesses in accurately forecasting the demand for spare parts, and other supply chain challenges. Our work has shown that these factors have contributed to the accumulation of billions of dollars in spare parts that are excess to current needs' (GAO 2015, p. 2). Progress in inventory management has been made since then, especially with regard to the visibility of physical inventories, receipt processing, and cargo tracking (GAO 2019). These improvements in information systems have led to inventory management being removed from the list of high-risk areas. However, it is notable that no claims have yet been made for corresponding improvements in demand forecasting.

1.2.3 Economic Benefits

Moving beyond the after-sales industry, and the defence sector, we now examine the potential benefits that may result from intelligent intermittent demand forecasting for the wider economy. Purchased goods inventories and their management are significant concerns for firms wishing to remain competitive and survive in the marketplace. According to the 26th Annual State of Logistics report (CSCMP 2015, statistics referring to 2014), the United States alone has been sitting on approximately $2 trillion worth of goods held for sale. According to the same report, the inventory carrying costs (taxes, obsolescence, depreciation, and insurance) are estimated to be around $0.5 trillion (i.e. about 25% of the value of the goods). The total value of inventory was equivalent to approximately 14% of the US gross domestic product (GDP) in 2014. Although similar statistics have not been given in subsequent publications, the 30th Annual State of Logistics Report (CSCMP 2019) revealed that inventory carrying costs in the United States increased by 14.8% between 2014 and 2018.

These figures show that a huge amount of capital is tied up in warehouses. They also indicate that small improvements in managing inventories may be translated into considerable cost benefits. We should, therefore, not be surprised to learn that firms, from manufacturing to wholesale to retail, are currently intensifying their search for more efficient and effective inventory management approaches. Their aim is to minimise not only their direct investments in purchased goods inventory but also the indirect cost incurred in managing this inventory. In a make to stock (MTS) environment (discussed in Section 1.4.2), if there is no decoupling in terms of the ownership and location of the inventories, then these indirect costs become more significant the longer the stock remains unsold. The high volumes of stocks of intermittent demand items, and their high risk of obsolescence, should put them very high up the list of priorities for modern businesses.

1.2.4 Environmental Benefits

Obsolescence is a very important topic for supply chain management. The complexity of supply chains, in conjunction with increasingly reduced product life cycles, is resulting in high levels of obsolescence. Molenaers et al. (2012) discussed a case study where 54% of the parts stocked at a large petrochemical company had seen no demand for the last five years. Syntetos et al. (2009b) evaluated the inventory practices employed in the European spare parts logistics network of a Japanese manufacturer. They found one case, reported in Sweden, where some parts in stock had not 'moved' at all over the preceding 10 years. The value of the on-hand excess (spare parts) inventory of the US Air Force, Navy, and Army has been estimated to be of $1.7 billion, $1.4 billion, and $2.5 billion, respectively (GAO 2015). Much of this excess stock is at risk of obsolescence.

When obsolescent (or 'dead') stock is created, there is considerable environmental waste. Firstly, there is an environmental cost associated with producing goods that are never used. Secondly, there are environmental costs of transporting these goods to national, regional, or local stocking points. Finally, there are environmental costs of disposing of these stocks. The prevention of the accumulation of dead stock relies on accurate demand forecasts. Consequently, more accurate and robust forecasting methods may be translated to significant reductions in wastage or scrap, with considerable environmental benefits.

1.2.5 Summary

More accurate forecasting of intermittent demand presents organisations with a distinct opportunity to reduce costs and address major issues on their environmental agenda. In the after-sales context, intelligent intermittent demand forecasting is of paramount importance, as many items have demand patterns that are intermittent in nature. Other inventory settings that are dominated by spare parts (e.g. the military, public utilities, and aerospace) would also benefit directly from more accurate intermittent demand forecasting methods.

1.3 Intermittent Demand Forecasting Software

Given the relevance of intelligent forecasting methods in modern organisations, it is vital that they are included in software solutions. The continuous update of software to reflect research developments in the area of intermittent demand forecasting is of great financial and environmental importance. Forecasting software solutions are briefly reviewed in this section and revisited in greater detail in Chapter 15.

1.3.1 Early Forecasting Software

Early forecasting software solutions in the 1950s and 1960s were based on single exponential smoothing (SES) (a method that is discussed in detail in Chapter 6), meaning that intermittent demand items were not treated any differently from fast-moving items. SES is a method devised for fast-moving items that exhibit no trend or seasonality. It is a very practical forecasting method for these items, and is included in the vast majority of (inventory) forecasting software applications. It is still used for intermittent demand, although we shall see in Chapter 6 that it is not a natural method for these items and it does suffer from some major weaknesses.

1.3.2 Developments in Forecasting Software

Software packages have since moved on, with most, but not all, packages offering methods that are designed for intermittent demand. Croston's (1972) method, for example, was developed specifically for intermittent demand items, and is incorporated in statistical forecasting software packages (e.g. Forecast Pro), and demand planning modules of component based enterprise and manufacturing solutions (e.g. Industrial and Financial Systems, IFS AB). It is also included in integrated real-time sales and operations planning processes (e.g. SAP Advanced Planning and Optimisation [SAP APO] and SAP Digital Manufacturing).

Similarly, more recent developments in demand categorisation (rules that distinguish between various types of demand patterns and signify when a pattern should be treated as intermittent) have also been adopted in some commercial software (e.g. Blue Yonder, Syncron International), allowing their clients the capability to achieve some dramatic inventory cost reductions (Research Excellence Framework 2014). However, the adoption of recent developments has not been widespread, and there are many software packages that have limited functionality. Overall, there have been rather minor improvements in commercial software since around 2000 despite some major improvements in empirically tested theory since that time.

1.3.3 Open Source Software

Another important development, to be discussed in detail in Chapter 15, is the availability of open source software of recently proposed intermittent demand forecasting methods. This enables companies to incorporate them in their own in-house developed solutions, or for commercial software companies to extend their repertoire of methods more readily. Furthermore, sophisticated database systems are enabling companies to 'slice and dice' their data more easily. This means that data may be examined more readily by segments, such as geographical regions or product groupings, in forecasting and planning software (e.g. Forecast Pro, Smoothie). This provides the groundwork for implementing developments in forecasting at different levels of aggregation (to be discussed in detail in Chapter 6). However, whilst software solutions are moving ahead by embracing slicing and dicing, they do not do so in terms of new forecasting methods (including those that take advantage of slicing and dicing). There are significant opportunities offered by open source software and modern data analytics to improve the forecasting functionality of commercial software.

1.3.4 Summary

There have been some very promising advances in the area of intermittent demand forecasting, some of which have found their way into software applications. However, much still remains to be done in terms of software companies keeping up with important methods that have recently been developed and particularly those that have been empirically tested and shown to yield considerable benefits.

1.4 About this Book

In this section we briefly review the stance taken, the scope of discussion, and the structure of the book.

1.4.1 Optimality and Robustness

Intermittent demand patterns are very difficult to model and forecast. It is the genuine lack of sufficient information associated with these items (due to the presence of zero demands) that may preclude the identification of series' components such as trend and seasonality. Demand histories are also very often limited, which makes things even worse. Demand arrives sporadically and, when it does so, it may be of a quantity that is difficult to predict. The actual demand sizes (positive demands) may sometimes be almost constant or consistently small in magnitude. Alternatively, they may be highly variable, leading to 'erratic' demand. Intermittence coupled with erraticness leads to what is known as 'lumpy' demand. The graph in Figure 1.1 shows examples of intermittent and lumpy demand patterns, based on annual demand history for two service parts used in the aerospace industry.

From Figure 1.1, two things become apparent: (i) the annual demand history contains only five positive demand observations and (ii) variability refers to both the demand arrivals (how often demand arrives) and the size of the demand, when demand occurs. The

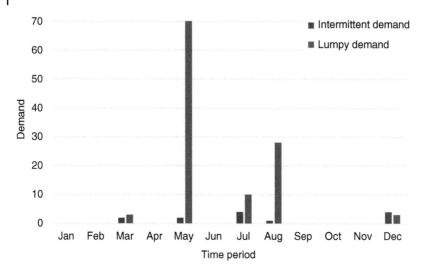

Figure 1.1 Intermittent and lumpy demand. Source: Boylan and Syntetos (2008). ©2008, Springer Nature.

lack of information associated with intermittent demand patterns coupled with this dual source of variability calls for simplifying assumptions when modelling these patterns. A common simplifying assumption is that the demand is non-seasonal. Such simplifications may impede the development of solutions that are optimal in a statistical sense, but do allow for the development of methods that potentially are very robust and easy to implement. Robustness is defined here as a 'sufficiently good' performance across a wide range of possible conditions. Optimality is defined, for particular conditions, as the 'best' performance.

We shall return to robustness and statistical optimality in later chapters but, for the time being, it is sufficient to say that robustness is essential in practical applications. While optimality is desirable, it should not be at the expense of robustness. Many of the methods to be discussed in this book have been found to be robust by such software companies as Blue Yonder, LLamasoft, Slimstock, and Syncron International, helping their customers to dramatically reduce inventory costs.

1.4.2 Business Context

With robustness in mind, this book presents a range of approaches to intermittent demand forecasting that are applicable in any industrial make to stock (MTS) setting. In addition to an MTS setting, unless otherwise specified, we focus on single stock keeping unit (SKU), single stocking location environments, as explained below.

Make to stock. In an MTS environment, customers are willing to wait no more than the time it takes to deliver the particular item to them and so the item needs to be available in stock, ready to be dispatched, or, in the case of retailing, it needs to be available on the shelf. In this case, demand is not known and needs to be predicted. The alternative environment is known as make to order (MTO), where the products are not assumed to be in stock, and the customer must wait until the manufacturer assembles the product for them. In this case, customer demand is known and does not need to be predicted. This situation is common for some products (e.g. furniture) but not for others (e.g. automotive or aerospace spare parts). There is also a move to 3D printing of products in some industries, which is a form of MTO but with shorter delays (Technical Note 1.1).

Single stock keeping unit (SKU) approaches. We are looking at forecasting the requirements (and managing the inventories) of single SKUs. Although some of the methods to be discussed in this book rely upon collective considerations (across a group of SKUs), the rest of the material considers single SKU problems. This is because higher levels of aggregation are, typically, not associated with intermittent demand. Consider, for example, 10 intermittent demand items, all of which are replenished from the same supplier. It makes sense to consider the aggregate demand of those items to facilitate efficient transportation arrangements. However, although demand at the individual SKU level may be intermittent, aggregate demand (across all 10 SKUs), most probably, will not be intermittent.

Single stocking location approaches. We focus on determining inventory replenishment requirements at each single location, without taking into account interactions between locations. As such, we do not consider the possibility of satisfying demand by lateral transshipments of stocks between stores. This is because these decisions relate explicitly to joint inventory-transportation optimisation, which is beyond the scope of this book. Further, and as discussed above, aggregate demand (across different locations in this case) is typically not associated with intermittence.

We should also mention that, although the term 'demand' is being used in this book when referring to forecasting, demand will not always be known and, in this case, actual sales must be used as a proxy. The terms 'demand' and 'sales' are used interchangeably in this book although, strictly speaking, the latter is often used as an approximation for the former.

1.4.3 Structure of the Book

This book starts by contextualising intermittent demand forecasting in the wider scholarship and practice of inventory management. We begin in Chapter 2 with a discussion of inventory management and some of its implications for forecasting. Then, in Chapter 3, we examine the service drivers of inventory performance. The focus shifts in Chapters 4 and 5 to the characterisation of intermittent demand patterns by demand distributions. This forms a natural foundation for the next two chapters, which focus on forecasting methods. Chapter 8 takes us back to inventory replenishment and the linkage between forecasting and inventory control. In the next chapter, we move on to the measurement of forecasting accuracy and inventory performance. Forecasting accuracy assessment is a notoriously difficult problem for intermittent series, and the chapter highlights the traps for the unwary and gives some pointers to good practice.

Although the main emphasis of this book is on forecasting, classification methods are also important in practical applications. In Chapter 10, we lay some of the groundwork for classification methods, discussed in Chapter 11, which have been designed specifically to address intermittence. In the next chapter, we turn our attention to obsolescence and forecasting methods that are particularly suited to this stage of the life cycle. Chapter 13 presents an alternative perspective on demand forecasting, concentrating on methods that do not assume any particular form of demand distribution. By contrast, Chapter 14 delves more deeply into methods that are based on demand distributions. The book closes with Chapter 15, which contains a discussion of software solutions for intermittent demand forecasting.

1.4.4 Current and Future Applications

Recent IT developments have greatly expanded the areas of application of intelligent intermittent demand forecasting methods. Data at a very low level of granularity have become available, which means that environments where traditionally intermittence would not be a problem now become natural candidates for further consideration. Take the retailing sector as an example: this is a traditionally fast demand environment where even the slower moving items sell in considerable volumes every day, making intermittent demand forecasting redundant. However, the current availability and utilisation of data for replenishment purposes, as often as three times per day, means that more items have intermittent demand. Although daily demand may not be intermittent, half-daily demand could be, and demand over a third of a day most probably will be.

Another factor in retail, highlighted by Boylan (2018), is the broadening of product ranges in larger retail outlets, with grocery stores introducing more clothing lines, for example. These items will often be slower moving than staple food ranges, thereby increasing the proportion of intermittent items. Recent discussions with major supermarkets in the United Kingdom such as Sainsbury's and Tesco indicate that intermittent demand forecasting has become one of their major problems.

Intermittent series occur in many other settings. For example, the planning of inventories for emergency relief must address highly intermittent and lumpy demand. Indeed, the benefits of good forecasting and planning (for any type of series) apply just as much to charitable and not-for-profit organisations as they do for profit-making wholesalers and retailers. Support for the promotion and realisation of these wider benefits is being offered at the time of writing by the 'Forecasting for Social Good' (www.f4sg.org) and 'Democratising Forecasting' initiatives launched in 2018 by Dr Bahman Rostami-Tabar.

Nikolopoulos (2021) made a strong case for the use of intermittent forecasting methods for series that are not intermittent but have sporadic peaks. These time series can be decomposed into two subseries: a baseline series and one containing more extreme values. Standard time series or causal methods can be used for the former. The latter include rare but expected events ('grey swans') and truly unexpected special events ('black swans') (Taleb 2007) and can be addressed using intermittent forecasting methods, at least as a benchmark against which other methods may be compared. Methods to address intermittence have their origins in inventory planning, but Nikolopoulos (2021) argued that these forecasting methods can be used more widely in business, finance, and economics or, indeed, in any other discipline. This line of enquiry will not be pursued in this book, although it seems a very promising direction for future research.

1.4.5 Summary

The material presented in this book reflects the authors' emphasis on robust solutions that may perform well under a wide range of differing conditions. We present the state of the art in intermittent demand forecasting, paying particular attention to the interface between forecasting and stock control. There is a very considerable market for the application of those methods, and this can only expand as more highly granular data become available.

1.5 Chapter Summary

The associated cost of inventories of purchased goods has been estimated to be between 25% and 35% of the value of those goods (e.g. Chase et al. 2006): a firm carrying $20 million in purchased goods inventory would, accordingly, incur additional costs of $5–7 million. These are costs that, once reduced, can significantly improve the firm's net profits (Wallin et al. 2006). The total cost of purchased goods inventory can be quite alarming, calling for innovative approaches to cut it down. Intelligent intermittent demand forecasting offers such opportunities.

In the defence environment, Henry L. Hinton Jr, Assistant Comptroller General, National Security and International Affairs Division, stated, 'Our work continues to show weaknesses in DoD's inventory management practices that are detrimental to the economy' (GAO 1999, p. 1). Sixteen years later, only minor improvements were reported (GAO 2015), and public announcements on the poor management of defence inventories and the resulting detrimental impacts on the economy constitute a recurring issue in the news. Similarly, the expansion of the after-sales industry and the increasing importance of commercial service operations have not been adequately reflected in the development of ERP and supply chain software packages, the functionality of which has often been judged to be inadequate (Syntetos et al. 2009b). In addition to the after-sales and MRO environment and the military sector, intermittent demand items dominate the inventories in a wide range of industries, calling for improved solutions for their cost-effective management.

There have been rather minor improvements in practical applications in this area since around 2000, but there have been major improvements in empirically tested theory since that time. Many of these theoretical advancements have not yet been incorporated in commercial software, and hence, there are major opportunities for improving real-world applications. We hope this book will help towards moving in that direction.

Technical Note

Note 1.1 3D Printing

An alternative form of MTO, enabled by advances in additive manufacturing, is 3D Printing (3DP) an item on demand. In this case, decision-making relates to the level of investment in 3DP machinery/technology that may 'print' the requested number of items upon demand. Potentially, this is very appealing in the case of spare parts and is currently being explored by various organisations seeking to cut down their inventories. For example, in 2018 the Dutch Army initiated a collaboration with the 3DP company DiManEx to examine spare part supply challenges. At the time of writing, there is no empirical evidence on the effect of 3DP on spare parts inventory management and how this compares with MTS approaches.

2

Inventory Management and Forecasting

2.1 Introduction

In the previous chapter, we showed that the management of intermittent demand items is an important task for many organisations. These items require certain operational decisions to be taken at the level of an individual stock keeping unit (SKU) including whether to stock the item at all and, if so, how much to stock. Both of these decisions will be addressed in this chapter. We discuss the major inventory replenishment policies and their appropriateness for intermittent demand items. This is the foundation for inventory forecasting and is an essential component of all software dedicated to inventory management. We also consider what forecasts are important when demand is intermittent. The interface between forecasting and stock control has been rather neglected in the academic literature although it is vital in real-world inventory applications.

2.2 Scheduling and Forecasting

Before discussing the integration of forecasting and inventory control for intermittent demand items, a distinction needs to be made between the inventory management practices required for dependent and independent demand items.

2.2.1 Material Requirements Planning (MRP)

The design and construction of any physical product is captured in its bill of materials (BoM) which, as illustrated in Figure 2.1, shows the product's assemblies (middle level) and components (bottom level). Demand at the top level, corresponding to the end product, is defined as 'independent', whereas demand at lower levels in the hierarchy is dependent on demand at higher levels.

If a company has a 'make to stock' policy, then immediate availability and thus shipment of the end products (also known as "finished goods") is promised to the customers. If a company operates a 'make to order' (MTO) policy, then immediate availability of the end products is not offered, but rather a delivery date is promised. In both policies, all the

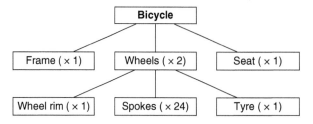

Figure 2.1 Bill of materials (BoM) example.

components and assemblies are produced or procured in time for the end product to reach the client by the promised time.

To meet delivery targets, a scheduling procedure is required and this is the backbone of the principal inventory methodology for dependent demand items, called material requirements planning (MRP) (see, for example, Ptak and Smith 2011). MRP will give a full BoM, showing all the elements needed for the final product, together with the required quantities. This is illustrated in Figure 2.1 for the example of a bicycle (end product, highlighted in bold type) comprising a frame, two wheels, and a seat (assemblies) and with each wheel comprising a wheel rim, 24 spokes, and a tyre (components).

MRP will give a full schedule of requirements, including quantities and dates by which all elements of the product must be produced or procured. In the example above, two wheel rims, 48 spokes, and two tyres would be required. Lead times for these components would also be specified, allowing all required delivery dates to be calculated. By following an MRP procedure, it is clear that if we know or can forecast the demand for the end product, then the requirements for all the lower levels can be calculated immediately.

2.2.2 Dependent and Independent Demand Items

In theory, all SKUs that appear at a level below the end product level are dependent demand items and should be treated using MRP-type procedures. However, there are two exceptions to this rule.

If a company is operating a MTO policy, then everything must be assembled during the time window from receipt of order to the delivery date. Not all the components will necessarily be produced or procured in this time frame, though. Therefore, stocks of the relevant components must be held. Ordering will no longer be based on demand that is completely known over the lead time. Instead, stock levels must be informed by forecasted demand.

The second exception relates to spare parts. Parts may be dependent demand items as far as manufacturing is concerned, but they are independent demand items as far as after-sales service is concerned. They are subject to unknown demand that varies over time, partly due to chance; such demand is known as 'stochastic'. Because spare parts demand is not known in advance, it needs to be forecasted, taking into account that spare parts are often subject to intermittent demand.

2.2.3   Make to Stock

Generally, demand is not known in advance in a make to stock environment, where the products need to be in stock when the customer orders are received. The lead time in these cases is expected (as far as the customers are concerned) to be equal to the time taken to ship the product to the customers' premises or, in the retailing sector, the lead time is expected to be zero: it is on-the-shelf availability that drives business.

In this book, we consider the case of stochastic demand in make to stock environments. (For an interesting discussion on how intermittent demand may be treated in MTO environments, please refer to the work of Bartezzaghi and Verganti 1995, briefly summarised in Technical Note 2.1.) But given the fact that demand is inherently slow moving, is it always worthwhile keeping an item in stock? This issue is discussed in Section 2.3. In practice, it should be addressed before determining ordering policies and their forecasting requirements.

2.2.4   Summary

There is great scope for advancing the inventory control practices for intermittent demand items. We treat intermittent demand as independent and do not expand further on MRP because the principal forecasting task relates to independent demand items. Dependent demand items present challenges relating to the planning of manufacturing but do not require a forecasting system if orders are known in advance and the items can be obtained within the requisite time frame.

In Section 2.3, we address a fundamental problem in this area, which is whether to stock an item or not. Given a positive stocking decision, follow-up decisions relate to determining how much to stock and when to replenish. These decisions depend on the stock rules that are in use, and we continue with an overview of appropriate inventory control rules for intermittent demand items. We conclude that, in general, the periodic order-up-to (OUT) level policy is appropriate for managing intermittent demand inventories. In the next chapter, we distinguish between systems that are driven by service and cost considerations. In Chapters 4 and 5, we determine what needs to be forecasted to allow inventory decisions to be made.

2.3   Should an Item Be Stocked at All?

A considerable amount of effort is expended by organisations to optimise inventory levels. This is expected, if we consider the huge inventory investments made in industry. Consider, for example, a car manufacturer investing £10 million in inventories of service parts to sustain their after-sales operations in Europe. A mere 5% reduction of their stock levels translates automatically to £500 000 savings that may be invested in other business areas, or account towards an increase in their profit margin. There are two ways of achieving such savings: (i) ceasing to replenish stock for some items; (ii) continuing to replenish stock for other items but reducing the quantities held. Sometimes, an organisation may become preoccupied with the second option, drawing their attention away from the equally important problem, for SKUs with intermittent demand, of whether the item should be kept in stock at all. The decision to stop replenishing an item does not necessarily coincide with the decision to write off stock from the accounts (Technical Note 2.2).

Of course, management of spare parts is often subject to very specific contractual agreements, such as the obligation to service a piece of equipment by carrying items in stock for an agreed length of time. In these cases, ceasing to replenish an item is obviously not an option. Similarly, the life cycle phase of a product or a service part often dictates inventory decisions beyond cost optimisation. For example, even if it is potentially cost-optimal not to stock an item in the introductory phase of its life cycle, high service requirements may result in always keeping some stock to satisfy demand.

Moreover, it is important to note that service levels are often targeted and measured on an 'order' rather than individual SKU basis. An order consists of a number of units requested for a number of items, and some organisations target the percentage of orders (rather than items) completely satisfied directly from stock on hand. (This is the 'order fill rate', which is further discussed in Chapter 3.) In this case, a non-stock decision, taken on the basis of individual SKU requirements only, may be reversed based on collective considerations.

2.3.1 Stock/Non-Stock Decision Rules

Having taken contractual and other constraints into account, a careful evaluation of whether an item should be stocked at all is needed. Such decisions typically rely upon an evaluation of the cost of keeping an item in stock, and the cost of not having an item in stock (see, for example, Croston 1974; Tavares and Almeida 1983). These are the two pillars upon which much inventory theory has been built, and so a detailed discussion of them is warranted.

The cost of keeping an item in stock is typically estimated based on the inventory holding charge (h), which is used to calculate the cost of keeping one unit of a particular item in stock over a specified time interval (unit time). The inventory holding charge is invariably expressed as a fraction applied to the unit cost of an item (C). Suppose for example that we operate with monthly time units and the inventory holding charge for a particular item is $h = 1\%$ for each item unit per unit of time (one month in this case). Further assume that the cost of this item is $C = £1000$. Then it costs £10 (h multiplied by C) to keep one unit of this item in stock for a month. The inventory holding charge is typically determined in an approximate manner to reflect such costs as the opportunity cost (i.e. the cost of not being able to invest the money, tied up in stock, elsewhere), warehousing space costs, potential pilferage and spoilage, and cost of obsolescence.

Usually, the inventory holding charge is set to be the same across an entire stock base. (At the time of writing, inventory holding charges in the range 10%–25% over a year reflect a good proportion of real-world cases.) However, this ignores the fact that intermittent demand items have a higher risk of obsolescence. This should be reflected by inventory holding charges that are higher than those imposed on faster-moving SKUs. Better informed inventory systems do distinguish between non-intermittent and intermittent SKUs, fixing the inventory holding charge for the former category and appropriately inflating it for the latter. The necessary degree of inflation depends on the industry and the nature of the products, which determines both the cost and environmental implications of disposing of an obsolete item. In our experience, it would vary between 3% and 5% over and above the inventory holding charge assumed for the faster-moving SKUs (see, for example, Trimp et al. 2004). The inventory holding charge does not take into account ordering costs, which are often omitted from stock/non-stock rules. Ordering costs do tend to feature in determining inventory replenishment policies, to be discussed later in this chapter.

The cost of not having an item in stock is typically estimated based on a charge that specifies the penalty cost of running out of stock. Such a charge will be different for cases where sales are lost and those where unsatisfied demand may be backordered (i.e. satisfied as soon as some stock becomes available again). Let us focus on the backorder case here; we return to the differences between lost sales and backordered demand later in the chapter. The backordering charge (b) may take different forms: (i) a specified fractional charge (of the unit cost) per unit short (regardless of the duration of the stockout) or (ii) a specified fractional charge per unit short per unit time.

In the first case, the backordering charge is typically set subjectively to reflect costs arising from expediting orders, loss of customers' goodwill, and negative word of mouth publicity. Expediting charges arise by ordering emergency replenishments from suppliers, which come at a (considerably) higher cost than normal replenishments.

The second case is more relevant in a maintenance spare parts context, as each unit short could result, for example, in a machine being idled, with the idle time being equal to the duration of the shortage. So, for the example considered above (with monthly time units and $C = £1000$), if $b = 20\%$/unit short/unit time, it costs £200 per unit short per month.

In both cases, the backordering charge is typically in the range of 5 up to 30 (or even more) times higher than the inventory holding charge, and this reflects the asymmetric costs of under-stocking and over-stocking. All else being equal, it always costs more to run out of stock by one unit than to keep in stock one unit that remains unused over a unit time period.

Then, why do we consider the possibility of not stocking an item at all? This is because, over time, it may indeed be more beneficial to allow for a potential (forthcoming) shortage, rather than having to carry an item in stock for a very long time. For example, if b is five times h, and (for monthly time buckets) unit sized demands occur on average every six months or more, then it is cost beneficial not to stock that particular item.

Early work in this area by Tavares and Almeida (1983) proposed a rule, along the lines discussed above, for the stock control of very slow moving spare parts in large production systems, such as ship repair yards and light steel mills. The decision rule was developed in order to decide whether it is economic to have one item in stock or none. In particular, a threshold level of the mean demand was proposed, equal to h/b, the ratio of the holding charge (h) to the backordering charge (b), with the latter covering additional delivery and penalty costs. The mean demand per unit time (λ) is then compared to that threshold value in order to make a decision. If the mean demand is less than the threshold, then the recommended stock (S) is zero; if the mean demand is greater than (or equal to) the threshold, then the recommended stock is one, as shown in Eq. (2.1).

$$S = \begin{cases} 0 & \text{if } \lambda < \dfrac{h}{b} \\ 1 & \text{if } \lambda \geq \dfrac{h}{b} \end{cases} \qquad (2.1)$$

For the example offered above, $h/b = 1/5 = 0.2$. So if the mean demand is $\lambda = 1/6 = 0.167$ (one unit is requested for that item every six months, on average), then we should not stock that item. (The symbol λ [lambda] is often used to denote the mean demand per unit time, and it is the standard symbol for the mean of the Poisson distribution, to be discussed in Chapter 4.)

Johnston et al. (2011) examined the inventory system at Euro Car Parts and demonstrated that, for practical purposes, stock/non-stock decisions may rely upon the number of movements over a particular time interval. 'Movements' are demand incidences that lead to an issue of stock. For unit sized demands, the number of demand incidences is equal to the demand over the same time interval.

The rule offered by Johnston et al. (2011) was derived empirically, following a comprehensive analysis of the stock base of the company. The researchers evaluated the stockout and inventory implications associated with alternative stock/non-stock cut-off points and found that a boundary of three movements (over a year) offered the best results: if there are three or more movements per year, then stock this item; else, do not keep it in stock. The implementation of the new rule at Euro Car Parts resulted in a 29% improvement in stock turn, at a time when no other major changes were made to the distribution system. (Stock turn, also known as inventory turnover, measures how many times an organisation has sold and replaced inventory during a given period and is discussed further in Chapter 3.)

2.3.2 Historical or Forecasted Demand?

In both of the papers discussed above, historical demand was employed. However, it has been argued that forecasted demand is more relevant for the stocking decision (Boylan 2018). It is the demand that is anticipated over the future that should determine an item's viability. The decision rules do not change their form as a consequence of this different perspective. All that changes is that forecasted mean demand (or number of movements) is used instead of the historical mean demand (or number of movements). The focus on the mean value is natural as the rules are based on the expected (mean) costs associated with stocking or not stocking an item.

The problem of whether to stock becomes particularly important when either products or spare parts reach the end of their life cycle, become obsolete, and are not being requested often or, eventually, at all. In Chapter 12, we return to this issue and discuss, in more detail, forecasting methods that have been proposed to estimate mean demand whilst allowing for explicit linkages to be made between the forecasting task and inventory obsolescence. More common methods for intermittent demand forecasting will be discussed in Chapter 6.

2.3.3 Summary

Before setting stock levels for intermittent demand items, a decision should be taken as to whether an item should be stocked at all. In some situations, keeping zero stock is not an option. Otherwise, an evaluation of demand is required to determine whether the item should be stocked. Such decisions are typically based on a forecast of the mean demand (discussed in Chapter 6), requiring no estimates of the variability of demand (discussed in Chapter 7), which may be required when deciding on replenishment quantities.

2.4   Inventory Control Requirements

Assuming that it is cost beneficial to keep replenishing a particular item in stock, the next important decision relates to how much to keep in stock for that item. Stock levels depend on the size of replenishment orders and how often these orders are placed on the supplier(s). Raising an order is not cost free. Therefore, in addition to the costs previously discussed, of holding inventories and the cost of running out of inventories, another cost factor comes into the equation, that of ordering inventories, as shown in Eq. (2.2).

Total Inventory Cost = Ordering Cost + Holding Cost + Backorder Cost

$$\text{TIC} = C_o + C_h + C_b \tag{2.2}$$

The ordering cost is usually a fixed cost per order, reflecting such things as raising invoices, cost of the personnel working in relevant organisational departments (e.g. purchasing, supplier management), and transportation and logistics costs, depending on whether customers, suppliers, or both assume such expenses. The true ordering costs sometimes depend on the size of the replenishment orders. For example, if logistics and transportation costs are shared between customers and suppliers, then a large order would attract a higher cost than a smaller one. However, these costs are customarily assumed fixed for modelling purposes.

Different stock control policies balance ordering, holding, and backorder costs in different ways, depending on the priorities and constraints set in the system, resulting in different decisions as to how much to stock and how often to replenish. The policies most relevant to managing intermittent demand inventories are discussed in Section 2.5. In this section, we focus on two precursors of the operation of any policy, namely:

1. How often an accurate indication is available of the stock levels for a particular item (which depends on how the stock status is maintained).
2. How often a test for reordering is made, to determine whether an order should be placed or not.

These issues constitute fundamental decisions in inventory management, and are integral to the selection of an appropriate stock rule.

2.4.1   How Should Stock Records be Maintained?

With regard to the first question, there are only two ways of 'posting' the stock status records. One is to add receipts and to subtract sales as they occur. In this case, each transaction triggers an immediate updating of the status and, consequently, this type of control is known as 'transactions reporting' (Silver et al. 2017) or as a continuous recording system. The second method of updating the stock status records is to do it periodically so that an interval of time elapses between the moments at which the stock level is updated.

Once the stock status records have been updated, the inventory control system can then check the stock status against one or more inventory parameters, so that a decision can be made about when and how much to order. Inventory parameters are essentially control numbers that tell us what actions are required. For example, in certain inventory policies if the stock levels drop at, or below, some minimum critical point, most often called an order point, then a replenishment order will be placed. In this case, the order point is the inventory parameter of interest. We discuss inventory parameters in detail in Section 2.5.

It is important to consider the relationship between continuous recording of transactions and continuous review of inventory. It is certainly true that we cannot have continuous review without continuous recording. However, a continuous recording of each transaction does not necessarily mean that there will be a continuous review of the stock requirements. Porteus (1985, p. 145) commented, 'What really matters is not how the inventory levels are monitored but the relationship between recognising that an order should be placed, placing the order, and receipt of that order. Many, if not most, transactions reporting systems are equivalent to periodic review systems.' The same is true at the time of writing, over 30 years later. For example, if the inventory records are up to date online continuously but the orders to a given supplier are issued at the end of the day (or at the end of any unit time period) then the system is one of periodic review with inventory levels being reviewed once a day (or once per time period). Transactions reporting systems are often referred to as continuous review systems although, strictly speaking, they are not the same thing.

There are two fundamental differences between continuous and periodic review systems. These differences relate to the following: (i) what triggers a new test for reordering and (ii) the time interval over which uncertainties in demand need to be taken into account.

With regard to the former, in periodic review systems an elapsed fixed time interval (the review interval) is what triggers an assessment of the stock status to decide whether a replenishment order should be raised. The test for reordering is triggered by time-interval considerations, and this is the reason why periodic review systems are also referred to as reorder interval systems. In continuous review systems, a reduction of the stock level (when a new transaction occurs, regardless of its magnitude) is what triggers the assessment of whether a new order should be placed on the supplier(s). So, the test for reordering is triggered by inventory level related considerations, and this is the reason why continuous review systems are also referred to as reorder level systems. The difference between the two types of systems is depicted graphically in Figure 2.2. This issue is further discussed in Section 2.4.2.

With regard to the time interval over which uncertainties need to be compensated, there are two major sources of uncertainty. The first one is that demand is 'stochastic'. This means

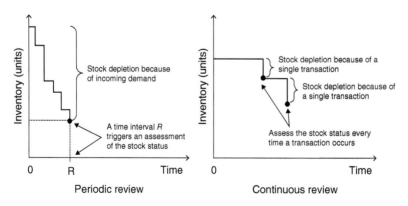

Figure 2.2 Periodic review and continuous review systems.

its occurrence and magnitude are subject to variations due to chance; demand can take on different values, each with an associated probability. This issue is discussed in detail in Chapter 4. Stochastic demand varies over time and is uncertain, and thus needs to be predicted. If demand were 'deterministic' (i.e. constant or non-constant over time but known with certainty), then it would be straightforward to decide how much we need to keep in stock to satisfy future demands.

The second source of uncertainty relates to the passage of time during which uncertain demand poses a risk of a stockout. This time lapse differs between continuous and periodic review systems. For continuous review, it is the time interval between placing an order and the received order being available for customers. This time interval is called the lead time, of length L, and includes not only the external lead time (until receipt of order) but also the internal lead time (until availability for customers). (See Technical Note 2.3 for further discussion.) If the lead time were zero, and inventory review continuous, then inventory control would be redundant because there would be no need to keep anything in stock. However, the lead time will never be zero in practice and so enough needs to be held in stock to satisfy demand from the point in time when an order is placed to the point in time when the order is received and available for customers.

For continuous review, the lead time is called the protection interval, because stocks are held to protect against a stockout during that period of time. (See Technical Note 2.4 for a discussion of an exception to this rule.) If the lead time is constant and known to be L, then we have the problem of forecasting stochastic demand over lead time (D_L). So if the lead time is, say, two months then the uncertainty we need to account for every time we place an order is the magnitude of the demand over the subsequent two months. In many real-world applications, the lead time varies, as demand does, contributing further to the uncertainty underlying the inventory control system. We assume for the time being (as often happens in practice when modelling inventories) that the lead time is known and constant, but we will relax this assumption in Chapter 7.

For periodic review systems, the protection interval not only includes the lead time but also an additional amount of time that needs to be taken into account. If orders are placed at the end of the review interval, of length R, the uncertainty of the demand over this period also needs to be accounted for. For example, if the review interval in a periodic stock control system is one month and the lead time is two months then the following will happen. At the end of, say, December, let us suppose that the stock is at the order-up-to level, S. Over what period of time does this stock level need to offer protection? At the review at the end of January, if stock has been depleted, then any order placed will not arrive until the end of March. Therefore, the stock level at the end of December needs to take into account uncertainty in demand during the review interval (January) as well as over the lead time (February and March). This explains why, in periodic stock control applications, we are interested in forecasting the stochastic demand over lead time plus the review interval ($L + R$). Because of the greater uncertainty that we need to compensate for in periodic review systems, more needs to be kept in stock, everything else being equal, than in continuous review systems.

What is the more appropriate review system for intermittent demand items? Although this is discussed in more detail in Section 2.5, at this stage it is sufficient to say that practical considerations point to the periodic systems being preferred. Often, items may be produced on the same piece of equipment, purchased from the same supplier, or shipped using the same transportation mode. In any of these situations, co-ordination of replenishments may be attractive (Silver et al. 2017). Periodic review is appealing because all items in the co-ordinated group can be given the same review interval. Sani (1995) noted that reorder interval or product group review systems are the most commonly used in practice for intermittent demand items (see also Teunter and Sani 2009a).

The main advantage of continuous review is that, to provide the same level of customer service, it requires less stock than periodic review. As previously discussed, this is because, in a periodic review system, stock is used to compensate for any uncertainties regarding demand over the review interval as well as the lead time. Under continuous review, the stocks are determined by considering lead time demand requirements only. Moreover, for intermittent demand items very little costs are incurred by continuous review as updates are made only when a transaction occurs. The relationship between ordering cost and inventory holding charge can be further explored so as to decide on the appropriateness of each type of system.

Quantifying the advantages and disadvantages of periodic and continuous review is not straightforward. However, periodic policies are more simple and convenient than continuous policies, which is a very important point from a practical perspective. So we may conclude that the practical advantages of periodic review explain its popularity in real-world applications.

2.4.2 When are Forecasts Required for Stocking Decisions?

So far, we have seen that the nature of a stock control system (periodic or continuous) affects the time interval over which a forecast is required. The second question we posed in the beginning of this section (and which has already been partly addressed), is: 'How often should the test for reordering be made?' Considering that question further reveals the difference between periodic and continuous review systems and the times when forecasts are needed for stocking decisions.

Before we address this question, it is essential to introduce the concept of inventory position. The inventory position is defined as the actual stock on hand (i.e. what we physically have in stock) for a particular SKU, plus any orders for that SKU pending to arrive, minus any demand that has not yet been satisfied and is to be satisfied as soon as some stock becomes available. This is expressed in Eq. (2.3).

$$\text{Inventory Position} = \text{Stock On Hand} + \text{Stock On Order} - \text{Backorders}$$
$$IP = SOH + SOO - BO \tag{2.3}$$

In *continuous review systems*, inventory parameters are not recalculated until the inventory position has fallen below a critical point or reached that critical point. This is known as the 'order point' but is also called a base stock or a minimum (Brown 1959). In this type of system, orders can be triggered only by a demand because the inventory position will not decline otherwise. (Exceptions may arise if the stock on hand (SOH) or backorders (BO) are found to be incorrectly recorded, or some of the stock on order (SOO) has been cancelled.) The triggering of an order is immediate with continuous review. Therefore, the issuing of stock, if available, at 'issue points', is generated immediately after demand has occurred.

Continuous systems require, as far as stock replenishment is concerned, forecasts at issue points only. Even if forecasts are automatically generated at other times, they are not relevant to ordering decisions; it is only those made immediately after a demand occurrence that affect orders. The decision may be to order nothing if demand has not been sufficiently large to deplete the inventory position to a level at, or below, the order point.

We have already noted that a continuous recording of each transaction, leading to inventory records that are 'live' continuously, does not necessarily mean a continuous review of the stock requirements. Indeed, such reviews take place most commonly periodically, at the end of fixed time intervals. Let us suppose that the stock requirements are reviewed at the end of every day, and that daily demand data are used for the calculation of forecasts. If an item were demanded at 13:00 during the day, reducing the inventory position to below the order point, then in a strict continuous system, an order would be automatically generated immediately after 13:00. However, if stock requirements are not reviewed until close of business, then the order would be generated at the end of the day. From a stock replenishment perspective, this is not continuous review. It is, in fact, a periodic system, to which we now turn.

In *periodic review systems*, the simplest case is when stock is reviewed at the end of every period ($R = 1$). In that case, if no items were demanded during a period, then the inventory position at the end of that period would be no lower than at the end of the previous period, and could be higher if a new order has arrived (as for continuous review, and with the same exceptions). Also, the required inventory level will not increase after zero demand, unless demand is forecasted to increase because of factors such as promotions, which are very much the exception for intermittent demand items.

Generally, then, the inventory position will not reduce and the required inventory level will not increase after zero demand, meaning that an order will be triggered only if there has been some demand. Hence, it is only those forecasts that are made immediately after the end of a period with a demand occurrence which may generate an issue point and initiate an issuing of stock.

Now suppose that stock is reviewed at the end of every second period ($R = 2$). For an order to be generated, there must have been some demand in the preceding two periods. However, this may not have occurred in the most recent period but in the period before that. So, in this case, we cannot restrict our attention to those periods with some demand. Forecasts affecting ordering decisions may be generated after a period of zero demand as well as after a period with some demand. The same argument applies for any length of review interval (R) of two periods or more. In the general case, the condition for an order to be able to be triggered at the end of a review interval of length R is that there has been some demand in the last R periods. It is only at the end of those review intervals satisfying this condition that forecasts may generate an issue point.

Stocking/non-stocking reviews are not generally undertaken on an individual item basis; more commonly, the stock range is reviewed collectively. This is done periodically, usually less frequently than the standard stock replenishment reviews, and not always at regular intervals. As discussed earlier, forecasts of mean demand are required whenever such reviews are conducted. At the level of the individual SKU, this may be at any point in time: it may or may not coincide with the previous periods having had some demand. No conditioning on previous periods experiencing demand is needed in this case. So, it does not matter whether stock/non-stock reviews are conducted at the end of every period, or at regular or irregular intervals, or whether it is done collectively or individually. As long as reviews are not triggered by demand occurrences, forecasts may be needed at any point in time for an individual SKU, to inform decisions regarding cessation of replenishment ('non-stock').

From a practical perspective, we will wish to use the same forecasting methods irrespective of the length of review interval and regardless of whether the forecast is used to decide how much stock to replenish or whether to continue stocking the item. Therefore, a forecasting method should provide good results when evaluated only after issue points (generated by review intervals containing some demand) or at any point in time. As we shall see in Chapter 6, this consideration is important in the evaluation of forecasting methods for intermittent demand.

Returning to the question of the frequency of testing for reordering, the ideal system from an inventory holding perspective is the continuous system with immediate reordering. However, this is not always desirable from a supplier perspective, and so a periodic system with reviews at the end of every period may be more realistic, and will probably incur a relatively small additional inventory cost when compared to the ideal system. Longer reviews may be suggested for some items, but an evaluation of the inventory costs should be performed before extending review intervals. Naturally, it is desirable that forecasting methods can perform well, whatever the length of review interval.

2.4.3 Summary

The fundamental purpose of any inventory control system is to provide answers to the following four questions (Brown 1967):

1. How should the stock status records be maintained?
2. How often should the test for reordering be made?
3. When should a replenishment order be placed?
4. How large should the replenishment order be?

In this section, we have been concerned with the first two questions. We have considered the relationship between recording of transactions and review of inventory and explained why 'true' continuous inventory review is less likely to be encountered in practice than periodic review. The differences between periodic and continuous review systems have also been discussed in detail with regard to their rationale, the time intervals over which uncertainties in demand need to be taken into account, and the forecasts that are relevant for replenishment purposes.

Having established the importance and forecasting implications of the first two questions, we now move to the second two questions. It will take a number of chapters to answer these questions fully, but the first step is to determine the most appropriate inventory policy. To inform this decision, we now provide an overview of stock control policies that may be used for intermittent demand items.

2.5   Overview of Stock Rules

Before we review stock rules, it is important to revisit the concept of inventory position. As discussed in Section 2.4, the inventory position is defined by taking the stock on hand, and adding any stock on order, and subtracting any backorders.

The opportunity of backordering demand is not always present. In retailing, for example, the lack of availability of an item usually leads to lost sales or sales of a substitutable product. Modelling 'lost sales' is far more difficult than assuming that demand may be backordered. This is because when customers are not willing to wait for their demand to be satisfied in the future, the amount of sales being lost is very hard to estimate. As we discussed in the previous chapter, sales are often used as a proxy for demand, when lost sales are not known. In a business-to-business context, where there is a record of the amount of items requested by the customer, lost sales will be known. However, these customers will often be willing to wait. So sales will not be lost, although there will be penalties that need to be paid for delaying the delivery of orders, and eventual loss of some customers, or adverse effects on their goodwill.

The measurement of the service level is affected by whether demand can be backordered or not. Achieved service levels reflect how often, or how much, demand is satisfied by the stock on hand, discussed in more detail in the next chapter. When sales are lost, the greater the uncertainty of the magnitude of that loss, the less clear the picture we have on the service our customers receive. Please note that service does not have any quality-related connotations in this book. It refers solely to availability of products.

In general, and unless we refer to the retailing sector, the case of backorders is far more relevant than the case of lost sales. The remainder of our discussion on inventory modelling, and its interface with forecasting, is focused on the case of backordering demand.

2.5.1   Continuous Review Systems

With regard to continuous review systems, the two most commonly encountered policies are of the (s, Q) or (s, S) form. After each transaction, the inventory position is compared with a control number, s, the order point. If the inventory position is less than s (or in some cases at or than s), a replenishment order is released. The replenishment order can be for a standard order quantity Q or, alternatively, enough may be ordered to raise the inventory position to the value S, the order-up-to level, or OUT level. (This is also known as the 'replenishment level'.) If all demand transactions are unit sized, the two systems are identical because the replenishment requisition will always be made when the inventory position is exactly at s (so that $S = s + Q$). If the demand sizes vary, then the replenishment quantity in the (s, S) policy also varies. In Figure 2.3, we show graphically the operation of the (s, Q) policy and its equivalence to (s, S), assuming unit sized transactions. We further assume, for ease of presentation, that no stockouts occur (i.e. backordered demand does not need to be accounted for).

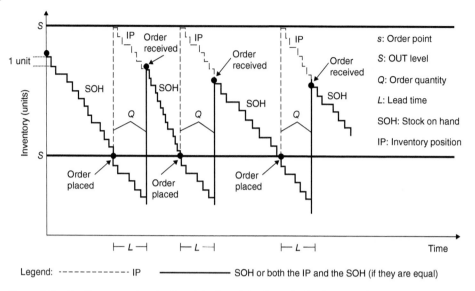

Figure 2.3 Continuous review (s, Q) and (s, S) policies for unit sized transactions.

When the inventory position drops to (exactly) the order point (s), then an order for a fixed quantity Q is placed or, equivalently, enough is ordered to raise the inventory position up to the OUT level S. Note that, at the time of ordering, the inventory position always equals the stock on hand because there are no pending receipts from the supplier(s). Once the order is placed, the inventory position increases to s (stock on hand) + Q (stock on order) (=S) and decreases thereafter in exactly the same way as the stock on hand. The quantity ordered is received after the lead time (L), at which point in time the inventory position equals again the stock on hand.

The problem is to find the optimal values of the control parameters s and Q. (See Technical Note 2.5 for discussion of equivalence with (R, S) optimisation.) Optimality here refers to a solution that has been explicitly developed based on minimising the total inventory cost (Ordering cost + Holding cost + Backorder cost). In theory, optimisation of the two control parameters, s and Q, should occur in parallel recognising that cost interactions exist between them. Alternatively, the parallel optimisation may be for s and S (rather than s and Q) (see, for example, Wagner 1975). In practice, though, in our experience, a separate (independent) optimisation of these parameters is the norm because of its relative simplicity. Further arguments in support of this approach relate to its near-optimal behaviour (Porteus 1985).

2.5.2 Periodic Review Systems

In periodic review systems, the inventory decision rules most usually take the form of a (R, S) or (R, s, S) policy, the former being the one to be discussed in more detail in this book. Under the regime of both policies, after every R periods (constant inventory review interval) enough is ordered to raise the inventory position up to the 'order-up-to level', S. The difference between the two policies is that the (R, s, S) policy requires the inventory position

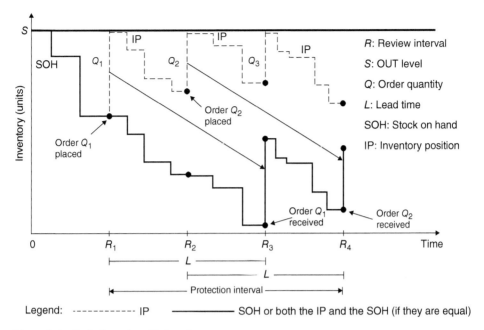

Figure 2.4 Periodic review (R, S) policy.

to be less than or equal to s (or in certain cases strictly less than s) before an order is placed. Therefore, the (R, S) policy always results in higher ordering costs because even a unit-sized transaction during the review interval will trigger a replenishment requisition, whilst the (R, s, S) policy will place an order only if the cumulative demand, over the review interval, exceeds some minimum level. The (R, s, S) can be viewed as the periodic implementation of the (s, S) system because the (R, s, S) reduces to (s, S) for $R = 0$.

In Figure 2.4, we show graphically the operation of the (R, S) policy. For ease of presentation, we assume that no stockouts occur (i.e. backordered demand does not need to be accounted for). We further assume that the review interval is shorter than the lead time (as is typically the case in practice in wholesaling), i.e. $R < L$. In particular, we assume that $L = 2R$.

At time R_1, the inventory position (which is assumed to be, for presentation purposes, at that point in time equal to the stock on hand (SOH)) is compared with the OUT level S and enough is ordered to raise it up to that level. Once the order has been placed, then the inventory position equals S and decreases thereafter in exactly the same way as the stock on hand. At time R_2, the stock on hand has been further depleted and the quantity ordered at R_1 is the stock on order; the inventory position is contrasted again to S and is raised up to that level. At time R_3, the order placed at R_1 is received and added to the stock on hand; the order placed at R_2 is the stock on order and the inventory position is raised again up to S.

The (R, S) system depicted in Figure 2.4 is based on a fixed OUT level, S, that does not change over time. The same is true for the control parameters s, Q, and S in Figure 2.3. Although it is actually common practice in industry for the control parameters to be fixed over long periods of time, more responsive inventory systems rely upon an update at each stock review occasion. So, for the (R, S) system, the OUT level S would be updated at every time interval R. This issue is discussed further later in this chapter.

With regard to the review interval, for both (R, S) and (R, s, S) systems, this can be either optimised or, as most often happens in practice, set to be equal to a convenient time unit. The review interval can be optimised by classical economic lot size computations. The expected time over which the economic order quantity (EOQ) will be demanded is used to determine the review interval, R (see, for example, Brown 1982). Alternatively, R may be set to a standard time unit such as, for example, half a day for a retailer, a week for a wholesaler, or a month for a manufacturer. The inventory review interval is usually decided by taking into account such factors as the nature of the business (the higher the volume of business the shorter the review interval will be to facilitate control), the lead times (if the lead time is one day it would not make much sense to set the review interval to one month), and inventory software related constraints. There is little guidance in the academic literature on setting appropriate inventory review intervals. Nevertheless, we remark that the forecast update interval is typically set to be equal to the inventory review interval, and this makes sense from a practical perspective.

As previously discussed, one may question the practical relevance of continuous review when most inventory control systems seem to be relying upon some sort of periodic review. However, continuous systems tend to be easier to analyse mathematically. In addition, as the review interval becomes shorter and shorter, periodic formulations become hard to distinguish from continuous ones. For daily or even half-daily review intervals commonly used by retailers, the continuous assumption is a reasonable one (e.g. Cattani et al. 2011).

Fixing the inventory review interval to be the same for a number of SKUs facilitates their collective replenishment from a common supplier, and introduces some stability in the inventory and purchasing organisational functions. We do not mean to imply here that all periodic inventory control systems are necessarily easy to implement, but in an intermittent demand context at least, where we deal with very high numbers of items, these are more realistic than continuous policies. In the subsections to follow, the literature on periodic inventory control for intermittent demand items is summarised and the main approaches to managing intermittent demand stocks are discussed.

2.5.3 Periodic Review Policies

The (R, s, S) inventory control systems have been claimed, on the basis of theoretical arguments, to be the best for the management of intermittent demand items (Sani 1995). Many (R, s, S) policies have been developed in the academic literature, some giving optimal solutions (e.g. Veinott and Wagner 1965), and some not (e.g. Wagner 1975; Naddor 1975; Ehrhardt 1979; Ehrhardt and Mosier 1984; Porteus 1985). The policies that are non-optimal are 'heuristic'. 'Heuristics' here refer to the use of some (more) easily implementable rules and calculations, which reach a solution that may be close to optimal but does not necessarily achieve optimality (Sani and Kingsman 1997; Babai et al. 2010). Optimality is sacrificed in favour of some increased practical applicability.

In practice, (R, s, S) systems are not used as much as (R, S) systems. This emphasis is reflected in the academic literature, where the latter has been researched more extensively. We now turn our attention to the (R, S) (or 'order-up-to') inventory policy and the reasons for its popularity.

Hadley and Whitin (1963) noted the differences, in the computational effort required, to generate results for the (R, S) system and (R, s, S) or (R, s, Q) type policies. They identified the circumstances under which the order-up-to policy is essentially optimal, meaning that the average annual costs differ so little from other policies that it is not worth making the additional computations. The answer depends on the relative magnitudes of the ordering and review costs. As previously discussed, the former comprises such things as raising invoices and the cost of the personnel working in relevant organisational departments. The latter reflects such things as inventory software investment and managerial time spent on reviewing SKUs' inventory positions.

When the ordering costs are low relative to review costs, an order-up-to policy should be almost optimal. All three policies ((R, S), (R, s, S), and (R, s, Q)) incur the same review costs (for the same review interval, R), but the (R, S) policy leads to more frequent ordering, everything else being equal. If the additional ordering cost is low, its impact on the relative cost performance of the (R, S) policy is only minimal, and worth incurring in light of the ease of implementation of such policies.

Sani (1995) developed a stock control model that reflected the main characteristics of a real inventory system. The model was of the (R, S) form where an overnight emergency delivery was offered in the case of a stockout. The model was used to conduct a sensitivity analysis of the inventory costs and customer service levels achieved by employing the real system. Sani argued that the (R, S) system represents many real-world cases and is intuitively and computationally more appealing to practitioners than the (R, s, S) system. Moreover, using R to coordinate ordering over multiple SKUs is preferable to using s (which would vary across SKUs). It is also easier to optimise the (R, S) system, as we know that the inventory position will be back up to S at every review point. Finally, (R, S) policies have been shown to be very robust (Bijvank et al. 2014) and that may help further explain their prevalence in real-world applications. Most of the empirical studies in the area of intermittent demand forecasting and stock control have considered an (R, S) system.

All three periodic review systems discussed in this chapter are possible candidates for implementation with intermittent demand items. Arguably, there are some disadvantages associated with the (R, s, S) and (R, s, Q) policies, but the evidence is not conclusive. (R, S) systems seem to be appropriate for intermittent demand. Although they may not be universally recommended for application, they are very appealing both in practical and theoretical terms. If the review interval has been determined, then there is only one parameter to optimise (S). This simplifies calculations and enables a more focused discussion about optimisation and the integration of forecasting into inventory calculations, than dealing with two parameters (which would be the case for (R, s, Q) and (R, s, S) policies).

The periodic order-up-to level system will be used for the remainder of this book. However, before we close this section some variations of this system should be discussed. This follows in Section 2.5.4.

2.5.4 Variations of the (R, S) Periodic Policy

The (R, S) can be viewed as a periodic implementation of the (s, S) policy or as a special case of the (R, s, S) policy for $s = S - 1$. The latter is an example of an $(S - 1, S)$ policy, which may be operated under continuous or periodic review.

Schultz (1987) discussed a periodic $(S - 1, S)$ policy for the control of intermittent demand items. At the end of every review interval, the inventory position is checked against the base stock level $S - 1$. If the inventory position is less than or equal to $S - 1$, an order is calculated to bring the inventory position up to S; otherwise, no order is needed. The policy's normal mode of operation is to place a replenishment order at the time the order is calculated, i.e. at the end of the review interval. Alternatively, a replenishment delay (of several periods) may be introduced with the aim of reducing inventory holding costs, if only minor increases in the cost of stockouts is expected. This modification was shown theoretically to offer considerable cost benefits (i.e. inventory holding cost savings that outweigh the increased cost of a stockout condition).

Schultz's proposition covers the inventory system against the possibility that one demand will occur during the lead time plus review interval. Necessary assumptions in this model's implementation are the following: (i) lead times are small, as compared to the average inter-demand interval and (ii) the cost of reordering is small relative to the cost of holding sufficient inventory to meet more than one order.

The first assumption is clearly very restrictive. However, some work has been conducted to exploit the fact that the lead time (plus review interval) may indeed sometimes be less than the average inter-demand interval. Syntetos et al. (2009a) developed a modified (R, S) policy that was shown empirically to perform very well for such cases. The database used for experimentation contained demand histories and lead times for 5000 SKUs from the Royal Air Force. About 50% of the sample met the qualifying condition for inclusion in the experiment (i.e. that the lead time plus review interval is less than the average inter-demand interval) showing that models exploiting this information may be very useful in practice. However, the fact remains that they cannot be used for all intermittent demand SKUs and we do not consider them further in this book.

2.5.5 Summary

From a practitioner's standpoint, robust and not overly complicated inventory control models are required for intermittent demand items. In this section, we first provided an overview of stock control policies, arguing for the consideration of periodic (as opposed to continuous) formulations for the management of intermittent demand items. Not all such policies are easy to implement and some of them are based on very restrictive assumptions. We view the (R, S) policies as being consistent with practical needs and we further consider their implementation in later chapters.

2.6 Chapter Summary

Intermittent demand items dominate the stock bases in many industries, and in their capacity as service parts constitute a major opportunity for financial gains in the after-sales market. In this book, we treat service parts as independent demand items and discuss estimating their future requirements and appropriately replenishing their inventories.

Owing to their inherent slow movement, an important decision relates to whether intermittent demand items should be kept in stock at all. Simple rules that rely upon a forecast of the mean demand may be employed to reach such decisions.

Assuming that an item is stocked, an appropriate policy is needed to decide when to replenish its inventory and by how much. We have argued for the relevance of periodic stock control policies, including the use of the periodic (R, S) policy (also known as the order-up-to (OUT) level rule) to manage intermittent demand items. The operation of this policy depends on the service measure employed and the distribution of demand, to be discussed in detail in the next three chapters. We return to the question of forecasting in Chapters 6 and 7.

Technical Notes

Note 2.1 Order Overplanning

Bartezzaghi and Verganti (1995) (see also the work by Verganti 1997; Bartezzaghi et al. 1999) proposed the order overplanning forecasting method to assist MTO manufacturers in dealing with intermittent demand. The method aims at fully exploiting early information that the prospective and regular customers generate during their purchasing process. It uses as forecasting unit each single customer order instead of the overall demand for the master production schedule (MPS) unit. So, the forecast unit is distinguished from the MPS planning unit. The expected requirements for a module (that belongs to a particular order) are overestimated. This is to take into account the sources of uncertainty within the planning horizon, namely order acquisition, actual due date, system configuration (number and types of apparatus), and apparatus configuration (modules) by implicitly incorporating in them the slack necessary to handle those uncertainties. This is done by introducing redundant configurations, so as to satisfy any request that may actually be received. The demand forecast for the MPS unit is obtained by adding up the requirements included in the individual forecast orders.

In order overplanning, forecasting is not the numerical result of an algorithm for analysing historical data but rather an organisational process, closely linked to the purchasing practices of the customer. In fact the method relies upon the capabilities of Sales to anticipate future requirements by continuously gathering information from customers and to exchange this subjective information with Manufacturing. The benefits associated with the use of this method can be realised only in an industrial MTO context, when (i) there is a certain amount of information available on customers' anticipated future requests and (ii) the information provided by the customers, during their purchasing process, has some predictive power.

Note 2.2 Cessation of Replenishment and Stock Write Off

The inventory decision of ceasing to replenish an item does not necessarily imply an immediate action from the accountancy department in terms of writing the item off the assets, which is needed for financial reporting. Rather, there will typically be some time elapsing between ceasing to replenish an item and (officially) writing the item off. Further, writing off an item does not necessarily imply an immediate disposal of any remaining stock for that item. Again, there may be some time elapsing between writing an item off and committing to the disposal of any remaining stock. Although the processes of writing an item off and disposing of any remaining stock are very important, any reference in the book to not stocking an item relates only to the inventory decision to cease replenishment.

Note 2.3 External and Internal Lead Times

An implicit assumption often made in inventory theory is that there is no time elapsing between receiving an order from the supplier(s) and making that order available for customers. The reality, though, is different as there are many situations when that time difference not only exists but is quite significant too. Unloading goods upon receipt, incoming goods inspection, moving the received items to their allocated space (especially in large warehouses), and updating the information system to reflect the receipts, are not necessarily trivial exercises, time-wise, and this should be taken into account when calculating lead times.

In summary, lead times consist of two time components: (i) external supply lead time (time difference between placing an order and receiving it); (ii) internal lead time (time difference between receiving an order and making it available for customers). However, the latter is usually ignored and the terms 'lead time' and 'supply lead time' are (wrongly) used interchangeably.

Note 2.4 Renewal Processes

In continuous review inventory control, it is only necessary to consider making replenishment decisions just after a demand has occurred. This is true for Poisson and Bernoulli processes, where the time between demands is exponentially and geometrically distributed, respectively, and hence the demand process is memoryless (see Chapter 4). However, for renewal demand processes, including Erlang arrival processes that are not memoryless, this is no longer true in general (see Chapter 5). Rather, for these processes the passage of time itself may carry information about the demand process. Thus, it may be optimal that a certain time span should trigger a replenishment order, even if a demand has not occurred. Therefore, an order may not only be triggered by a change in the inventory position (defined in the usual way). Heuristically, and for practical purposes, replenishment orders may, of course, be allowed only at the time instances just after a demand has occurred (or at predetermined time intervals, as in a periodic review system). This issue has implications for the kind of information that is useful for inventory control purposes but is not discussed further in this book.

Note 2.5 Optimisation of (R,S) and (s,Q) Systems

For optimisation of control parameters, the results obtained for the (R, S) system can be easily transferred to an (s, Q) system by substituting s for S, L for $L + R$, and Q for D/R (where L is the lead time and D the annual demand). The (R, Q) combination does not take into account the variability of demand and hence should not be applied in a probabilistic demand context.

3

Service Level Measures

3.1 Introduction

In Chapter 2, we reviewed inventory rules that may be used to manage the stock of inter-mittent demand items, paying particular attention to the (R, s, S) and (R, S) policies. In both of these policies, the inventory position is reviewed every R periods, and enough stock is ordered to raise it to the order-up-to level, S, also known as the OUT level. We noted that (R, S) is often used for intermittent demand items because of its simplicity and robustness.

The (R, S) policy requires the determination of the review interval and OUT level for each individual stock keeping unit (SKU). In practice, the review interval is usually set to be the same for all SKUs or for whole classes of SKUs, for reasons that were discussed in Chapter 2. The setting of the review interval varies according to industry sector. In grocery retail, this may be every day or half day, whereas in automotive spare parts, the review may be weekly or monthly.

The OUT level, S, should be set separately for each SKU, to take account of its demand uncertainty. The determination of an OUT level for an individual SKU is an important issue for 'mission-critical' items, for example spare parts without which a grounded plane cannot fly. For other SKUs, the determination of OUT levels may be less critical but is still important because of its effect on aggregate inventories. As discussed in Chapter 1, a whole range of SKUs may account for significant stock holding, the level of which is influenced by the OUT levels.

The setting of the OUT level in service-driven inventory systems depends on three main factors:

1. Service measure.
2. Demand distribution.
3. Forecasting method.

The first factor, the service measure, is analysed in this chapter. Chapters 4 and 5 focus on the second factor, with discussion of various demand distributions and the criteria they should satisfy. The following two chapters are concerned with the third factor: Chapter 6 concentrates on methods to forecast the mean demand, while Chapter 7 is devoted to fore-casting the variance of demand and its associated forecast error. All of these elements are

Intermittent Demand Forecasting: Context, Methods and Applications, First Edition.
John E. Boylan and Aris A. Syntetos.
© 2021 John Wiley & Sons Ltd. Published 2021 by John Wiley & Sons Ltd.
Companion Website: www.wiley.com/go/boylansyntetos/intermittentdemandforecasting

brought together in Chapter 8, which explains how, for a given service measure, the OUT level can be found for intermittent demand items.

In this chapter, we begin by arguing against using rules of thumb for setting OUT levels, and by stressing the strategic significance of aggregate level financial and service targets. The choice of SKU-level service measures is examined, noting their links to inventory costs, before moving on to the calculation of the two operational service level measures that are most commonly employed in inventory systems. Then, we return to the setting of aggregate service targets, emphasising the importance of 'what-if' modelling capabilities. The chapter concludes with comments on the use of judgement and points to the need for reliable demand distributions to assess the service implications of different ordering policies.

3.2 Judgemental Ordering

In this book, we argue for a systematic and analytical approach to forecasting and inventory management. This should be based on inventory replenishment rules and forecasting methods that are well grounded statistically and have solid evidence of good performance in practice. From our work with a variety of organisations, we are aware that practitioners may use ordering rules that are ad hoc, or may adjust computer-generated orders using their own judgement. In this section, we make some brief remarks on these practices.

3.2.1 Rules of Thumb for the Order-Up-To Level

Suppose that the review interval is one week and the lead time is two weeks, giving a total protection interval of three weeks. Suppose, further, that our forecasted mean demand is two units per week, and the demand is non-trended and non-seasonal. It may be tempting to set the OUT level as the forecasted mean demand over the protection interval, namely six units. This would be correct if it were certain that demand would be for the exact mean demand predicted, but this is rarely the case. More commonly, the demand will be fluctuating. Not taking account of these fluctuations can lead to frequent stockouts.

An alternative calculation, which attempts to address this issue, is to multiply the forecasted demand per week by a period that is longer than the protection interval, to allow for demand uncertainty. For example, we could multiply the forecasted demand, of two per week, by four weeks, instead of three, to give an OUT level of eight units. The problem now is that the setting of four weeks is arbitrary. Why not use five or six weeks instead of four? There is no guarantee of hitting service level targets using this type of calculation. For highly unpredictable demand, we may set the OUT level too low and, for more predictable demand, we may set it too high. Therefore, although this rule of thumb has the merit of simplicity, it risks service level targets being missed or targets being achieved with excessive stocks.

3.2.2 Judgemental Adjustment of Orders

Some demand planners exercise judgement by adjusting stock orders directly, whilst others do so by adjusting demand forecasts. Judgemental ordering has been the subject of some research, mainly through studies of behaviour in simulated environments. An early study of a simulated inventory distribution system (known as the 'beer game') showed that participants in the game often misperceived the feedback they received in multiple-stage supply chains. This leads to ordering decisions that can be far from optimal (Sterman 1989) and can cause amplification of order variability throughout the supply chain, known as the 'bullwhip effect'. In a different setting, based on a single-stage supply chain, Tokar et al. (2014) found that participants tended to over-order in anticipation of a spike of demand, relative to the optimal orders that would minimise the total inventory costs.

Although the experimental evidence on judgemental ordering is not encouraging, there are situations when it can be beneficial. A prime example is to take advantage of discounts from suppliers that are available only for a limited period of time. In making a judgemental adjustment to the order, the demand forecast should be left untouched if no change in demand from end-customers is anticipated. In other circumstances, it may be appropriate to adjust the forecasts themselves. We shall return to forecast adjustments in Chapter 10, where there is a detailed discussion of the subject.

To summarise, judgemental adjustment of orders may have positive effects in gaining price discounts but can also contribute to the bullwhip effect, leading to additional inventory holdings. The effect of order adjustment may not be as great as the impact of forecast adjustment, as shown by a system dynamics investigation (Syntetos et al. 2011b) and a further empirical study (Syntetos et al. 2016b). Nevertheless, any price benefits should be weighed against increased inventory costs. If order adjustments are frequent, it would be good practice to keep records of the original recommended orders, as well as the adjusted orders. In this way, an organisation can monitor the effect of judgemental adjustments and evaluate whether they are beneficial or, more specifically, the circumstances under which they are beneficial.

3.2.3 Summary

Order-up-to (OUT) levels are sometimes set by using a rule of thumb of multiplying the forecasted demand (per period) by a set number of periods. This ignores the degree of demand uncertainty, leading to a misdirection of inventory investment. Consequently, rules of thumb like this are not recommended.

Judgemental adjustment of orders may be worthwhile in some situations. These adjustments should be continually monitored, to evaluate their effects on price benefits and inventory costs.

3.3 Aggregate Financial and Service Targets

Organisations should assess their inventory performance with respect to financial and service targets. While service targets are needed at SKU level, assessment of service targets at higher levels of aggregation elevates an operational task to a strategic issue. A strategic view of service and costs is essential because there is often a trade-off between these two aspects of performance and looking at just one aspect may lead to poor decisions.

3.3.1 Aggregate Financial Targets

A financial target can be set in a variety of ways. One way to express it is in terms of the average inventory valuation, obtained by recording the financial value of inventories at a number of times during the year and averaging them. Sufficient times during the year should be included to obtain a reliable average, especially if inventories are seasonal. The exact method of valuation depends on the accounting rules employed; for further discussion see, for example, Muller (2019).

An important issue to be addressed is the 'write off' of obsolescent stock if it has no residual value or its 'write down' if it still has some value, for example as scrap. Once stock becomes so slow moving that it is unlikely to be ever sold, then these adjustments to the balance sheet are necessary. The record of inventory written off, or written down, is useful in two ways. Firstly, it can be used to assess the additional percentage inventory holding cost to allow for the potential obsolescence of slow moving SKUs, as discussed in Chapter 2. Secondly, the write-off and write-down values can be monitored to assess the effectiveness of measures to prevent the build-up of obsolete inventory.

Inventory turnover is another useful financial measure. It is calculated as the ratio of the cost of goods sold (COGS) to the average inventory valuation. For example, if the annual COGS is £8 million and the average inventory valuation is £2 million, then the inventory turns four times a year. This measure is useful because it takes into account the growth or decline of sales. If COGS rises by 20% but inventory value increases by only 10%, then the inventory turnover will improve. It is possible to benchmark a company's performance on inventory turnover against competitors, but care is needed in drawing conclusions from the comparison. Inventory turnover is strongly influenced by the breadth of products in the stock range. If it is necessary to include slower-moving stocks, because of contractual obligations, then the inventory turnover will necessarily be lower. If required, inventory turnover can be assessed for categories of SKUs (e.g. by volume of sales) or at the level of an individual SKU. It is most commonly measured at the aggregate level and provides a useful headline figure. It should be monitored over time, so that the effect of any changes in policies or practices can be assessed.

A full financial assessment of the impact of stockouts can be difficult to achieve. If stockouts lead to backorders, then it may be possible to estimate the costs of expediting orders to minimise the delay in satisfying the order. It is more challenging to assess the costs of lost goodwill from clients. For this reason, aggregate financial targets are usually complemented by aggregate service level targets, to which we now turn.

3.3.2 Service Level Measures

Johnson et al. (1995, p. 57) observed, 'The rhetoric on customer service has grown from a quiet whisper to a deafening roar'. Twenty-five years later, customer service is still a prominent issue in supply chain management and is likely to remain so. There are many aspects of service relating to customer orders, including user-friendly ordering systems, availability of accurate order status information, delivery of the correct goods at the promised time, and the prompt and courteous response to customer queries or complaints. In this book, we are concerned with just one aspect of customer service, namely the availability of stock to satisfy customer demand. We refer to this as the 'service level', whilst recognising that there are many other aspects of customer service.

Some organisations have formal service level agreements (SLAs) with their major suppliers. These usually specify target service levels and may include financial penalties for missing these targets. This highlights the importance of using appropriate forecasting and inventory management methods. Otherwise, as Willemain (2018) emphasised, suppliers will incur financial penalties much more frequently than they were expecting. An SLA will specify either lump-sum penalties or penalties proportional to underperformance. This choice needs careful consideration as it can influence 'gaming' behaviour by the supplier (Liang and Atkins 2013).

It is essential that the service level measure is clearly specified in an SLA, and that performance is regularly monitored against target. Indeed, even if an SLA is not in place, it is vital that there is a common understanding of how service is measured, and that the measure is appropriate for the business. A number of measures have been proposed and we now proceed to review how these measures are calculated and how they should be used.

From a customer perspective, it would be ideal if all of their orders could be met in full, immediately from stock. Consider the example of a single customer order shown in Table 3.1.

There are three levels at which service may be evaluated:

1. *Orders*: In this example, the order is not completely filled because the order lines for SKUs B and E are not fully satisfied, and the order line for SKU C is not satisfied at all. To calculate the proportion of orders completely filled (the order fill rate [FR]) would require data on all relevant orders. If the order in Table 3.1 were included, it would be counted as unfulfilled.
2. *Order lines*: Two out of the five order lines are completely filled, for SKUs A and D, giving an order-line fill rate of 40%.
3. *Units*: Table 3.1 shows that 18 out of 25 units are filled from stock, giving a unit fill rate of 72%. Alternatively, this could be calculated according to value. A value of £5100 is filled from stock, out of a total value requested of £6000, giving a value fill rate of 85%.

This example is restricted to a single order, but each of the measures can also be calculated at the aggregate level, over a whole collection of orders. We can find the total number of orders completely filled, the total number of order lines (over all orders) completely filled,

Table 3.1 Order comprising five order lines.

SKU	Ordered	Filled	Ordered (£)	Filled (£)
A	5	5	500	500
B	10	8	1000	800
C	4	0	500	0
D	1	1	3000	3000
E	5	4	1000	800
Total	25	18	6000	5100

and the total number of units filled (over all order lines and all orders). These totals can then be divided by the total orders, order lines, and units demanded, respectively.

To perform well on the order and order-line fill rate measures requires good service on a wide spectrum of SKUs, including slow-moving and intermittent items. The unit fill rate is an important measure as it can be applied straightforwardly at both the aggregate and SKU levels. For an individual order line, the value fill rate is the same as the unit fill rate, but these measures may differ when calculated for a whole order, as illustrated in Table 3.1. Full satisfaction of the most expensive order line, for SKU D, has resulted in the value fill rate, of 85%, being somewhat higher than the unit fill rate of 72%.

Although complete order fulfilment is ideal from a client perspective, the percentage of orders completely filled should not be the only service level measure. Retailers usually submit numerous order lines in an order on a wholesaler. Even if the wholesaler improves the availability of stock, this will not necessarily be reflected by the complete order fill rate. For example, if the order lines for SKUs A, B, C, and D were filled completely but only four out of five units were filled for SKU E, then the order would still be counted as unfilled. The order-line fill rate and the unit fill rate would be raised to 80% and 96%, respectively, thereby reflecting the improved stock availability.

The measures discussed here may be embedded in a broader framework of order fulfilment metrics. Johnson and Davis (1998) described how Hewlett-Packard augmented inventory holding and fill rate metrics with a measure of customer delivery reliability. This helped to identify the impact of stockouts on delivery delays, including some cases where there was no impact because non-available stock became available in time for the dispatch of the last truck.

3.3.3 Relationships Between Service Level Measures

Occasions may arise when an organisation needs to change from one service level measure to another, and new service level targets are required. If service levels have not been monitored according to the new measure, then a relationship between the old and new measures can help to set new targets. Boylan and Johnston (1994) showed how relationships may be obtained between order-line and order fill rates, and between unit and order-line fill rates. The relationship between the unit fill rate, FR_{Unit}, and the order-line fill rate, FR_{Line}, is given by Eq. (3.1).

$$FR_{Unit} = 1 - (1 - FR_{Line})\frac{u_u}{l_u}\frac{l_d}{u_d} \tag{3.1}$$

where u_u/l_u is the average number of units unfilled per unfilled order line and l_d/u_d is the reciprocal of the average number of units demanded per order line. In Table 3.1, seven units are unfilled over three order lines, giving an average of $u_u/l_u = 7/3 = 2.33$, to two decimal places. Also in Table 3.1, 25 units are demanded over five order lines, giving an average of $u_d/l_d = 25/5 = 5$ and a reciprocal of $l_d/u_d = 0.2$. In this example, the product of the two ratios in Eq. (3.1) is $2.33 \times 0.2 = 0.466$. Applying Eq. (3.1) to an order-line fill rate of 0.40 yields a unit fill rate of $1 - ((1 - 0.4) \times 0.466) = 1 - 0.28 = 0.72$, agreeing with our original calculation.

Equation (3.1) is useful when the original calculation cannot be performed. This situation can arise when backorder (BO) records are maintained but data is not retained on the quantity filled for each order line. Boylan and Johnston (1994) described such an application at Unipart, a large UK-based manufacturing, logistics, and consultancy company. In this case, new unit fill targets were determined, based on old order-line fill targets. This was done separately for each of the company's major logistics clients and for each of the movement classes (fast, medium, and slow moving automotive spare parts) and led to a smooth introduction of the new measure.

3.3.4 Summary

In this section, we have stressed that aggregate service and financial targets both need to be attained. Aggregate service level measures may be recorded at order, order line, or unit level and monitored accordingly. It may be beneficial to use more than one measure, so that service can be assessed from a variety of perspectives. If there is a need to convert from one measure to another, then relationships are available for this purpose. In all situations, it is important to gauge the financial implications of hitting service targets, to ensure that the targets are set at an appropriate level.

3.4 Service Measures at SKU Level

Financial and service performance at the aggregate level are ultimately determined by the performance at SKU level. In this section, we begin with a brief discussion of financial measures, before moving on to potential service measures, at the level of the individual SKU, and when they may be most appropriately applied.

3.4.1 Cost Factors

Inventory holding costs can be assessed at SKU level based on the opportunity cost of capital, warehousing space costs, costs of potential pilferage and spoilage, and costs of stock obsolescence. Of these components, the opportunity cost of capital is generally the largest. Gardner (1980, p. 43) remarked on the difficulty of assessing the cost of capital, describing it as: '…a highly subjective measure, which depends on the risk environment of the firm and management goals for rates of return on investment'. The difficulty of measuring inventory holding costs is well recognised, although there may be benefits of organisations thinking through these costs as thoroughly as they can.

The costs of stockouts can be assessed at SKU level, based on a penalty cost for backordering and the delay of fulfilment of an order line for a period of time. As mentioned in Chapter 2, there are two ways of estimating these costs. There can be a fractional charge of the unit cost per unit short (regardless of the duration of the stockout), or there can be a fractional charge per unit short per unit time. Both approaches suffer from the difficulty of making the charge reflect loss of customer goodwill, which is just as hard to quantify at SKU level as at an aggregate level.

For some decisions, such as to stock or not to stock an item, it is common to use an approach based on holding and backordering costs, notwithstanding the difficulty in measuring them. To set OUT levels, we suggest that it is more straightforward to adopt a service-driven approach, which will be the focus for the remainder of this chapter.

3.4.2 Understanding of Service Level Measures

Whilst the concept of inventory service is well understood, the same cannot always be said for the details of its measurement. Some managers and planners are well informed but others are not, as observed by Silver et al. (2017, p. 246): '...an inventory manager, when queried, may say the company policy is to provide a certain level of service (say 95%) and yet not be able to articulate exactly what is meant by service'.

There are various reasons for this. The measurement of inventory service may appear to be self evident, leading managers to take it for granted, not realising that there are numerous ways of measuring it. Moreover, the measure employed at an aggregate level may not be the same as the measure used at SKU level to determine OUT levels. Again, managers may not appreciate that there is such a difference and assume that it is measured in the same way at all levels. This is just one example of the need for training and development of staff involved in inventory management and demand forecasting. We return to this important issue in the final chapter of the book.

3.4.3 Potential Service Level Measures

There are three main service level measures that are employed at SKU level:

1. *Cycle service level*: The fraction of replenishment cycles in which all of the demand can be satisfied directly from stock (denoted as P_1).
2. *Unit fill rate*: The fraction of the total volume of demand that can be satisfied directly from stock (denoted as P_2).
3. *Ready rate*: The fraction of time during which the net stock (stock on hand (SOH) minus backorders) is positive (denoted as P_3).

In the definition of the cycle service level (CSL), a 'replenishment cycle' is the interval between two consecutive replenishment decisions (see, for example, Çetinkaya and Lee 2000). For a periodic review system, the replenishment cycle is the same as the review interval (R) because a replenishment decision is made every R periods.

The unit fill rate measure translates naturally from the aggregate level to the level of the individual SKU. It is defined in the same way, as the fraction of the total volume of demand that can be satisfied directly from stock. It is an intuitive measure and allows all the necessary calculations to be made to inform the setting of OUT levels.

The ready rate and the cycle service level assess conditions for order-line and order fulfilment but they do not measure them directly. Starting with the ready rate, if the net stock is positive for 90% of the time, then there is the possibility of fulfilling all order lines during this portion of time. However, there is no guarantee that there will be sufficient stock to satisfy the entire quantity requested for every order line. For example, if the net stock is at two units, but four units are requested by a customer, then their order line cannot be fully satisfied.

Turning now to the cycle service level, suppose that in 10% of the review intervals, not all demand can be met from stock. This does not mean that all of the order lines will be unfulfilled in these review intervals; it is possible that some, at least, may be filled completely.

So, neither the ready rate nor the cycle service level measure the order-line fill rate directly. However, they do offer alternatives that are more convenient for the calculation of

OUT levels than the order-line fill rate (or the order fill rate). This does not mean that we should stop monitoring fill rates at the aggregate level, either for orders or order lines, but it does mean that these aggregate measures do not correspond exactly to any of the three main SKU-level measures.

In considering the selection of an SKU service level measure, it is helpful to distinguish between wholesaling and retailing environments. A wholesaler is in a business-to-business relationship, and should have reliable records of well-defined orders for specific volumes of specific SKUs. In this case, the cycle service level (P_1) and the unit fill rate (P_2) are measurable. These measures can also be calculated by retailers if their customers submit orders, for example through an online platform. However, the situation is not the same for 'walk-in' customers to a retail store. When customers enter the store, they may have only a rough idea of what they intend to buy. When the customers leave the store, the retailer knows what was bought, but not what was not bought because of stockouts, unless specific requests were made and recorded. So, in this case, the cycle service level and the unit fill rate are not measurable. On the other hand, the ready rate, P_3, is measurable, making it a useful measure of stock availability in retail stores.

These general considerations now need to be addressed in the light of inventory control for intermittent demand items. Such items are generally far more prevalent at wholesalers, especially where a wide range of stocks is held, including SKUs with very slow demand rates. In retailing, intermittent items are becoming more common, as discussed in Chapter 1, but are still less prevalent than in wholesaling. Demand on retailers, from individual customers, is generally for much smaller quantities than demand on wholesalers. This means that demand on retailers for slow-moving items tends to be intermittent rather than lumpy (see Chapter 1). For such items, the fill rate and the ready rate may be identical (Axsäter 2015) or the latter may act as an approximation to the former.

In summary, both the P_1 and the P_2 measures are measurable at wholesalers, where intermittent demand items are more common. In retail, intermittent SKUs are less common. Where they do occur, the P_2 measure can often be approximated by P_3, which is measurable. In the remainder of this chapter, we focus on the P_1 and P_2 measures, with some discussion on the variety of ways in which these measures may be calculated in practice.

3.4.4 Choice of Service Level Measure

The choice between the P_1 and P_2 measures depends on the immediate consequences of a stockout and the financial impacts of these consequences. If the customer is prepared to wait for the SKU to come into stock (as is common in wholesaling), then a backorder will be generated and there are two possible courses of action for the organisation:

1. Place an emergency order on the supplier for all the units of the item that have not been satisfied. The supplier is requested to satisfy this order in a shorter lead time than normal, to mitigate the poor service provided to the client(s).
2. Advise the client(s) to wait until the next replenishment order is due to arrive, after the usual lead time has elapsed. When the order arrives, the backorders will be released, subject to sufficient stock having arrived.

On the other hand, if the customer is not prepared to wait for the SKU to come back into stock (as is common in retailing), then there are two possible outcomes:

1. Sales of a substitute product.
2. A complete lost sale, with no substitute items sold.

In the backorder case, for the first course of action, there will usually be an additional price to be paid to the supplier for expediting the goods in a shorter time than normal. If this additional price is fixed, and not proportional to the number of units short, then the P_1 service measure may be appropriate. This is because it is based on the proportion of replenishment cycles for which expediting is necessary, rather than on the proportion of items not satisfied from stock.

For the second course of action in the backorder case, there is no expediting cost for the organisation, but there is a potential cost in terms of loss of goodwill. This also applies if the customer is not prepared to wait, although the loss may be mitigated if the customer is prepared to buy a substitute product. It was mentioned earlier that loss of goodwill is very difficult to quantify. However, a fixed cost does not seem appropriate. It is surely worse to be short by four units, with two client orders for two units not being satisfied, than to be short by one unit for one client. Instead, a cost that is proportional to the fraction of unsatisfied demand seems more suitable, as reflected by the P_2 measure.

If the customer is not prepared to wait and does not purchase a substitute product then, in addition to the indirect cost of loss of goodwill, there is also a direct cost of loss of profit to take into consideration. Again, a cost that is proportional to the fraction of unfilled demand seems appropriate, making the P_2 measure suitable.

3.4.5 Summary

In this section, we have seen that, although there may be real costs associated with inventory holdings and shortages, they can be very difficult to measure reliably. For this reason, we have advocated a service level measure approach at the SKU level.

We have found that both the cycle service level (P_1) and fill rate (P_2) are measurable in a wholesaling environment, and the fill rate may be approximated by the ready rate (P_3) for non-lumpy intermittent items in a retail environment.

There is a link between the cost-driven approach and the service-driven approach. If the main costs are in expediting orders, then the cycle service level is a better reflection of the costs. On the other hand, if the main costs are in loss of immediate profit or loss of goodwill, then the fill rate is a more appropriate measure.

3.5 Calculating Cycle Service Levels

If we decide to proceed with a cycle service level (CSL) measure at SKU level, then we need to be able to assess the CSL implications of alternative OUT levels. The calculation of CSLs depends on the probabilities of demand over the protection interval and so, before going further, we start this section with a discussion on demand probabilities.

Table 3.2   Distribution of demand over one week.

Demand	Probability
0	0.5
1	0.3
2	0.2
3 or more	0.0

3.5.1   Distribution of Demand Over One Time Period

A 'demand distribution' assigns a probability to each of the possible values of demand over a specified period of time. An example of a distribution of demand for an SKU over one week is shown in Table 3.2. The distribution assigns a probability of 0.5 to 0, indicating that the SKU is intermittent and we expect 50% of future weeks to contain no demand, and similarly assigns probabilities of 0.3 and 0.2 to demands of one and two units, respectively. According to this distribution, there will never be demand for three or more units over a period of one week, as the probability of this eventuality is zero.

The distribution in Table 3.2 may be represented physically by an icosahedral die of 20 faces, with the numbers on the faces representing the possible demand values. The values should be shared out amongst the 20 faces in direct proportion to the probabilities shown in Table 3.2. So, there would be 10 faces showing zero, six faces showing one, and four faces showing two.

The icosahedral die is a convenient way to visualise probabilities but suffers from the limitation that a 20-sided die can represent only those chances that are multiples of 0.05, because each side represents a chance of 1/20. Probabilities such as 0.02 cannot be represented. In practice, we can replace a physical die with a virtual one, and use software to generate random numbers to the required level of resolution.

In this chapter, we make two important assumptions, which correspond to the representation of chance events by a physical or virtual die:

1. *Independent*: The probability of demand in one period does not depend on the demand in previous periods (as each roll of the die is independent of previous rolls). This may not always be true in practice if 'streaks' of non-zero demands are observed more frequently than would be expected if demands were truly independent.
2. *Identically distributed*: The probabilities are not changing over time (as the faces on the die do not change). In practice, it is possible that the chance of a zero demand may decrease or increase over time. For example, as original equipment is withdrawn from production, the demand for spares will eventually decline, leading to a higher chance of zero demand.

For the remainder of this chapter, these two assumptions are maintained. In Chapters 6 and 7, we look at situations where demand is not identically distributed over time. In Chapters 13 and 14, we examine non-independent demand processes leading to streaks of demand.

In addition to the two assumptions of independence and identical distribution over time, we also make a third assumption:

3. *Non-negative*: Demand cannot be negative, although it can be zero.

This is a natural assumption for demand itself, although it is not appropriate for 'net demand', which is found by subtracting returns from demand (Kelle and Silver 1989). This is relevant in closed-loop supply chains where items are returned for refurbishment or remanufacturing.

3.5.2 Cycle Service Levels Based on All Cycles

In Chapter 2, we indicated why the distribution of demand over the whole protection interval $(R + L)$ is needed to determine OUT levels in periodic review systems. To recap, suppose that the stock on hand is at the OUT level just after a review and no order is triggered. In that case, the stock must last not just until the time of the next review (an interval of R time units), but until any stock is received after that review. This necessitates a further delay of L time units, to allow for the supplier's lead time. Care is needed in counting the length of the lead time. The use of an $R + L$ protection interval assumes that an order placed at the end of period t arrives in time to satisfy demands of period $t + L + 1$. If it arrives in time to satisfy the demands of period $t + L$, then the effective lead time is $L - 1$ and, for review intervals of length one period, the protection interval is of length L rather than $L + 1$ (Teunter and Duncan 2009).

Suppose that the demand distribution in Table 3.2 accurately represents the probabilities of future demand values over a single week, and that demand is independent and identically distributed. We are using a periodic review system, with a review interval of one week and a lead time of one week. Therefore, the protection interval is two weeks, and the distribution of demand over two weeks is shown in Table 3.3.

Table 3.3 Probability distribution of total demand over two weeks.

Total D_{R+L}	Week 1 D_R	Week 2 D_L	Week 1 $\mathbb{P}(D_R)$	Week 2 $\mathbb{P}(D_L)$	Product	Total $\mathbb{P}(D_{R+L})$
0	0	0	0.5	0.5	0.25	0.25
1	1	0	0.3	0.5	0.15	
	0	1	0.5	0.3	0.15	0.30
2	2	0	0.2	0.5	0.10	
	1	1	0.3	0.3	0.09	
	0	2	0.5	0.2	0.10	0.29
3	2	1	0.2	0.3	0.06	
	1	2	0.3	0.2	0.06	0.12
4	2	2	0.2	0.2	0.04	0.04

Table 3.4 Cumulative distribution of total demand over two weeks.

Demand	Probability	Cumulative probability
0	0.25	0.25
1	0.30	0.55
2	0.29	0.84
3	0.12	0.96
4	0.04	1.00

In Table 3.3, D_R denotes demand over the review interval (Week 1), D_L demand over the lead time (Week 2), and D_{R+L} demand over the protection interval (Weeks 1 and 2). Probability is denoted by the symbol $\mathbb{P}$.

To find the probabilities in Table 3.3, we first consider all the possible ways of achieving the demand values over two weeks. For example, a total demand of two can be achieved in three ways (two in Week 1, zero in Week 2; or one in Week 1, one in Week 2; or zero in Week 1 and two in Week 2). The full listings are given in the second and third columns of Table 3.3.

The probabilities in the fourth and fifth columns are taken directly from Table 3.2. The product of these probabilities in the sixth column represents the chance of a particular sequence of demands in Weeks 1 and 2 (assuming independence of demands). In the final column, the probabilities are summed appropriately, for each potential value of total demand over two weeks. For example, the probability of having a total demand of two is the sum of 0.10, 0.09, and 0.10, giving a value of 0.29. Now that the probabilities of demand over two weeks have been calculated, we can find the cumulative probability distribution, which represents the probabilities of observing particular demand values, or less than those values, as shown in Table 3.4.

The cumulative distribution of total demand over the protection interval is often used as an approximation to the cycle service level in (R, S) inventory systems (Cardós and Babiloni 2011). (The reasons why this is approximate, rather than exact, will be explained in Section 3.5.3.) Therefore, the approximate service levels may be read directly from the cumulative probabilities in Table 3.4, which shows a CSL of 84% if the OUT level is set at two units and a CSL of 96% if the OUT level is set at three units. So, knowledge of all the probabilities of demand (the demand distribution) is sufficient to allow the calculation of the approximate CSL for different OUT levels if demand is independent and identically distributed.

3.5.3 Cycle Service Levels Based on Cycles with Demand

The CSL measure is appropriate for non-intermittent demand but suffers from some drawbacks for intermittent demand. Cardós et al. (2006) gave the example of a product, without any stock at all, facing a demand once every 10 weeks. Even with no stock, there would be no stockouts in 90% of the weeks because there is no demand in 90% of the weeks. If the replenishment cycle is one week, then this would mean that the CSL is 90%. However, as the authors commented, with no stock, there is no service!

Examples such as this motivate the development of a revised method of calculating the cycle service level for intermittent demand items. Instead of looking at all replenishment cycles, we focus on those replenishment cycles that contain some demand. In this book, the revised cycle service level will be denoted as CSL^+, where the plus sign indicates restriction to review intervals with a positive (non-zero) demand. Cardós et al. (2006) argued that the usual calculation of demand probabilities would require amendment to recognise this restriction. Teunter and Duncan (2009) also took this into account in their non-parametric analysis, to be discussed in Chapter 13. Finding CSL^+ will require separate evaluation of:

1. The probability of demand over the review interval, conditional on this demand being strictly positive.
2. The (unconditional) probability of demand over the lead time.

These calculations are illustrated in Table 3.5.

The notation in Table 3.5 is the same as in Table 3.3. The probability in the fifth column is unconditional, and may be written as $\mathbb{P}(D_L)$, as there is no restriction on demand during lead time. The probabilities in the fourth and final columns are conditional, as they are subject to the condition that D_R is strictly positive ($D_R > 0$), and are written as $\mathbb{P}(D_R|D_R > 0)$ and $\mathbb{P}(D_{R+L}|D_R > 0)$, where the vertical lines indicate 'subject to the condition that'.

In Table 3.5, the review interval (Week 1) and the lead time (Week 2) are considered separately. In the second column, we exclude the possibility of zero demand, as the CSL^+ measure is restricted to review intervals with non-zero demand. The values in the fourth column have also changed. In the long run, only half of the weeks have non-zero demands, according to Table 3.2. Therefore, although only 30% of weeks have a demand of one unit, 60% of weeks with some demand have a demand of one unit. Similarly, 40% of weeks with some demand have a demand of two units. The fifth column uses the same probabilities as in Table 3.2 because the possibility of zero demand is not excluded in Week 2. The final two columns in Table 3.5 are calculated in the same way as in Table 3.3.

Table 3.5 Distribution of total demand over two weeks conditional on non-zero demand in first week.

Total D_{R+L}	Week 1 D_R	Week 2 D_L	Week 1 Probability	Week 2 Probability	Product	Total Probability
1	1	0	0.6	0.5	0.30	0.30
2	2	0	0.4	0.5	0.20	
	1	1	0.6	0.3	0.18	0.38
3	2	1	0.4	0.3	0.12	
	1	2	0.6	0.2	0.12	0.24
4	2	2	0.4	0.2	0.08	0.08

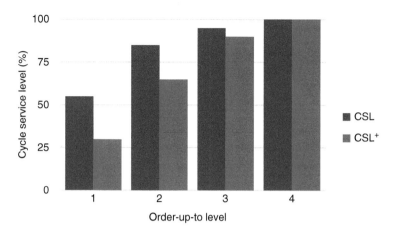

Figure 3.1 Comparison of CSL and CSL$^+$.

Now that the conditional probabilities have been calculated, it may be asked if they can be used to estimate CSL$^+$. Cardós and Babiloni (2011) pointed out that, strictly speaking, we are interested in the probability that demand over a replenishment cycle does not exceed the stock on hand at the beginning of the cycle. This value would give an exact cycle service level but it is very difficult to calculate and Cardós and Babiloni (2011, p. 64) concluded, 'The exact method to compute the CSL is not an appropriate procedure to be widely used in a business context'. Consequently, they recommended basing calculations on the cumulative conditional probabilities of demand over the protection interval, in order to estimate the revised cycle service level (CSL$^+$). Returning to our example, the results are given in Figure 3.1, and are compared with the original CSL values for different potential OUT levels.

In this example, there is a large difference between the two cycle service level measures, for OUT levels of both one and two units. The difference between the two measures for three units is smaller (96% for CSL, 92% for CSL$^+$) but would lead to a disagreement on the OUT level needed to ensure that a 95% cycle service level target is met. For an OUT level of four units, there is no difference: all demand is satisfied, as the maximum demand over two weeks is for four units (see Table 3.4). It does not matter whether cycles with no demand in the review intervals are excluded or not; there can be no stockouts in either case.

In our example, the calculations were manageable because the protection interval was only for two periods and the OUT level did not need to exceed four units. The calculations can become more involved for longer protection intervals and higher OUT levels, and approximate formulae have been given to simplify the calculations (Cardós and Babiloni 2011). In Chapter 8, we explain how other formulae can be used if the demand follows certain demand distributions. If no demand distributions can adequately represent the real demand, then another option is to use non-parametric approaches, to be discussed in Chapter 13.

3.5.4 Summary

There are two approaches to measuring the cycle service level. These methods produce the same results for non-intermittent demand. They differ for intermittent items because the second method excludes those cycles with no demand during the review interval. This makes more sense for intermittence, but it complicates the calculation, which depends on combining two different demand distributions, one for the review interval and one for the lead time.

3.6 Calculating Fill Rates

The unit fill rate is defined as the proportion of demand satisfied directly from stock on hand, as noted earlier. It can be calculated at both aggregate and SKU levels, and can be defined in terms of volume filled or value filled. At SKU level, volume and value fill rates will be the same (unless calculated over a period of time in which there has been a price change) but will usually differ at an aggregate level. In this section, we look at some of the issues that need to be addressed in finding the unit (volume) fill rate, and discuss how demand distributions can be used in its calculation.

3.6.1 Unit Fill Rates

The basic unit fill rate calculation is straightforward. For example, if in a particular period we satisfy three units out of four demanded directly from stock, then the fill rate is 75%. Let us now consider an example of four periods with each period showing some demand, as shown in Table 3.6.

How should we define the overall fill rate? There are two possible approaches. The first is to total the satisfied demand (8 units) and divide by the total demand (16 units) to give an overall fill rate of 50%, as shown in Table 3.6. The second approach is to average the fill rates over all four periods, giving an overall fill rate of 56.25%, which is somewhat higher than the first calculation. If all four periods had a fill rate of 50%, then the two calculation methods would agree. The disagreement arises because the average of the fill rates in the second and third periods is 62.5%, whereas only 50% of the total demand over these two periods is fulfilled. The second method can be applied to intermittent demand only if periods with zero demands are excluded from the calculation. For further discussion of this method, please refer to Guijarro et al. (2012). We will base our analysis on the first method, as it is simpler for intermittent demand, and is the standard method in the literature and in practice.

Table 3.6   Fill rates per time period.

Period	Demand	Satisfied	Fill rate
1	2	1	0.50
2	4	1	0.25
3	2	2	1.00
4	8	4	0.50
Total	16	8	0.50

3.6.2   Fill Rates: Standard Formula

To calculate the unit fill rate (FR), we need to evaluate how much demand is satisfied, over a given period of time, as a proportion of the demand over the same period. Equivalently, we can evaluate the average unsatisfied demand per period, as a proportion of the average demand per period, and subtract this ratio from one, as shown in Eq. (3.2).

$$FR = 1 - \frac{\frac{1}{n}\sum_{t=1}^{n}(d_t - SOH_t)^+}{\frac{1}{n}\sum_{t=1}^{n}d_t} \qquad (3.2)$$

where SOH_t represents the stock on hand at the start of time period t, after receipt of any orders and dispatch of any outstanding backorders, d_t is demand during time period t, and n is the number of time periods over which the fill rate is being measured. The superscript + indicates a result of zero if the expression in the brackets is negative, and unchanged otherwise. For example, $(2 - 6)^+ = 0$ and $(6 - 2)^+ = 4$.

In Eq. (3.2), the expression $(d_t - SOH_t)^+$ represents the backorders generated at the end of period t as a consequence of demand in that period not being satisfied. If there is sufficient stock (d_t less than or equal to SOH_t), then there are no backorders. If there is insufficient stock (d_t strictly greater than SOH_t), then $d_t - SOH_t$ units are backordered. In the numerator of the ratio in Eq. (3.2), the backorders are summed over all periods and divided by the number of periods (n) to give the average unsatisfied demand per period. In the denominator, we have the average demand per period. The ratio represents the average unsatisfied demand per period as a proportion of the average demand per period.

For ease of exposition, from this point on, we assume that the review interval is one period ($R = 1$). At the end of this section, we return to the more general case when it can be longer.

Equation (3.2) is an exact calculation of the fill rate. It can be used to find the historical fill rates, providing that we maintain records of the demands in each period, and the backorders in each period. Suppose that, for a particular SKU, the average demand per period was for 10 units and the average backorder quantity per period was one unit. Then, it follows immediately that the historical fill rate for that SKU was 90%.

Now suppose that we wish to experiment with different OUT levels. Equation (3.2) is not helpful because, even if the average demand per period remains unchanged, the equation does not reveal the effect on backorders of changing the OUT level (S). To assess the effect of different OUT levels (S) on the fill rate (FR(S)), the formula given in Eq. (3.3) is often used.

$$FR(S) = 1 - \frac{\sum_x \mathbb{P}(D_{R+L} = x)(x - S)^+}{\mu} \qquad (3.3)$$

where D_{R+L} is the demand over the protection interval ($R + L$) and μ is the long-run average demand per (single) period. We shall refer to this as the traditional fill rate calculation.

As we shall see later, this traditional fill rate calculation suffers from some drawbacks, whether demand is intermittent or not. However, it is often used in practice, and so it is important to understand its calculation, including its flaws and how they can be rectified.

To illustrate the traditional calculation of fill rates, we now look at another example. The review interval is set as one week and the lead time as two weeks. The distribution

Table 3.7 Distribution of lumpy demand over one week.

Demand	Probability
0	0.5
1	0.3
4	0.2
5 or more	0.0

Table 3.8 Traditional fill rate calculation ($S = 7$ and $S = 8$; $R + L = 3$).

Demand (x)	Probability $\mathbb{P}(D_3 = x)$	Not satisfied $(x - 7)^+$	Expected $S = 7$	Not satisfied $(x - 8)^+$	Expected $S = 8$
1	0.225	0	0.000	0	0.000
2	0.135	0	0.000	0	0.000
3	0.027	0	0.000	0	0.000
4	0.150	0	0.000	0	0.000
5	0.180	0	0.000	0	0.000
6	0.054	0	0.000	0	0.000
8	0.060	1	0.060	0	0.000
9	0.036	2	0.072	1	0.036
12	0.008	5	0.040	4	0.032
		Total	0.172	Total	0.068
		Fill rate ($S = 7$)	84.4%	Fill rate ($S = 8$)	93.8%

of demand is similar to the example in Table 3.2, except that it is lumpier, with a spike of demand at four units, as shown in Table 3.7.

Continuing this example, we summarise in Table 3.8 the probabilities of demand over a protection interval of three weeks (first two columns) and traditional fill rate calculations for OUT levels of seven units (middle two columns) and eight units (final two columns).

The first column of Table 3.8 lists all of the possible total demands over three weeks, given possible demands of zero, one, and four units in one week. The possibility of zero demand over the whole three weeks has not been included. It is not relevant from a fill rate perspective because there is no demand to be fulfilled. Some demand values are omitted, such as seven, as there is no combination of three weeks of demand, in this example, that can give this number. The detailed calculations for the second column are not given but they follow exactly the same approach as in Table 3.3, where all combinations of demands are identified, and probabilities are calculated accordingly.

The third and fifth columns of Table 3.8 show how much demand would not be satisfied for the specified OUT levels. For example, for an OUT level of seven units, a demand of six units can be fully satisfied, but demands of eight, nine, or twelve units will be only partly satisfied, with unsatisfied demand of one, two, and five units, respectively.

The fourth and sixth columns contain the expected shortages, corresponding to different demand values. These expected shortages are calculated by multiplying the number of items not satisfied (third and fifth columns) by the probability of demand over the protection interval (second column). The values in the fourth and sixth columns are summed to give the total expected shortages for OUT levels of seven and eight units.

The final calculation of fill rates uses Eq. (3.3). The mean value, μ, is found as a weighted average of the probabilities of demand in a single period (see Table 3.7). The calculation is: $\mu = (0.5 \times 0) + (0.3 \times 1) + (0.2 \times 4) = 1.1$. This value, and the overall values for expected unsatisfied demand per period are substituted into Eq. (3.3) to give the fill rates of 84.4% and 93.8% for OUT levels of seven and eight units, respectively.

3.6.3 Fill Rates: Sobel's Formula

Johnson et al. (1995) pointed out that the traditional fill rate calculation can suffer from double counting. This arises from the same shortage being counted in two separate periods. To appreciate how this happens, we continue with our example in Table 3.8.

Let us look again at the results corresponding to a demand of 12 (over three weeks), shown in the bottom row of the middle section of Table 3.8. For $S = 7$, the traditional formula gives a shortage of five units at the end of the third week. However, this is not accurate. A total demand of 12 can have arisen only from a demand of four in each of the three weeks because the distribution in Table 3.7 shows that four is the maximum weekly demand. Therefore, the demand in the first two weeks must have been for eight units, giving a shortage (and backorder) of one unit at the end of the second week if $S = 7$. The shortage of five units at the end of the third week is actually the sum of one unit backordered in the second week and a further four units backordered in the third week. To count this as five would be to double count the unit that was short in the second week and is still short in the third week.

More generally, the traditional fill rate formula is appropriate if there are no backorders at the end of L periods (still assuming that $R = 1$). However, if there are some backorders, then these should not be added on to any further backorders that may arise in the next period. This motivated the development of a revised formula, proposed by Sobel (2004), for calculating the fill rate when the review interval is of one period:

$$\text{FR}_{\text{Sobel}}(S) = 1 - \frac{\sum_x \sum_y \mathbb{P}(D_L = x)\mathbb{P}(d_{L+1} = y)(y - (S - x)^+)^+}{\mu} \tag{3.4}$$

where D_L is the demand over the lead time, d_{L+1} is the demand in the single period just after the completion of the lead time, and the other notation is unchanged. This formula overcomes the problem of double counting if demand is always non-negative, and is independent and identically distributed. To show how the formula works in practice, we recalculate the fill rate for $S = 7$ using Sobel's formula, keeping the lead time as two weeks, as shown in Table 3.9.

Table 3.9 Sobel's fill rate calculation ($S = 7, L = 2, R = 1$).

Demand, D_2 (x)	SOH $(7 - x)^+$	Demand, d_3 (y)	Not satisfied $(y - (7 - x)^+)^+$	Probability $\mathbb{P}(D_2 = x)$	Probability $\mathbb{P}(d_3 = y)$	Expected not satisfied
0	7	1	0	0.25	0.3	0.000
0	7	4	0	0.25	0.2	0.000
1	6	1	0	0.30	0.3	0.000
1	6	4	0	0.30	0.2	0.000
2	5	1	0	0.09	0.3	0.000
2	5	4	0	0.09	0.2	0.000
4	3	1	0	0.20	0.3	0.000
4	3	4	1	0.20	0.2	0.040
5	2	1	0	0.12	0.3	0.000
5	2	4	2	0.12	0.2	0.048
8	0	1	1	0.04	0.3	0.012
8	0	4	4	0.04	0.2	0.032
					Total	0.132
					Fill rate ($S = 7$)	88.0%

In Table 3.9, the first and third columns give all the potential combinations of demands during the lead time (two periods) and the review interval (one period), excluding the possibility of zero demand in the review interval, as this cannot yield unsatisfied demand in that period. The second column shows the stock on hand (SOH) for $S = 7$, after depletion of the lead time demand (zero if the lead time demand is for eight units).

The fourth column shows the unsatisfied demand, given the stock on hand in the second column and the review interval demand in the third column. Let us return to the case of a demand of eight units in the first two weeks and four units in the third week, shown in the bottom row of the middle section of the table. Now, the unsatisfied demand in the third period is shown as four units, avoiding double counting of the one unit of unsatisfied demand in the second week.

The probabilities in the fifth and sixth columns are multiplied together to give the chance of the combination of demand values in the lead time and the review interval (assuming independence of demands over time). This is then multiplied by the unsatisfied demand, in the fourth column, to give the expected unsatisfied demand. (The probabilities of demand over two weeks, shown in the fifth column, are calculated in the same way as for Table 3.3. The probabilities in the sixth column are taken directly from Table 3.7.) Finally, the overall expected unsatisfied demand per period of 0.132 and the mean demand of 1.1 per single time period are substituted into Eq. (3.4) to give a fill rate of 88.0%. As anticipated, Sobel's formula gives a higher fill rate than the traditional formula (84.4%) because it avoids the problem of double counting of backorders.

It is instructive to repeat these calculations for an OUT level of eight units. In this case, Sobel's formula gives a fill rate of 93.8%, which is exactly the same as the traditional formula (see Table 3.8). The reason is that, in this case, the maximum demand over the lead time (eight units) can deplete the stock to zero but cannot result in a backorder situation. Therefore, there will be no double counting of backorders from past periods.

Sobel's formula (Eq. (3.4)) is based on reviews every period ($R = 1$). Zhang and Zhang (2007) presented a fill rate formula which applies for any whole-number length of review interval (R). This formula is given in Technical Note 3.1, together with an explanation of its components. The formula applies for the (R, S) periodic inventory policy, which has been our main focus of attention. Teunter (2009) extended this analysis to the continuous (s, Q) policy. There are further refinements to fill rate calculations for normally distributed demands that are not independent or when negative demands are permitted (interpreted as returns). The interested reader is referred to Disney et al. (2015) for a more detailed discussion.

3.6.4 Summary

In some ways, the fill rate is the most natural service measure for intermittent demand. The concept is straightforward to explain to managers and is often used in practice. However, the implementation of the fill rate calculation raises some technical issues. Adjustments are needed to avoid double counting of backorders. Although these adjustments do make the calculation more complex, they may be beneficial, particularly for those items with lumpy demand patterns. The formulae given in this section and in Technical Note 3.1 require distributions of demand over the lead time or longer. If the demand is assumed to be independent and identically distributed, then these distributions may be obtained from the distribution of demand per period. Selecting this distribution will become our focus of attention in Chapters 4 and 5.

3.7 Setting Service Level Targets

Once a choice of measure has been made, there is a need to set targets that appropriately reflect the organisation's broader goals. These may be applied universally, across all SKUs, or differentially, for different categories of SKUs. The setting of these targets is the subject of this section.

3.7.1 Responsibility for Target Setting

Who should be responsible for setting service level targets? Often, the sales department is allocated this responsibility. Snapp (2018) suggested that this may be misguided because sales people may not be fully aware of the supply chain implications of a change in the target service level. Similarly, the supply chain department may be unaware of the competitive implications in the market. Snapp recommended a cross-functional approach, for example in a sales and operations planning (S&OP) process, to overcome silo-oriented target service level setting. (Please refer to Jandhyala et al. 2018, for further information on S&OP.)

3.7.2   Trade-off Between Service and Cost

At what levels should service level targets be set? This is not an easy question to answer. Nevertheless, if an organisation is clear on the priority level of inventory service as part of its positioning, and the costs it is prepared to bear, then it is in a good position to set service level targets strategically.

An assessment of service level options should be informed by an evaluation of the trade-off between service level and cost. It is here that well-designed inventory systems can be very helpful. An early example was given by Johnston (1980), who designed an interactive stock control system for builders' merchants. He included a facility to allow managers to experiment with alternative stocking strategies, using the system to provide estimates of the anticipated average stock values, stock turns, service levels, and expected lost sales per annum. This type of analysis can enable exchange curves to be drawn, such as that illustrated in Figure 3.2.

Figure 3.2 shows an example of the trade-off between fill rates and average inventory values. Curves such as this can be drawn for whole categories of stocks for which different service level targets may be applied. For example, separate analyses could be conducted for fast, medium, and slow-moving SKUs and service level targets set accordingly for each stock category.

Exchange curves can be drawn only if the inventory system allows the simulation of inventories with different service level targets. At a higher strategic level, it is possible to design systems to allow experimentation on service level targets at a stocking location, or to examine the stock implications of merging two stocking points (Johnston et al. 1988).

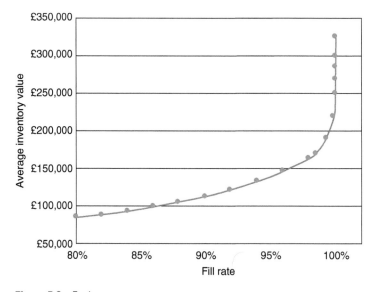

Figure 3.2   Exchange curve.

3.7.3 Setting SKU Level Service Targets

It is natural to define fill rates in the same way at aggregate and SKU levels. Then, it is clear that fill rate targets set at an aggregate level can also be applied at SKU level. As previously mentioned, these targets can be set differentially by stock category.

An alternative approach is to treat the items in a class separately if they have different unit costs. Thonemann et al. (2002) presented a model to reduce the overall stock costs by assigning higher fill rate targets to lower cost items and lower fill rate targets to higher cost items, while ensuring that the overall fill rate target is met. Other authors (Zhang et al. 2001; Teunter et al. 2010, 2017) have proposed approaches based on ranking SKUs, using various criteria, and then treating the SKUs differentially. Some of these approaches will be reviewed in Chapter 11.

Systems having the facility to experiment with service level targets at the level of the individual SKU are available (for example, at the time of writing, RightStock from DBO Services and the Inventory Planner of Arkieva). In Figure 3.3 we show a screenshot of the Inventory Strategist function from RightStock.

In the example given in Figure 3.3, the current system target cycle service level is set to 95% (fifth row of the 'Current parameters' column). Managers may experiment with the setting of different targets for a particular SKU. In the example given above, these experiments are shown as three scenarios (target service levels of 93%, 97%, and 99.5%). The bar chart shows the effect of varying the target, with respect to the average cycle stocks (to cover expected demand) and safety stocks (to allow for uncertainty of demand). This

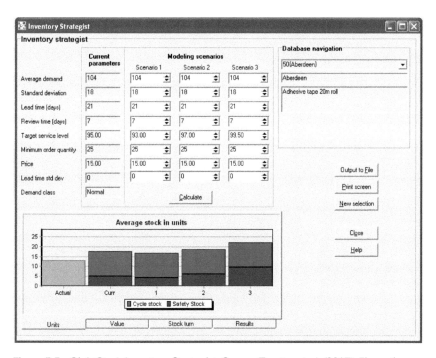

Figure 3.3 RightStock Inventory Strategist. Source: Teunter et al. (2017), Figure 1.

enables managers to make more informed judgements as to the most appropriate service level for a specific SKU.

In conclusion, we can use the 'what if' facilities of software packages to experiment with different target service levels, at the level of an individual SKU. This experimentation will show the predicted effect of different targets on inventory levels and, hence, on inventory investment. It is then a matter for managers to make a judgement about the most appropriate target, taking into account the investments that would be required.

3.7.4 Summary

In this section, we have seen that judgements need to be made before setting aggregate service targets. The choice of service level targets should be informed by the service offered by others and the degree to which inventory service is prioritised as a source of competitive advantage. Service targets may then be set for whole classes of SKUs or differentially for each individual SKU.

Software can be used to conduct experiments at aggregate or SKU level, to show the inventory consequences of different service level targets. It is important to undertake such evaluations to ensure that the balance being struck between service and costs is one that reflects the aims of the organisation as a whole.

3.8 Chapter Summary

In this chapter, we started by arguing for a more analytical approach to inventory management and not relying on ad hoc rules. Nevertheless, there is still room for managerial judgement. In fact, such judgement is essential for

1. Selecting an aggregate service measure (or set of measures) against which performance will be monitored.
2. Selecting an appropriate service measure at SKU level, which best reflects the costs to the organisation of backordering and not satisfying demand from stock.
3. Deciding on the best target service levels.

Judgement may also be exercised at the level of the individual SKU, by making adjustments to demand forecasts (to be discussed further in Chapter 10) or by making adjustments to orders, without adjusting demand forecasts. These adjustments can be beneficial in certain circumstances but may also worsen performance. If such adjustments are frequent, then ongoing assessments should be made to check that performance is being improved.

We have also reviewed issues in calculating cycle service levels and fill rates. Some of these issues are quite technical but it is important that they are resolved and the measures are calculated correctly, so that inventories are set at the right levels.

The usual calculation for cycle service levels, as given in many textbooks, has some limitations for intermittent demand. It will lead to an inflated assessment of customer service, as it will count a review interval with no stockouts as a success even if there has been no demand. For intermittent demand, we saw how an alternative measure can be calculated, based on a restriction to those review intervals in which there has been some demand.

The traditional calculation for fill rates is an approximation, as it can double count some stockouts. This can lead to an underestimate of the fill rate that may, in turn, lead to excessive stocks being held. The double counting problem is particularly concerning for SKUs with lumpy demand patterns. In fact, it is an issue for particularly volatile non-intermittent demand as well. The formulae of Sobel (2004) and Zhang and Zhang (2007), although somewhat more complicated, can address this issue and give more reliable fill rate calculations.

The calculations for both the cycle service level and the fill rate rely on demand probabilities. These may be over the review interval, the lead time, or the whole protection interval, and can be found from the probabilities of demand in a single period. The estimation of these probabilities is central to supply chain forecasting. Over the next two chapters, we examine different probability distributions that can be used to represent demand, and then move on to their forecasting requirements.

Technical Note

Note 3.1 Fill Rate Expression of Zhang and Zhang

Zhang and Zhang (2007) gave a formal mathematical justification for their measure. Here, we give a more informal explanation. Zhang and Zhang's fill rate measure for periodic review systems with review interval R, and OUT level S, is given in Eq. (3.5).

$$\text{FR}_{ZZ}(S) = 1 - \frac{\sum_{j=0}^{R-1}\sum_x\sum_y \mathbb{P}(D_{L+j} = x)\mathbb{P}(d_{L+j+1} = y)(y - (S-x)^+)^+}{R\mu} \tag{3.5}$$

where $D_{L+j} = d_1 + \cdots + d_{L+j}$, x denotes possible total demand values over the periods up to $L+j$, and y denotes possible demand values in the next period, $L+j+1$.

The amount subtracted from 1 represents the proportion of demand that is not satisfied. The denominator represents the average demand over the whole review interval (length R), recalling that μ is the average demand per unit time period.

In the numerator, each unit of time in the review interval is analysed separately. For the first unit of time, denoted by $j = 0$ in Eq. (3.5), backorders are generated if the demand d_{L+1} is in excess of the remaining stock, after taking into account the cumulative demand over L periods, D_L. The same argument applies for the second unit of time, denoted by $j = 1$: backorders are generated if the demand d_{L+2} is in excess of the remaining stock, after taking into account the cumulative demand over $L+1$ periods, D_{L+1}. This argument holds for every unit of time in the review interval. In each case, the backorders are weighted by the probability of demand in the unit of time and the probability of cumulative demand in the preceding periods, and are summed appropriately. The results are totalled over the whole review interval to give the expected total backorders.

4

Demand Distributions

4.1 Introduction

If demand over lead time were certain, then inventory replenishment would be a straightforward task. Hypothetically, suppose we know with certainty that demand never varies and is always for two units per day. Also, we know that, whenever we place an order with our supplier, then the order will always arrive in a fixed lead time period of five days without fail. If we review stock levels continuously, and place an order for 10 units whenever stocks drop to 10 units exactly, then we will be able to satisfy all customer demand while we are waiting for the order to arrive.

Of course, things are never so straightforward in real life. Firstly, the lead time may not be fixed but may vary according to the situation at the supplying company. Shortage of labour, equipment, or materials, unexpected transportation problems, or simply poor management may result in the supplier failing to meet the promised lead time. Secondly, even if the supplier does keep to the promised lead time, it is very unlikely that demand would be fixed. Instead, it is much more likely to vary over time and follow a demand distribution, as discussed in Chapter 3, with some periods showing higher demand than others. The reasons for this variability may be explainable. For example, it may be due to promotions or seasonal effects. Often, the reasons elude any convincing explanation.

In summary, we may need to address variability in lead time as well as variability in demand. The focus of this chapter is on demand variability, but supply variability is also important and should be minimised whenever possible. Indeed, working with suppliers to ensure reliable and consistent deliveries, according to planned lead times, is an essential part of inventory management. If lead times are unreliable and inconsistent, then demand variability will be magnified by lead time variability. We return to lead time variability in Chapters 7 and 8, while concentrating on the characterisation of demand variability in this chapter and in Chapter 5.

Demand variability may be severe when demand is intermittent. Suppose we have a demand history of 5, 0, 0, 20, 0, 1, 0, 10, 0, 1 (a pattern that is not untypical in practice). Predicting such highly variable demand over the next few periods is a daunting task. We cannot know what the demand will be, even in the next period, unless we have advance demand information, which is usually not available. However, as we saw in the previous

Intermittent Demand Forecasting: Context, Methods and Applications, First Edition.
John E. Boylan and Aris A. Syntetos.
© 2021 John Wiley & Sons Ltd. Published 2021 by John Wiley & Sons Ltd.
Companion Website: www.wiley.com/go/boylansyntetos/intermittentdemandforecasting

chapter, an exact forecast of demand is not required for inventory control. The requirement is for estimates of the probabilities of demand. Then, we can also estimate the cycle service levels or fill rates that will follow from using different order-up-to levels.

In this chapter, we look at how probabilities of demand may be characterised in the form of a demand distribution. We begin by discussing two different approaches to estimating a demand distribution, noting their advantages and disadvantages. Then, we give four criteria against which any proposed demand distribution may be judged.

We introduce the Poisson distribution, which is one of the most frequently recommended distributions for intermittent demand. It was also one of the earliest to be applied in stock-control systems for slow-moving items (see, for example, the work of Boothroyd and Tomlinson 1963, on engineering spare parts in the coal industry). The general properties of the Poisson are outlined, followed by a more specific investigation of its application to intermittent demand.

We make a careful distinction between demand, demand incidence, and demand occurrence, as a foundation for the formulation of compound distributions, to be discussed in Chapter 5. We reappraise the Poisson as a distribution of demand incidence, rather than as a distribution of demand itself, before turning to the Bernoulli distribution, which can be used to represent demand occurrence. We conclude with a summary of the chapter and some pointers towards the material on demand forecasting in future chapters.

4.2 Estimation of Demand Distributions

In the previous chapter, it was assumed that the demand distribution is known. In practice, the distribution is never known exactly and has to be estimated. In this section, we look at two approaches to estimating demand distributions. One approach (called 'empirical') is based on straightforward calculations of probabilities, based on past data. The other approach (called 'fitted') is based on fitting a mathematical function, known as a probability mass function, to the past data. The 'fitted' approach is often used in commercial software packages.

4.2.1 Empirical Demand Distributions

Figure 4.1 shows a time plot of the demand for a spare part from the automotive industry over the last 24 months.

The data is not particularly sparse. In fact, there is only one zero demand observation in Period 8. In the next plot, Figure 4.2 shows the frequency with which each of the observed demands (including zero) appears in the demand history. For example, there were five periods when the demand was for one unit. Frequencies may also be presented in relative terms. Relative frequencies measure the proportion of historical periods having each of the observed values of demand. For example, the relative frequency of zero demand is 1/24 = 0.0417 (=4.17%), as there is one period out of 24 with no demand.

Figure 4.2 shows the number of time periods containing each of the demand values from 0 to 12. It is an exact representation of demand frequencies in the past 24 months. Ideally, our

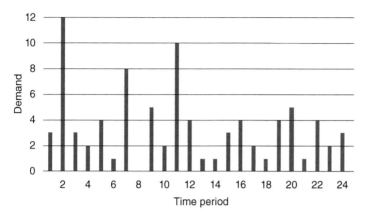

Figure 4.1 Monthly demand time series for an automotive SKU.

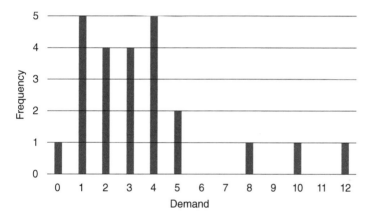

Figure 4.2 Demand frequencies for an automotive SKU.

inventory replenishment decisions should be based on demand relative frequencies in the near future, over the protection interval. Of course, these relative frequencies are unknown. Therefore, we must rely on estimates of demand probabilities in the future. There are two ways of turning past relative frequencies into future probabilities.

In the first (empirical) approach, we assume that the demand probabilities over the forthcoming protection interval may be represented by relative frequencies in the past, showing the proportion of historical periods having each of the observed values of demand. Referring to Figure 4.2, this would mean that our estimate of the probability of observing demand for eight units in the next period is $1/24 = 4.17\%$ and the probability of nine units is zero. However, having observed demand for 8 and 10 units in the past, it may seem unreasonable to assume that 9 cannot be demanded in the future.

In the second (fitted) approach, we begin by assuming that future demand probabilities will be similar to past relative frequencies, but not necessarily the same. This can be achieved by using a fitted demand distribution. In this case, the probability estimates should be close to the past relative frequencies but they are allowed to differ.

4.2.2 Fitted Demand Distributions

Using fitted demand distributions, we try to mimic the main features of the demand series without matching the observed relative frequencies exactly. Returning to Figure 4.2, if future probabilities are to resemble the pattern of past demand frequencies, then we would expect a low probability of zero demand, higher probabilities within the range of demand values from one to four, and lower probabilities for demand values of five or higher.

These features may be illustrated, at least in part, by superimposing two lines over the relative frequencies, one rising (for lower demand values) and one falling (for higher demand values), as shown in Figure 4.3.

The bold lines in Figure 4.3 are merely illustrative. The only demand values that take probabilities are whole numbers. It is meaningful to speak of a probability of a demand of two units but not usually of 2.33 units. (An exception would be goods that are purchased by weight and any weight is permitted.) The bold lines are included to highlight the shape of the distribution, known as a 'triangular distribution' because it resembles a triangle, with the base shown as a dashed line. Later, in Figure 4.4, the distribution will be drawn more precisely, showing probabilities at whole numbers only.

It is immediately obvious that the two sloping lines are far from a perfect fit to the past relative frequencies (which can be read from the right-hand vertical axis of Figure 4.3). Indeed, we shall see that other shapes may be better but, for the moment, we proceed with the idea of a triangular demand distribution. The upward sloping line in Figure 4.3 indicates a steep increase in the probabilities for lower demand values. The downward sloping line in Figure 4.3 shows a steady decrease between each of the probabilities for higher demand values.

To fully describe a triangular distribution, we need to specify three values, known as parameter values:

1. The lowest demand value to be assigned a probability.
2. The highest demand value to be assigned a probability.
3. The demand value at which the apex of the triangle is attained.

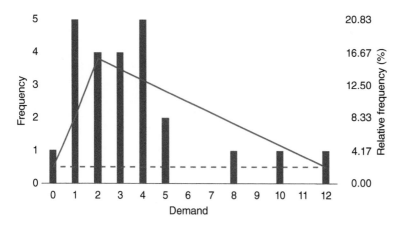

Figure 4.3 Demand relative frequencies with triangle superimposed.

We know that demand is sometimes zero, and cannot be negative, so the lowest possible demand value is zero. This, then, is our lowest demand value requiring a probability.

We also know that the highest value observed in the last 24 periods is 12, but it is possible that higher values may be observed in the future. This presents a difficulty with using the triangular distribution to represent demand, as it is far from obvious what a future maximum value may be. In our case, we assume that the maximum demand is 13, but recognise that this choice is arbitrary and other values could have been chosen.

The apex of the triangle is also hard to identify. In Figure 4.3, it has been drawn at the demand value of two but it could have been drawn at other neighbouring values. The difficulty of identifying an apex is an indication that the triangular shape may not be the best for this data. However, to make further progress with this example, we shall assume that the apex is at a demand value of two.

The triangular distribution between 0 and 13, with apex at two, is shown in Table 4.1. (The probability calculations are explained in Technical Note 4.1.)

The demand distribution shown in Table 4.1 allows for the possibility of demand for 6, 7, 9, or 11 units, which are within the range of previous observations, although not previously observed. It also allows for the possibility of demand of 13 units, which lies beyond the previously observed range. All of these features are potentially beneficial, but we now need to check the 'fit' of the distribution to the relative frequencies. How closely does the triangular distribution match the relative frequencies of previous actual values? This may be observed in Figure 4.4.

The first criterion that must be met by any hypothesised distribution is that it should be a 'good fit' to the observed data. In Figure 4.4, we should be very doubtful about this.

Table 4.1 Triangular distribution example.

Demand	0	1	2	3	4	5	6	7	8	9	10	11	12	13
Probability	$\frac{4}{90}$	$\frac{8}{90}$	$\frac{12}{90}$	$\frac{11}{90}$	$\frac{10}{90}$	$\frac{9}{90}$	$\frac{8}{90}$	$\frac{7}{90}$	$\frac{6}{90}$	$\frac{5}{90}$	$\frac{4}{90}$	$\frac{3}{90}$	$\frac{2}{90}$	$\frac{1}{90}$

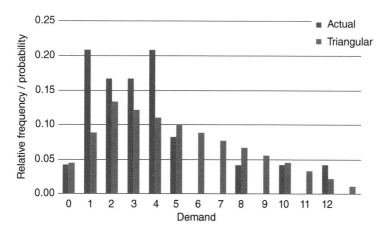

Figure 4.4 Actual relative frequencies and triangular probabilities.

The triangular distribution probabilities seem to be too low for demand values from one to four units and too high for demand values between five and nine units. In Section 4.4, we examine an alternative distribution to see if a better fit can be obtained.

4.2.3 Summary

In this section, we have noted the difference between empirical and fitted demand distributions. Empirical distributions make no assumptions about the shape of the demand distribution except that the demand probabilities over the protection interval will be the same as the relative frequencies observed in the historical data. This has the advantage that it does not force an inappropriate shape on the distribution. However, if the empirical method is not adapted (to be discussed in Chapter 13), it has the disadvantage that demand values not observed in the past are automatically assigned zero probabilities for the future. Fitted distributions, on the other hand, have the flexibility of allowing non-zero probabilities for demands not observed in the past, but may sometimes force a shape on the demand pattern that does not provide a good fit. In this section, we used the triangular distribution for the purposes of illustration and explanation. It is rarely used for intermittent demand in practice and so we proceed to review distributions that are much more commonly applied. To do this, we need criteria against which the distributions may be compared.

4.3 Criteria for Demand Distributions

In Section 4.2, we focused, quite naturally, on how closely the triangular distribution conformed to the relative frequencies of demand values observed in the past. This is known as the distribution's 'goodness of fit'. This is the first requirement for a demand distribution and we shall say more about it shortly. However, it is not the only criterion for a good demand distribution and, in this section, we discuss three further criteria that should be taken into consideration.

4.3.1 Empirical Evidence for Goodness of Fit

The discussion in Section 4.2 illustrated the idea of goodness of fit by checking the triangular distribution's fit for one time series (shown in Figure 4.1). In practice, we usually want to check that a particular distribution is appropriate for a whole set of stock keeping units (SKUs) (e.g. all slow-moving items). To do this, we can look at the demand histories for each SKU in the set, fit a distribution to the frequency data for each series, and then check the goodness of fit. This gives us empirical evidence that is directly relevant to the application of a distribution in practice. The checking can be challenging if the demand is highly intermittent or the history is short. Some alternative checking approaches will be reviewed later in this chapter.

4.3.2 Further Criteria

It is desirable that the distribution has properties that are consistent with the known features of the demand pattern. For example, if demand data cannot be negative, then the demand distribution should not be defined for negative values. Such features may be determined prior to any statistical analysis of goodness of fit, and are known as 'a priori' grounds for choosing a distribution.

There are also some practical issues to consider. It would be convenient to have a small number of distributions that, collectively, cover the whole range of SKUs. For this to be achieved, each of the distributions chosen must be sufficiently flexible to cover a wide variety of demand patterns, and the distributions should be complementary. Also, the distributions should have forms that can be computed easily and quickly. This enables demand planners to check probability calculations and the implications of any changes to distributions or their parameters.

4.3.3 Summary

In summary, we recommend four criteria for a good demand distribution:

1. Empirical evidence in support of its goodness of fit.
2. A priori grounds for its choice.
3. Flexibility to represent different types of demand patterns.
4. Computational ease.

The first three criteria for demand distributions were suggested by Boylan (1997), with the fourth criterion added by Lengu et al. (2014).

In this chapter and in the next, each of the demand distributions will be assessed against these four criteria to judge their suitability for intermittent demand. We start by looking at a priori grounds, in advance of any data being available. We ask how easy it is to calculate probabilities using the distribution. Then, we examine the flexibility of the distribution, as this may help us to understand the results from the final stage, which is the assessment of goodness of fit using real data.

4.4 Poisson Distribution

Events follow a Poisson process if the following conditions are satisfied:

- The numbers of events in non-overlapping time intervals are mutually independent.
- The probability of an event within a certain length of time interval does not change over time.
- The probability of two or more events in a small time interval is negligible.
- The probability of observing a single event over a small time interval is approximately proportional to the length of that interval.

These are general conditions for a Poisson process, which can be used to represent a wide range of phenomena. In the case of intermittent demand, an 'event' may be interpreted as an incidence of demand for a single unit of a product. If demand incidences satisfy the four conditions given above, then the probabilities of demand, over a unit period of time, follow the Poisson distribution, whose formula is given in Eq. (4.1) for non-negative whole numbers ($x = 0, 1, 2, \ldots$).

$$\mathbb{P}(x) = \frac{\lambda^x e^{-\lambda}}{x!} \tag{4.1}$$

In this formula, e is Euler's number; e = 2.718 to three decimal places. The distribution is controlled by a single parameter, denoted by the Greek letter λ (lambda), which is the mean number of demand incidences per unit time. The factorial function, denoted by an exclamation mark, is the product of a positive number and all the positive whole numbers below it (e.g. 3! = 3 × 2 × 1 = 6). An example of this formula's application will follow in Section 4.5.2.

4.4.1 Shape of the Poisson Distribution

Figure 4.5 shows how the shape of the Poisson distribution varies according to its mean value (λ).

In this figure, the mean values are all whole numbers (1, 4, and 10). This need not be the case. Although the number of events is a whole number, the mean number of events per unit time may be fractional. This is respected by the Poisson distribution, which allows fractional values of the lambda parameter. On the other hand, the Poisson distribution is defined only for whole numbers, including zero. It is meaningless to speak of the Poisson probability of a value such as 1.9. Consequently, the dotted lines joining the points in Figure 4.5 are merely for illustration, to give a better idea of the shape of the distribution.

In Figure 4.5, the three Poisson distributions are represented by points in blue, red, and green. For each of these distributions, we can read the probabilities associated with different demands. For example, for a mean value of one ($\lambda = 1$), the blue point above zero (on the horizontal axis) is at a probability value of 0.37 (on the vertical axis), meaning that there is a 37% chance of observing no demand in a unit period of time.

For high values of its mean, the Poisson resembles the symmetric 'bell shape' of the normal distribution (to be discussed in Chapter 5); see, for example, the distribution in green ($\lambda = 10$) in Figure 4.5. For lower mean values, the distribution is more asymmetric.

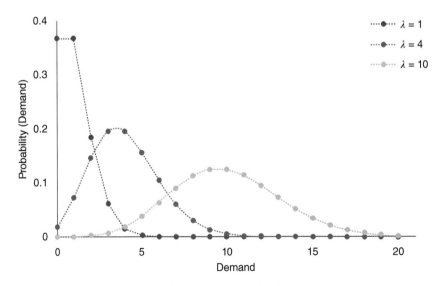

Figure 4.5 Poisson distribution for varying mean (λ) values.

For $\lambda = 1$, the Poisson distribution becomes highly asymmetric and diverges from a bell shape quite markedly. Therefore, the Poisson can take on a wide variety of shapes, depending on its mean value.

4.4.2 Summary

In this section, the Poisson distribution has been defined and the shape of the distribution has been illustrated for different mean values. The shapes vary, but the probabilities always decline after a certain point. In Section 4.5.1, a justification for the Poisson is given in terms of the occurrence of rare events, which is particularly relevant for intermittent demand.

4.5 Poisson Demand Distribution

In this section, we scrutinise the Poisson distribution, to assess its suitability for our work with intermittent demand items. To do so, we use the four criteria outlined in Section 4.3, namely a priori grounds, ease of calculation, flexibility, and goodness of fit.

4.5.1 Poisson: A Priori Grounds

Demand is usually defined only for non-negative whole number values. Therefore, the Poisson distribution is appropriate on the grounds of being discrete, and not defined for fractional or negative values. Intermittent demand may arise from a combination of rare events. For example, a particular SKU may be a spare part in a large number of independently maintained machines. Whenever one of these machines breaks down, there is a small chance that a single unit of the SKU is required for repair. Such a process is likely to obey the first condition for a Poisson distribution (the numbers of events in any non-overlapping time intervals are mutually independent) and the third condition (the probability of two or more events in a very small time interval is negligible). Providing the other two conditions also hold, the combination of rare events provides an a priori justification for the Poisson distribution. In fact, it also provides a justification for a broader family of distributions, known as compound Poisson distributions. These arise when the demands for the SKU may not be for a single unit but for several units, and will be discussed in detail in Chapter 5.

　If demands arise from a Poisson distribution, then the intervals between demands are memoryless. This means that the waiting time to the next demand does not depend on how much time has elapsed since the last demand (Technical Note 4.2). This property is shared by the Bernoulli distribution, to be discussed in Section 4.8.

4.5.2 Poisson: Ease of Calculation

If demand is Poisson distributed, with mean value λ, then the probability of observing a particular value, x, denoted by $\mathbb{P}(x)$, was given by Eq. (4.1), $\mathbb{P}(x) = \lambda^x e^{-\lambda}/x!$ for $x = 0, 1, 2, \ldots$ To appreciate the formula in more detail, we examine the special case of the mean demand being two units per unit time ($\lambda = 2$). In this case, the probability calculations are shown in Table 4.2.

Table 4.2 Poisson probabilities ($\lambda = 2$).

x	λ^x	$e^{-\lambda}$	x!	$\mathbb{P}(x)$
0	1	0.135	1	0.135
1	2	0.135	1	0.271
2	4	0.135	2	0.271
3	8	0.135	6	0.180
4	16	0.135	24	0.090
5	32	0.135	120	0.036

In Table 4.2, the first column indicates the potential demand values. Values of six or higher have been omitted because the probabilities of observing them are small. The second column shows the powers of the mean value. The third column shows $e^{-\lambda} = e^{-2} = 0.135$. The fourth column shows the factorial function which, as noted earlier, is the product of a positive whole number and all the positive whole numbers below it; by convention, zero factorial is taken to be equal to one. The final column shows the Poisson probabilities, calculated using Eq. (4.1).

Once the probabilities have been calculated, the cumulative probabilities may also be found. These represent the chance of demand being less than, or equal to, a predetermined number. For example, if we want to know the chance of demand being less than or equal to two, then we add the probabilities of demand being zero, one, and two. In the example shown in Table 4.2, this is $0.135 + 0.271 + 0.271 = 0.677$, giving a 67.7% chance that the demand will not exceed two units. Cumulative Poisson probabilities may often be found quickly using built-in software functions. Consequently, the Poisson distribution is easy to work with computationally and satisfies this criterion for a 'good' demand distribution.

In the above discussion, it is clear that the probability of observing any particular value depends only on the value itself (x) and the mean demand (λ). To focus on the calculations, we assumed that the mean demand is known and unchanging over time. In Chapter 6, we make the more realistic assumption that the mean demand is not known and may be changing over time. Hence, it will need to be forecasted. If demand is Poisson distributed, it is the only parameter that needs to be forecasted.

4.5.3 Poisson: Flexibility

In general, it is desirable for intermittent and lumpy demand distributions to be flexible in two respects: (i) the ability of a distribution to take a variety of shapes (including symmetrical or asymmetrical shapes) and (ii) the ability to take a wide range of values of the variance to mean ratio.

As we saw in Figure 4.5, the Poisson distribution can take quite a wide variety of shapes, depending on the value of its parameter λ (mean demand). It is right-skewed (right tail longer than the left) and becomes more symmetrical for higher mean values. It cannot represent left-skewed distributions (left tail longer than the right), but such intermittent demand distributions are not often encountered in practice.

The variance measures the spread of a distribution, with a high variance showing a wider spread of demand values. By looking at the variance divided by the mean (the 'variance to mean ratio'), we can compare distributions with different means more consistently. For example, a distribution with variance of 20 and mean of 5 is more variable, relative to its mean, than a distribution with variance of 50 and mean of 25, and this is reflected by the variance to mean ratios of four and two, respectively.

In practice, we do not know the exact variance of any demand distribution and so it must be estimated (to be discussed further in Chapter 7). If we assume that both the mean and the variance are unchanging over time, then the estimated variance may be calculated as follows: (i) take the difference between each observed value and the sample mean; (ii) square these differences; and (iii) take the average of the squared differences. The idea behind this calculation is to treat negative and positive differences the same and to weight higher differences much more heavily than lower differences.

To illustrate the calculation of variance, we use the time series shown in Figure 4.1. The sample mean is the average of the 24 demand observations $(3, 12, \ldots, 3)$, which is 3.54 (to two decimal places). The sample variance is found by calculating the squared difference of each observation from the sample mean, and then averaging these squared differences. For example, the first observation is 3, giving a squared difference of $(-0.54) \times (-0.54) = 0.29$, and the second observation is 12, giving a squared difference of $8.46 \times 8.46 = 71.57$. Repeating these calculations for all of the 24 observations, and averaging the results gives a sample variance of 8.08. Note that demands with large deviations from the sample mean, such as the second observation, have a particularly strong influence on the overall sample variance.

Returning to Figure 4.5, we can see that the distribution with the highest variance of observations from the mean is the (almost) symmetrical distribution with a mean of 10, and the one with least variance is the asymmetrical distribution with a mean of one. It is clear from the figure that the variance increases as the mean increases. In fact, the Poisson has the property that the variance is always the same as the mean, giving a variance to mean ratio of one.

In summary, the Poisson distribution is flexible with regard to its shape but inflexible with regard to its variance to mean ratio. Actually, it is completely inflexible in this respect, as the ratio must always equal one. The implications of this restriction on the distribution's goodness of fit are explored in Section 4.5.4.

4.5.4   Poisson: Goodness of Fit

We saw, in Section 4.2, that the triangular distribution was not a good fit to the demand data presented in Figure 4.1. For the Poisson distribution, we can find the predicted demand probabilities, for $x = 0, 1, 2, \ldots$ by using the calculations shown in Table 4.2, but now with a mean value of 3.54. The results are shown in Figure 4.6, side by side with the observed relative frequencies.

It is apparent from Figure 4.6 that the Poisson is mimicking the relative frequencies in the centre of the distribution rather better than the triangular distribution. Unfortunately, this is at the cost of a poor fit at the higher demand values. Further reflection on the demand variance shows why the Poisson fits the higher demand values so badly. The sample variance (8.08) is much higher than the sample mean (3.54), giving a variance to mean ratio

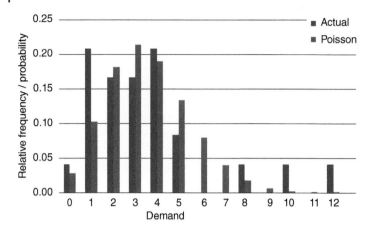

Figure 4.6 Poisson probabilities and actual relative frequencies.

of 8.08/3.54 = 2.28. However, the Poisson's variance to mean ratio is always equal to one. Because the mean value is 3.54, the Poisson's variance is also fixed at 3.54, whereas the data is showing a sample variance of 8.08. Consequently, the Poisson distribution does not spread out widely enough and the higher demand values are under-represented by it.

Intermittent and lumpy demand patterns vary considerably from one SKU to the next. They differ in terms of their shape, and in their degree of variability. This example highlights a general weakness of the Poisson distribution in representing these demand patterns. Whilst the Poisson may be a good fit to demand data with identical variance and mean, it lacks the flexibility to represent demand when the variance exceeds the mean (or is below the mean). This is borne out by empirical evidence. In Chapter 5, we review a large-scale empirical study, using real data from three organisations, showing that the Poisson was a good fit for less than a quarter of the SKUs for two datasets, and for less than a half of the SKUs for the third dataset.

Real-world data often exhibit very high variability, leading to higher demand values having larger probabilities than would be anticipated by the Poisson distribution. This is particularly concerning from an inventory management perspective, as it is important to represent the higher values realistically. Suppose that we have estimated the probabilities of demands of 10, 11, and 12 as 0.9%, 0.4%, and 0.2%, respectively (and probabilities of higher demand values are so small as to be negligible). Totalling these values gives the probability of a demand of 10 or more to be 1.5%. Now suppose that the true probabilities are 3.1%, 1.4%, and 0.5% (and the probabilities of higher demands are still negligible). Then the true probability of a demand of 10 or more is 5.0%. Differences such as these can be significant in determining inventory requirements. In the example given, if we rely on our (incorrect) probability estimates, then we will underestimate the risk of stockouts from high demands and may therefore stock too little. More accurate representation of higher demand values is required if availability of stock is to be maintained.

4.5.5 Testing for Goodness of Fit

In Section 4.3, we referred to empirical evidence in support of goodness of fit, but did not explain how goodness of fit can be tested. Kwan (1991), Boylan (1997), and Eaves (2002) all

Table 4.3 Calculation of chi-square goodness of fit statistic.

Monthly demand	Observed months	Expected months	Chi-square components
0 or 1	10	5.964	2.731
2	12	9.901	0.445
3	12	13.614	0.191
4	10	14.040	1.162
5	5	11.583	3.741
6	8	7.963	0.000
7	8	4.693	2.331
8 or 9	7	4.243	1.792
Total			12.394

Source: Adapted from Eaves 2002.

analysed real data series, using chi-square tests to assess the goodness of fit of the Poisson distribution. This testing procedure may be illustrated by an example of an SKU analysed by Eaves.

In Eaves' example, 72 months of data were available. The first two columns of Table 4.3 show the number of months for which each demand value was observed. For monthly demands between two and seven, inclusive, the observed numbers of months are given exactly. For monthly demands of zero and one, the observed numbers of months have been combined; the same has been done for monthly demands of eight and nine. The reason for these amalgamations is to allow the chi-square test to proceed (to be discussed in more detail later).

To calculate the sample mean, we take into account the original data, which showed two months with zero demand, eight months with demand of one unit, three months with a demand for eight units, and four months with demand for nine units. Then, we can calculate the sample mean, giving a value of 4.125. Using this value in the Poisson formula (Eq. (4.1)) and multiplying by 72 enables the third column (expected months) to be calculated. The expected number of months for demands of zero and one are calculated separately, and then added to give 5.964; the same applies for demands of eight and nine.

The number at the bottom of the final column shows a measure of the difference between the observed and expected values, and is called the 'chi-square' statistic. In each row, the difference between the observed and expected values is squared, and then divided by the expected value. For example, in the first row, $((10 - 5.964) \times (10 - 5.964))/5.964 = 2.731$. Then, these values are totalled across all the rows to give the chi-square statistic of 12.394 (with a small rounding error of 0.001 in the table). The higher this value, the greater the evidence that the Poisson is not a good fit to the data. In this example, the chi-square value was sufficiently low to accept that the Poisson was a satisfactory fit. (Statistical tables are available to quantify 'sufficiently low'; see Technical Note 4.3 for further explanation.)

The reason for the amalgamation of demand values zero and one (and eight and nine) is to ensure that the expected frequency is not too low. In these circumstances, the chi-square test cannot be used. A good rule of thumb is that the expected value should be at least five, but this is not a hard and fast rule. (In the example above, the expected values are 5.964 for zero and one, and 4.243 for eight and nine.)

The requirement that expected values should not be too low results in two difficulties. Firstly, it is not always obvious how best to amalgamate the data. Eaves (2002) pointed out that another alternative in the above example is to amalgamate demands of seven, eight, and nine to form a separate category. The amalgamation gives a different chi-square value and, in this case, a value that is sufficiently high to reject the Poisson as a satisfactory fit. Eaves discussed strategies for addressing this problem, by choosing data groupings with similar frequencies throughout the whole distribution. The second difficulty arises when there are few historical observations. This can result in insufficient non-zero data points to conduct a meaningful chi-square analysis, especially if the data is highly intermittent.

4.5.6 Summary

The Poisson distribution has often been used to represent slow-moving and intermittent demand. It is relatively straightforward to use, and readily implemented in computer code. It is also used in many software packages. The Poisson arises as a combination of rare independent events, giving it an a priori justification for the representation of intermittent demand.

The Poisson is flexible with regard to its shape, but not with respect to its variance to mean ratio, which must always equal one. However, intermittent and lumpy demand patterns vary considerably from one SKU to the next. They differ in terms of their shape, and in their degree of variability. Whilst the Poisson may be a good fit to demand data that has identical (or at least very similar) variance and mean, it lacks the flexibility to represent demand when the variance exceeds the mean, as often observed in practice.

Detailed empirical evidence on the goodness of fit of the Poisson distribution will be reviewed in Chapter 5. This evidence will confirm the preliminary findings in this chapter. The Poisson provides a good fit to the demand distributions of some SKUs but, for others, it does not offer a good fit, primarily because the distribution is not sufficiently variable, and can underestimate the probabilities of higher demand values. In Chapter 5, we look at a generalisation of the Poisson distribution which retains its flexibility to take different shapes but is more flexible in terms of the variance to mean ratio. We also revisit the question of how to test for goodness of fit, with some suggestions for overcoming the difficulties of using the chi-square test when demand histories are relatively short or the data is highly intermittent.

4.6 Incidence and Occurrence

In this section, we clarify the distinction between the terms 'demand incidence' and 'demand occurrence', and explain why each of these concepts is important in intermittent demand forecasting and inventory management.

4.6.1 Demand Incidence

Suppose that, over a period of 10 weeks (each of seven working days), we recorded the demands given in Table 4.4.

Table 4.4 Example of demand incidences.

Week	Day and time	Elapsed days	Intervals (days)	Demand (units)
4	Day 23, 11:09	22.24		2
4	Day 26, 15:45	25.75	3.51	1
6	Day 39, 13:12	38.47	12.72	1
10	Day 65, 09:33	64.06	25.59	1
10	Day 65, 12:54	64.43	0.37	5
10	Day 67, 16:22	66.82	2.39	1
			Total	11

Table 4.4 shows an example of time-stamped data for a particular SKU. Such detailed data is often available from retail outlets, where it represents the purchases from individual consumers. At wholesalers, each row would represent an order from a business customer (or one order line as part of an order for a collection of SKUs). Whether the demand arises from consumers or businesses, each row describes a 'demand incidence'.

In this example, demand may occur on any day in the week. The elapsed days calculations, shown in the third column of Table 4.4, assume a nine-hour working day (09:00–18:00), equating to a working day of 540 minutes. So, for example, the first demand incidence is after 129 minutes in the 23rd day since we started counting. Therefore, 22 full days have elapsed, plus a fraction of the 23rd day, where the fraction is $129/540 = 0.24$. And so the elapsed days for the first demand incidence is 22.24. Then, the time intervals are calculated as the differences between successive elapsed days. For example, the first interval is of $25.75 - 22.24 = 3.51$ days.

The total demand over the 10 week period is 11 units, giving a mean demand of 1.1 units per week. We can also observe that there are six separate demand incidences over 10 weeks and so the mean number of demand incidences per week is 0.6. It is important to note the difference between these two figures. If we use the Poisson distribution to represent weekly demand (as in Section 4.5), it is the first figure of 1.1 that is relevant. If we use the Poisson to represent weekly demand incidence (as in Section 4.7), it is the second figure of 0.6 that must be used.

4.6.2 Demand Occurrence

The mean interval between demand incidences is the average of the five figures in the 'Intervals' column, which is calculated as 8.92 days. Now, as we shall see, the meaning of an average interval between demands depends on how demand is recorded. Suppose that, instead of the detailed data in Table 4.4, we have time-aggregated data, as shown in Table 4.5.

Table 4.5 shows the total demands in each of the weeks, together with the number of demand incidences. For example, there were two demand incidences in Week 4, giving a total demand of three units, whereas there was only one demand incidence in Week 6, giving a total demand of one unit.

Table 4.5 Weekly demand data.

Week	1	2	3	4	5	6	7	8	9	10
Incidence	0	0	0	2	0	1	0	0	0	3
Total demands	0	0	0	3	0	1	0	0	0	7

Table 4.6 Sequence of demand occurrences (1) and non-occurrences (0).

Week	1	2	3	4	5	6	7	8	9	10
Occurrence	0	0	0	1	0	1	0	0	0	1

We can now record whether there has been a demand occurrence (labelled as 1) or not (labelled as 0). If demand has occurred in a particular period, this may have arisen from one, two, or more demand incidences. This is why we refer to 'demand occurrences', rather than 'demand incidences', when we focus on time periods. Continuing with the example, the sequence of weekly demand occurrences is given in Table 4.6.

This sequence of demand occurrence variables is said to be a Bernoulli process if there is a constant probability of demand occurrence and the outcomes are independent (i.e. the outcome in one time period has no influence over the outcome in another time period). We return to this process in Section 4.8.

The calculation of the mean interval between weeks with demand occurrence is straightforward. The gap between Week 4 and Week 6 is two weeks and the gap between Week 6 and Week 10 is four weeks, giving a mean interval of three weeks. Notice that this is quite different to our earlier calculation, based on the same data (Table 4.4), which gave a mean interval of 8.92 days, or just over one week. The reason is that different things are being measured. The average of 8.92 days represents the average gap between demand incidences (of which there are six). The average of three weeks represents the average gap between weeks with demand occurrence (of which there are only three).

4.6.3 Summary

In this section, we have endeavoured to be precise in the distinction between demand incidence and demand occurrence. There are two reasons why this distinction is important.

Firstly, the forecasting of mean demand can be decomposed into forecasting of the mean size of demand (when demand occurs) and forecasting of the mean demand interval. This will be one of the major themes of Chapter 6. The forecasting method needs to take into account the distribution of demand intervals, which depends on the distribution of demand incidence or occurrence.

Secondly, the characterisation of the demand distribution can be decomposed into the specification of the distribution of demand size and the distribution of demand incidence or occurrence. If this approach is taken, it is important to use appropriate distributions for demand size and demand incidence or occurrence. The resulting 'compound' demand distributions will be analysed in Chapter 5, building on the distributions discussed in the remainder of this chapter.

4.7 Poisson Demand Incidence Distribution

Although the Poisson distribution has some limitations in representing the total demand, it has been found to be a good representation of demand incidence. In this section, we review the Poisson as a distribution for demand incidence, using the same criteria as we did previously when reviewing the Poisson as a distribution for demand itself.

4.7.1 A Priori Grounds

We commented earlier that the Poisson distribution has two a priori arguments in its support.

1. It is defined only for non-negative whole numbers. This is appropriate for demand and also for the number of demand incidences.
2. It may arise from the combination of rare events. This argument is, in fact, based on demand incidences. If each incidence of demand is for a single unit of an SKU, then the mechanism also gives rise to a Poisson distribution of demand.

It is clear, then, that these arguments provide support for the Poisson as a distribution of demand incidence.

4.7.2 Ease of Calculation

The calculations for the Poisson as a demand incidence distribution are the same as those shown earlier in Table 4.2 for a demand distribution, except that, now: (i) the figures in the first column (0, 1, 2, 3, 4, 5, etc.) refer to the number of demand incidences per period rather than the total demand per period, and (ii) the mean value refers to the mean demand incidence rather than the mean demand. Therefore, it is just as straightforward to calculate Poisson probabilities of demand incidences as it is to calculate Poisson probabilities of demand.

It is also possible to conduct calculations regarding the probabilities of the duration of time that elapses between one incidence of demand and the next. This is possible because of a link between the Poisson distribution of demand incidences and the negative exponential distribution of time intervals between incidences. In a nutshell, if demand incidences are Poisson, then demand intervals are negative exponential; and if demand intervals are negative exponential, then demand incidences are Poisson. The probability that the time interval between demand incidences will be less than or equal to a given value, t, is given by the cumulative probability of the negative exponential distribution, shown in Eq. (4.2).

$$\mathbb{P}(\text{Interval} \leq t) = 1 - e^{-\lambda t} \tag{4.2}$$

where λ is the mean number of demand incidences per unit time period (and the mean demand interval is equal to $1/\lambda$).

Calculations of probabilities relating to time intervals may be readily conducted using Eq. (4.2), if demand incidence is assumed to be Poisson distributed. For example, if the mean demand incidence is 0.5 per week then, using Eq. (4.2), the probability that the time interval will not exceed t is given by $1 - e^{-0.5t}$. If we wish to know the probability of the time interval not exceeding one week ($t = 1$), then this is given by $1 - e^{-0.5} = 1 - 0.607 = 0.393$. So, there is a 39.3% chance that the time interval between demand incidences will not exceed one week.

We revisit the negative exponential distribution in Chapter 5, and extend the discussion to distributions that allow for greater regularity in the time intervals between demand incidences.

4.7.3 Flexibility

The Poisson demand incidence distribution has flexibility of shape, as discussed earlier in this chapter, but inflexibility of the variance to mean ratio, which must equal one. This is less problematic than for demand itself because high variance to mean ratios are less common for demand incidence in practice. Sometimes, the variance to mean ratio for demand incidence may be less than one. In these cases, there are alternative demand distributions that may be more appropriate, to be discussed in Chapter 5.

4.7.4 Goodness of Fit

Kwan (1991), Boylan (1997), and Eaves (2002) all analysed real data series, at the level of the individual SKU. Their analyses were conducted by examining demand intervals to see if they were consistent with the negative exponential distribution, as would be required for Poisson demand incidence. Boylan and Eaves found a large majority of SKUs to be fitted by negative exponentially distributed intervals, while Kwan found less than half of her SKUs well-fitted by this distribution.

One of the challenges in conducting statistical goodness of fit tests is the paucity of non-zero observations when demand is intermittent. Kwan (1991) and Eaves (2002) addressed this issue by analysing long histories of data (10 and 6 years, respectively). There are two problems here. Firstly, such long histories are usually not available in commercial databases. Secondly, even if they are available, it is necessary to assume that the mean demand incidence is unchanging over time, and this assumption becomes less plausible as the demand history lengthens.

Boylan (1997) recognised this issue and restricted his empirical analysis to a history of one year. The organisation, an engineering supplies company, categorised their SKUs according to the number of customers requesting them over a year. In his analysis, Boylan included only those SKUs with at least four customers and, therefore, at least four demand incidences in a year. However, this limits the range of SKUs that can be examined and excludes very slow moving SKUs from the analysis.

To overcome this problem, Shale et al. (2008) proposed two ways of checking that demand incidences are Poisson, both of which relate to a collection of SKUs: (i) checking that the

variance and mean are the same; (ii) examining the overall distribution of demand incidences for SKUs that have the same total number of demand incidences in a year.

The variance and the mean should take the same values if demand incidence is Poisson.
Of course, they will not necessarily be exactly the same for all SKUs but a clear relationship
should be evident between these values. Shale et al. (2008) examined the weekly order frequencies of 500 SKUs from users of a computer system by Kerridge Computer Company,
over a period of 51 weeks (one whole year except the week containing Christmas, which was
highly untypical). The means and variances of order frequencies of these SKUs are shown
in Figure 4.7.

Figure 4.7 is shown on a logarithmic scale, on both axes, where the distance from 1 to 10
is the same as the distance from 10 to 100. This allows the results for the slower movers,
including intermittent items, to be seen more clearly on the left side of the graph. It does not
change the interpretation of the straight line. If the logarithm of the variance equals the logarithm of the mean, then it must follow that the variance equals the mean, as required for a
Poisson distribution. The diagram shows a good linear fit, with a reported correlation coefficient of 0.973 on the logarithm of the values. The dotted lines show the 95% prediction
interval, based on a Poisson model. The researchers remarked that the number of observations outside the dotted line (24) is in accordance with expectation (25, which is 5% of
500), but most (22) are above the upper limit, perhaps because of the additional variability
induced by statutory holidays and religious festivals.

Shale et al. (2008) proposed a test of the Poisson distribution for demand incidence, based
on the overall distribution of demand incidences over a collection of SKUs. They analysed
the demand histories for almost 52 000 SKUs held at 81 branches of an electrical wholesaler
and over 17 000 SKUs held at 10 branches of a builders' merchant. This led to an examination of over 2.3 million incidences of demands (orders) at the electrical wholesaler and
over 300 000 at the builders' merchant.

The analysis proceeded by identifying all the SKUs across all the branches with the same
number of orders per year and by examining the frequencies of the number of orders in
successive four-week periods over one year. For example, we may specify the number to be
13 orders per year, which would result in a sample mean of one order per four-week period.

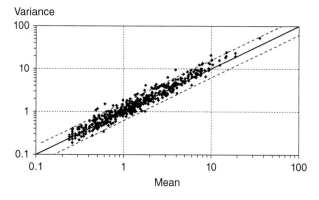

Figure 4.7 Variance and mean of weekly order frequencies. Source: Shale et al. 2008.

Then we count the number of four-week periods over the year with zero orders, one order, two orders, and so on.

If the orders (for each SKU and each branch) are Poisson distributed, and they are mutually independent, then the orders (regardless of SKU or branch) are also Poisson distributed. Mutual independence implies that the demand for one SKU is uncorrelated with the demand for another SKU, and the demand at one branch for a particular SKU is uncorrelated with the demand for the same SKU at another branch. This is not always true, particularly for fast-moving, seasonal, or promoted items, but it is often a more reasonable assumption for slow-moving and intermittent SKUs. So, if demands are mutually independent and the orders (regardless of SKU or branch) are not found to be Poisson distributed, then this casts doubt on the orders being Poisson distributed for each SKU and each branch.

The comparison undertaken by Shale et al. (2008), for the case of 13 orders per year, is shown in Table 4.7.

Table 4.7 shows a reasonably close agreement between the observed frequencies and those estimated from the Poisson distribution, at least for the lower order incidences (from zero to four, inclusive). (The calculations were subject to some adjustment to allow for 13 orders arising from different underlying mean order incidences. See Technical Note 4.4.) The chi-square analysis highlights the most noticeable discrepancies, which are at the highest order incidences (five and six or more). The Poisson predicts a markedly smaller frequency of high order frequencies (of five or more) than observed in practice ($171.3 + 45.1 = 216.4$ predicted, compared with $247 + 66 = 313$ observed). Because of this, if the Poisson distribution were subjected to a chi-square test, then the outcome would be to reject it.

The categories of five, and six or more, order incidences comprise only 0.8% of observations, with the remaining 99.2% of observations showing four orders or fewer. Hence, although we cannot conclude that the data is Poisson distributed, we can say that the Poisson provides a good approximation, at least for cumulative distributions up to 99.2%. This was sufficient for the electrical wholesaler and builders' merchant, whose data had been

Table 4.7 Observed and estimated order incidences over four weeks.

Orders in four week period	Observed frequency	Cumulative percentage	Estimated frequency	Chi-square components
0	15 826	39.0	15 753.5	0.33
1	14 096	73.7	14 340.7	4.18
2	6 990	90.9	7 075.3	1.03
3	2 604	97.3	2 503.2	4.06
4	770	99.2	710.0	5.07
5	247	99.8	171.3	33.45
6 or more	66	100.0	45.1	9.69
Total	40 599			57.81

Source: Shale et al. 2008. ©2008, Oxford University Press.

analysed, and would be sufficient for most real-world inventory applications. The only exceptions would arise in organisations with very high service level targets.

Shale et al. (2008) reported that similar results were obtained for many other SKU-branch combinations with different values (other than 13) of the total number of orders per year. Their study provides evidence that the Poisson distribution can be a good fit to demand incidence, assuming that the highest number of orders, in the extreme right-hand tail of the distribution, are not important for subsequent inventory decisions.

4.7.5 Summary

The Poisson has strong support as a demand incidence distribution. It is easy to calculate and has a priori grounds for representing demand incidence. The Poisson is restricted by its variance to mean ratio being equal to one. Nevertheless, it has empirical evidence to confirm its suitability as a demand incidence distribution. Testing for Poisson demand incidence is not always straightforward in practice. Two approaches have been proposed by Shale et al. (2008) to allow testing for the Poisson distribution, while circumventing the need to use long demand histories.

4.8 Bernoulli Demand Occurrence Distribution

In Section 4.6, we introduced the distinction between demand incidences and demand occurrences. In Section 4.7, we focused on demand incidences, and their representation by the Poisson distribution. In this section, we turn our attention to demand occurrences, and their representation by the Bernoulli distribution.

4.8.1 Bernoulli Distribution: A Priori Grounds

Referring back to Section 4.6, 'demand incidence' refers to individual transactions, whether they be consumer purchases or orders from a business. Periods with 'demand occurrence', on the other hand, refer to those periods where there has been some demand, no matter how many transactions have occurred. In each period with demand, there will have been at least one demand incidence, but there may have been more than one.

The Poisson distribution is based on representing incidences of demand separately. (In a business-to-business environment, each demand incidence corresponds to a different order line.) An alternative way of thinking about demand is to disregard individual demand incidences and focus on demand occurrence in a given time period. In this case, the Bernoulli distribution is more appropriate.

Table 4.5 showed 10 weeks of demand observations, which were then relabelled in Table 4.6 as one (demand occurred) or zero (demand did not occur). Such a sequence of demand occurrence variables is said to be a 'Bernoulli process' if there is a constant probability of demand occurrence and the outcomes are independent (i.e. the outcome in one time period has no influence over the outcomes in any of the later time periods). Intermittent demand may often be characterised as arising from combinations of rare events, with event occurrences in different time periods being mutually independent. This characterisation offers an a priori justification for the Bernoulli distribution, providing that the demand occurrence probability remains constant.

The Bernoulli process of demand occurrence leads to the intervals between periods with demand being geometrically distributed. The details of this distribution are discussed in Section 4.8.2 but, for now, it is sufficient to note that the Bernoulli process (and its associated geometric demand interval distribution) is memoryless; please see Technical Note 4.5 for further explanation. This property is shared with the Poisson process of demand incidence. Moreover, the resulting demand interval distributions, the geometric (Bernoulli process) and negative exponential (Poisson process), are the only memoryless interval distributions.

4.8.2 Bernoulli Distribution: Ease of Calculation

The Bernoulli distribution has only one parameter. This parameter is the probability of observing a demand occurrence, and it is also equal to the mean of the demand occurrence distribution. It is not difficult to estimate this parameter. If we assume that the probability has not been changing over time, then the probability may be estimated as the ratio of the number of periods with a demand occurrence to the total number of periods. If the probability is changing over time, other approaches may be required, but they are not difficult to implement. An example of such an approach is due to Teunter, Syntetos, and Babai (2011), and this will be discussed in Chapter 12.

If it is assumed that demand occurrence is Bernoulli distributed, then we can also estimate the probabilities of the number of periods with some demand occurrence over a longer period of time. The general formula for the probability of observing exactly r periods with demand occurrence out of n periods is given by Eq. (4.3) for $r = 0, 1, \ldots, n$.

$$\mathbb{P}(r) = \frac{n!}{r!(n-r)!}p^r(1-p)^{n-r} \tag{4.3}$$

This is known as the binomial distribution. It may be calculated straightforwardly, once the probability, p, has been estimated.

It is also possible to undertake calculations relating to the mean time between a period with a demand occurrence and the next such period. If the probability of demand occurrence is p, then the mean time between demands is $1/p$. For example, if the probability of a period showing some demand is 0.5, then the mean number of periods between demands is two. The chance of the time interval between such periods being t (for $t = 1, 2, \ldots$) is given by Eq. (4.4).

$$\mathbb{P}(t) = (1-p)^{t-1}p \tag{4.4}$$

This is known as the geometric distribution. The first thing to notice from Eq. (4.4) is that the geometric distribution is defined only for positive whole numbers. Unlike the negative exponential distribution, time is taken to be defined as buckets with whole numbers attached to them (e.g. Week 1, Week 2). Therefore, the times between these periods must also be whole numbers. The first part of the right-hand side of Eq. (4.4), $(1-p)^{t-1}$, represents the chance of the first $t-1$ periods all showing no demand at all. The second part, p, represents the chance of there being some demand in period t.

The probability that the time interval between periods with demands is no more than t, for $t = 1, 2, \ldots$ is given by Eq. (4.5).

$$\mathbb{P}(\text{Interval} \leq t) = 1 - (1 - p)^t \qquad (4.5)$$

In Eq. (4.5), the term $(1 - p)^t$ represents the chance of no demand in any of the first t periods. Therefore, the chance of there being some demand in the first t periods is given by $1 - (1 - p)^t$.

In summary, the Bernoulli has a natural a priori justification and is straightforward to calculate. The same applies to the geometric distribution of time intervals between periods with demand occurrences.

4.8.3 Bernoulli Distribution: Flexibility

The Bernoulli distribution has the flexibility to represent highly intermittent demand (with lower probability of demand occurrence) through to mildly intermittent demand (with higher probability values) and including non-intermittent demand (probability of one).

Bernoulli demand occurrences take a value of one when demand occurs (with probability p) and a value of zero when demand does not occur (with probability $1 - p$). The mean number of demand occurrences per unit time period is p and the variance is $p(1 - p)$. This gives a variance to mean ratio of $1 - p$. As the probability value, p, must be between zero and one, it follows that the variance to mean ratio must also be between zero and one.

It is evident that the Bernoulli distribution is unable to represent demand occurrences where the variance to mean ratio exceeds one. However, it is not restricted to being equal to one, and has the additional flexibility of being able to represent demand occurrences where the variance to mean ratio is less than one.

4.8.4 Bernoulli Distribution: Goodness of Fit

Boylan (1997) undertook an empirical investigation of demand occurrences on empirical data and found that approximately 90% of intermittent weekly demand items (with less than 50 demand incidences per year), had demand processes consistent with both Poisson and Bernoulli distributions. However, the sample of intermittent items was small (only 55 SKUs). Eaves (2002) analysed a much larger sample of data (6795 SKUs from the Royal Air Force) and included items with highly intermittent, mildly intermittent, and non-intermittent demand patterns. His findings agreed with those of Boylan (1997): approximately 90% of the SKUs were well fitted by Poisson and Bernoulli demand processes.

How should the Bernoulli distribution for demand occurrence be tested? There are two possibilities:

1. Bernoulli demand occurrence over one period translates to a binomial distribution of the number of periods of demand over a longer duration of time (see Section 4.8.2). For example, if we have daily data, then we can assess the distribution of the number of days in each week that have some demand. This can be checked using a chi-square

test (see earlier discussion). This test can be applied only if there are sufficient non-zero observations, and is not suitable for the slowest-moving SKUs.

2. Bernoulli demand occurrence translates to a geometric distribution of demand intervals. This can be assessed using a Kolmogorov–Smirnov (KS) test (to be discussed in Chapter 5). Some care is needed in applying this test because, strictly speaking, it applies to continuous data and not to whole number data, and this can lead to misleading results.

4.8.5 Summary

The Bernoulli demand occurrence distribution shares the advantages of the Poisson distribution. It is a memoryless distribution and is easy to use. It allows for the variance to mean ratio to be less than one (unlike the Poisson) but the ratio cannot exceed one (like the Poisson). Importantly, it has empirical evidence in its support.

The Bernoulli gives rise to a geometric distribution of times between periods with demand occurrences. Again, this is easy to work with, and will provide a foundation for the analysis of methods to forecast mean demand.

4.9 Chapter Summary

In this chapter, we have maintained that any proposed demand distribution should be assessed according to four criteria:

1. Empirical evidence in support of its goodness of fit.
2. A priori grounds for its choice.
3. Flexibility to represent different types of demand patterns.
4. Computational ease.

The Poisson demand distribution satisfies the second and fourth criteria quite straightforwardly. With respect to the third criterion, the distribution is flexible with regard to its shape, but is always constrained to have a variance to mean ratio equal to one. Empirical investigations, to be discussed further in Chapter 5, show that the Poisson is a satisfactory demand distribution, in terms of goodness of fit, for some SKUs but not for others. The reason for the lack of fit relates to its lack of flexibility to represent highly variable demand patterns.

For those SKUs where the Poisson is a good fit, it is to be recommended in preference to the more elaborate distributions that will be discussed in Chapter 5. All probability values can be calculated if a mean demand value is available. Therefore, a forecast of the mean demand is sufficient to make the probability calculations that will be required for periodic review (R, S) inventory systems.

In this chapter, we have also seen that intermittent demand incidences and occurrences may be represented by the Poisson and Bernoulli distributions respectively. These distributions form the foundation for the compound Poisson and compound Bernoulli distributions, which will be examined in Chapter 5. They are also useful in informing the development of methods for forecasting mean demand, as we shall see in Chapter 6.

Technical Notes

Note 4.1 Triangular Distribution Calculations

The probabilities in Table 4.1 are calculated as follows:

1. Start with the highest demand (13) and assign it a value of one.
2. Work backwards to the apex, adding one to the value each time, so that a demand of 12 gets a value of 2, and so on, up to a demand of 2 being allocated a value of 12.
3. Beyond the apex (Demand = 2), assign values of 8 (Demand = 1) and 4 (Demand = 0) to give equal levels of decline from the value of 12 at the apex.
4. Calculate the total of the values. In this case, the total is:
   $$1 + 2 + 3 + 4 + 5 + 6 + 7 + 8 + 9 + 10 + 11 + 12 + 8 + 4 = 90.$$
5. Divide each of the values by 90, to give probabilities that sum to one.

Note 4.2 Memoryless Property of the Poisson Process

The property of being memoryless is a fundamental feature of 'waiting times' arising from the Poisson distribution. Suppose the mean level of demand is λ per period. Then the mean level over s periods is λs, and the mean level over $s + t$ periods is $\lambda(s + t)$. In this case, the Poisson distribution of demand over $s + t$ periods is expressed in Eq. (4.6) for $x = 0, 1, 2, \ldots$

$$\mathbb{P}(x) = \frac{(\lambda(s + t))^x e^{-\lambda(s+t)}}{x!} \tag{4.6}$$

Therefore, the probability of no demand ($x = 0$) over $s + t$ periods is $e^{-\lambda(s+t)}$. Now, we want to find the chance of no demand in $s + t$ periods, given that there was no demand in the first s periods. If it is equal to a function which does not depend on s, then we will have shown that the demand process is memoryless.

If $\lambda = 1$, what is the chance of waiting for two further periods, given that we have been waiting for one period already? To answer this question, we should take ourselves back in time by one period. The chance of observing no demand in the next three periods is $e^{-3} = 0.0498$. The chance of observing no demand in the next period is $e^{-1} = 0.3679$. Another way of thinking about this is that if we had 10 000 SKUs all with the same mean value ($\lambda = 1$) and all following Poisson distributions, we would expect only 498 of them to show no demand by the end of three periods, i.e. a chance of 498 in 10 000. However, if we restrict our attention to those SKUs that had no demand after one period, then the chance is not 498 out of 10 000, but 498 out of 3679, or $e^{-3}/e^{-1} = 0.0498/0.3679 = 0.1353$. This is equal to e^{-2}, and so is a function of the further waiting time (two periods) but not of the initial waiting time (one period).

Some reflection shows why this argument works in general and not just for the specific example outlined in the previous paragraph. The general calculation for there being no demand in the next $s + t$ periods is $e^{-\lambda(s+t)}$, as noted above. Then, following the logic in the previous paragraph, the chance of waiting t further periods, given that we have already been waiting for a demand occurrence for s periods, is $e^{-\lambda(s+t)}/e^{-\lambda s} = e^{-\lambda t}$. This is a function of the further waiting time (t periods) but not of the initial waiting time (s periods). As this function does not depend on s, we see that a Poisson demand process is memoryless.

Note 4.3 Chi-square Test for Goodness of Fit

The full procedure for testing the goodness of fit of a distribution is as follows:

1. Formulate the null hypothesis and the alternative hypothesis. In our case, the null hypothesis is that the data are Poisson distributed. The alternative hypothesis is that the data are not Poisson distributed.
2. Decide on a significance level (e.g. 5%). The significance level is the maximum acceptable probability of rejecting the null hypothesis (of demand being Poisson distributed) if it were true.
3. Work out the number of 'degrees of freedom'. This is the number of categories (after amalgamation of demand values) minus two in the case of the Poisson distribution. The number to be subtracted is the number of parameters plus one. As the Poisson has just one parameter (mean demand) to be estimated, we subtract two. Hence, the number of degrees of freedom is eight minus two, equals six.
4. The 'critical value' of the chi-square distribution is read from Table 4.8. If the significance level is 5% and there are six degrees of freedom, then the critical value is 12.592 (highlighted in bold type).
5. The observed chi-square value (12.394, see Table 4.3) is compared with the critical value of 12.592. As 12.394 is less than 12.592, there is insufficient evidence to reject the null hypothesis of Poisson distributed data (at the 5% significance level). Therefore, we continue with our assumption that the demand is Poisson distributed. This may be reviewed again, at a future date, when more data have become available.

Note 4.4 Chi-square Calculations by Shale et al. (2008)

In the example given, the SKU-branch combinations were selected because they had 13 order incidences in a year. This gives a sample mean of the order incidences of 1.0 per

Table 4.8 Critical values of the chi-square distribution for degrees of freedom (df) from 1 to 10.

df	Significance levels		
	0.10	0.05	0.01
1	2.706	3.841	6.635
2	4.605	5.991	9.210
3	6.251	7.815	11.345
4	7.779	9.488	13.277
5	9.236	11.070	15.086
6	10.645	**12.592**	16.812
7	12.017	14.067	18.475
8	13.362	15.507	20.090
9	14.684	16.919	21.666
10	15.987	18.307	23.209

four-week-period. However, SKU-branch combinations with true means other than 1.0 have a chance of producing 13 order incidences in a year, and being included in the selection of combinations. Therefore, the theoretical frequencies should not come from a single Poisson distribution but from a weighted average of the frequencies of all SKU-branch combinations. The weights reflect the probability of observing 13 order incidences in a year, given an underlying mean of m_i orders per annum at the ith SKU-branch combination, and may be expressed as $\text{Poiss}(13|m_i)$. The weighted combination is shown in Eq. (4.7).

$$\mathbb{P}(k) = \frac{\sum_{i=1}^{N} \text{Poiss}(k|m_i/13)\text{Poiss}(13|m_i)}{\sum_{i=1}^{N} \text{Poiss}(13|m_i)} \tag{4.7}$$

where N denotes the number of SKU-branch combinations with 13 order incidences in a year. This approach may be generalised to any number of order incidences in a year.

Note 4.5 Memoryless Property of the Bernoulli Process

The memoryless property arising from a Bernoulli process becomes evident by following a similar argument to the Poisson process (Technical Note 4.2). The general calculation for there being no demand in $s + t$ periods is $(1 - p)^{s+t}$. The chance of no demand in a further t periods, given that there were no demand occurrences in the previous s periods, is $(1 - p)^{s+t}/(1 - p)^{s} = (1 - p)^{t}$. This is a function of the further time (t periods) but not of the previous time (s periods). As this function does not depend on s, we can see that a Bernoulli demand process is memoryless.

5

Compound Demand Distributions

5.1 Introduction

In Chapter 4, we reviewed the Poisson demand distribution and saw how it requires only one parameter to be forecasted, namely the mean demand over the protection interval. For those stock keeping units (SKUs) where the Poisson is a good fit to the demand, this will be sufficient. However, it was highlighted that the Poisson may not always be a good fit to real data because it is restricted to having its variance equalling its mean. In this chapter, we review some empirical evidence that shows the Poisson to be a good fit for a minority of SKUs only, albeit a significant minority. So, although the Poisson is useful, a stock control system for intermittent demand items should not be based on the Poisson distribution alone. Other distributions are needed.

In Chapter 6, we shall see how the forecasting of the mean demand of an intermittent series can be achieved by decomposing demand into two components: demand sizes (when demand occurs) and demand intervals (Croston 1972). This decomposition is also helpful for the characterisation of demand patterns using compound distributions, as will become evident in this chapter.

In Chapter 4, some evidence was reviewed showing that, even when the Poisson is not a good representation of demand, it may still be a good representation of demand incidence. This motivates the focus, in this chapter, on compound Poisson distributions, where demand incidence continues to be represented by the Poisson but demand size has its own distribution. We also saw that the Bernoulli distribution may be a good representation of demand occurrence, where an occurrence variable takes the value of one if there is some demand in a period, and zero if there is no demand. This can be extended to a compound Bernoulli distribution, where the size of demand in a period has its own distribution.

This chapter begins by examining the properties of compound Poisson distributions, showing that they are more flexible than the (non-compound) Poisson distribution. We proceed, in Sections 5.3 and 5.4, to look at two members of the compound Poisson family. In both cases, we see how they can be applied in practice and review the evidence on their goodness of fit. We then turn our attention to compound Bernoulli distributions, focussing on their general properties, and appropriateness for intermittent demand. In Section 5.6, we move on to discuss distributions that allow for more regular demand incidences

Intermittent Demand Forecasting: Context, Methods and Applications, First Edition.
John E. Boylan and Aris A. Syntetos.
© 2021 John Wiley & Sons Ltd. Published 2021 by John Wiley & Sons Ltd.
Companion Website: www.wiley.com/go/boylansyntetos/intermittentdemandforecasting

than the compound Poisson, and may therefore act as a complementary family of distributions.

It is important to look at the relationship between demand distributions over a unit period of time and over longer periods such as the lead time or protection interval. As well as exact relationships, we also explore approximate relationships, focussing on the normal distribution. Finally, we conclude with a review of our findings and some comments on the forecasting requirements for the main distributions discussed in the chapter.

5.2   Compound Poisson Distributions

In Chapter 4, the Poisson distribution was discussed as a distribution of demand incidence and also as a distribution of demand itself. If each customer demand is for a single unit, then the total demand is just the same as the number of demand incidences. So, if demand incidences are Poisson distributed, and all demands are for single units, then the total demand is also Poisson distributed. This situation is not always realistic, as some customers will require two, three, or more units of an SKU. Therefore, let us suppose instead that:

- Demand incidences for a single unit of an SKU are Poisson distributed, with a mean of $\lambda_1 = 0.2$ incidences per unit time period, or two incidences every 10 periods on average.
- Demand incidences for two units of the same SKU are Poisson distributed, with a mean of $\lambda_2 = 0.1$ incidences per unit time period, or one incidence every 10 periods on average.

This can be extended to as many units as are required at a single demand incidence. For explanatory purposes, we assume that the maximum number of units demanded is two. If the two streams of demand are independent of each other, then demand incidences overall will also follow a Poisson distribution. The mean number of incidences per unit time is the sum of the means from the individual streams. In our example, this sum is 0.3 (or three incidences in every 10 periods on average). When there is a demand incidence, the probability of the demand being for one unit is two-thirds, and for two units is one-third because the former occur twice as often as the latter.

This is an example of a compound Poisson distribution. Demand incidences are Poisson distributed, but the size of demand (when it occurs) follows its own probability distribution. More generally, a compound Poisson distribution represents demand patterns of the following form:

1. Total demand over a fixed period is the sum of the demands from a number of separate demand incidences. Each of these demands may be for a single unit or for several units.
2. Demand incidences follow a Poisson distribution.
3. The sizes of the demands follow their own distribution, which is independent of the demand incidence distribution.

The compound Poisson is actually a family of distributions, which restricts demand incidence to be Poisson but allows for any probability distribution of demand sizes. In this section, we look at its general properties, before turning to specific examples in the sections that follow.

5.2.1 Compound Poisson: A Priori Grounds

The structure highlighted in the three points above provides a justification for the compound Poisson as a natural separation of intermittent demand into its components of demand incidence and demand size. Also, if demand is compound Poisson, then demand incidences are memoryless, because they follow the Poisson distribution. This may be justifiable for intermittent demand, especially if it arises from failures of independent products, as discussed in Chapter 4. The compound Poisson is memoryless for demand, as well as demand incidence, if the demand sizes are independent of previous demand sizes and previous demand intervals.

5.2.2 Compound Poisson: Flexibility

A compound Poisson demand distribution may be characterised by its mean (μ) and variance (σ^2). These, in turn, are determined by the mean number of demand incidences per period (μ_N) and by the mean and variance of the demand sizes (μ_S and σ_S^2, respectively). The subscript N denotes the number of demand incidences and the subscript S denotes the demand sizes. The relationships between these variables are given in Eqs. (5.1).

$$\mu = \mu_N \mu_S$$
$$\sigma^2 = \mu_N(\mu_S^2 + \sigma_S^2) \tag{5.1}$$

The variance to mean ratio for a compound Poisson distribution is given by Eq. (5.2).

$$\frac{\sigma^2}{\mu} = \mu_S + \frac{\sigma_S^2}{\mu_S} \tag{5.2}$$

If all the orders are of unit size, with no variability, then $\mu_S = 1$ and $\sigma_S^2 = 0$, and the variance to mean ratio is one. Because there is no compounding, we have returned to the case of a non-compound Poisson distribution for which it is known that the variance and the mean are identical. If, on the other hand, not all orders are of unit size, then we will have some orders for two units or more and this will result in μ_S being strictly greater than one. So, in this case, the variance to mean ratio can take values strictly greater than one, unlike the Poisson. Therefore, the compound Poisson is more flexible than the Poisson in terms of its variance to mean ratio.

5.2.3 Summary

The compound Poisson distribution is more flexible than the Poisson as it allows for variance to mean ratios greater than one. This is particularly beneficial when the mean demand size (μ_S) is large or the variance to mean ratio for demand sizes (σ_S^2/μ_S) is high. The latter will often occur for lumpy demand patterns with occasional large spikes in demand. The compound Poisson retains the memoryless property of the Poisson for demand incidences and, under some additional conditions, is memoryless for demand as well.

We have not yet commented on the ease of calculation of the compound Poisson or its goodness of fit. These properties depend on the form of the distribution of demand sizes. In Sections 5.3 and 5.4, we look at these characteristics for two members of the compound Poisson family that have been recommended for intermittent demand, namely the stuttering Poisson distribution and the negative binomial distribution (NBD).

5.3   Stuttering Poisson Distribution

One of the earliest proposals for a distribution to represent slow-moving demand was the stuttering Poisson distribution (Galliher et al. 1959), which is a member of the family of compound Poisson distributions (Adelson 1966). The stuttering Poisson distribution is based on Poisson demand incidences and geometrically distributed demand sizes (when demand occurs), which are independent and identically distributed, and independent of demand incidences. It is, therefore, also known as the geometric Poisson distribution (Sherbrooke 1968), and is sometimes called the Pólya–Aeppli distribution, after the authors who first described and commented on it.

The geometric distribution of demand sizes is shown, for $S = 1, 2, \ldots$, in Eq. (5.3). It is not defined at $S = 0$ because if a demand occurs, then it must be for at least one unit.

$$\mathbb{P}(S) = (1 - \rho)^{s-1} \rho \tag{5.3}$$

The geometric distribution can also be used to represent the length of intervals between demands. This application was discussed in Chapter 4 and will be useful in the derivation of forecasting methods in Chapter 6, but is not relevant here.

The geometric distribution is controlled by a single parameter, denoted by the Greek letter rho (ρ), which is a positive decimal number less than one. It has a natural interpretation as the reciprocal of the mean demand size ($\rho = 1/\mu_S$). In some applications of the geometric distribution (such as demand intervals), this parameter may be interpreted as a probability and is denoted by the letter p. This is not a natural interpretation in the representation of demand sizes and so we have used a different letter (ρ) as its symbol. The effect of the ρ parameter on the distribution is shown in Figure 5.1.

In Figure 5.1, the mean demand sizes for the three distributions are quite different ($\mu_S = 5.00, 2.00, 1.25$ for $\rho = 0.2, 0.5, 0.8$, respectively). For all distributions, though, a demand size of one unit has the highest probability. Thereafter, the demand size probabilities decline at varying rates, depending on the value of ρ. If the value of ρ is low (e.g. $\rho = 0.2$), the decline

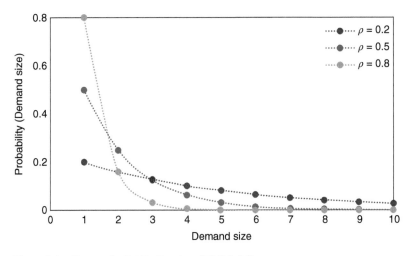

Figure 5.1   Geometric distribution ($\rho = 0.2, 0.5, 0.8$).

is quite slow, allowing for a higher mean and variance than the other two distributions. For high values of ρ (e.g. $\rho = 0.8$), there is a rapid decline of probabilities from one unit to three units, with probabilities very close to zero for four units or more. Therefore, the geometric distribution is flexible with regard to its rate of decline. It is less flexible in that the highest probability must be for a demand size of one unit, with the probabilities declining thereafter as demand sizes increase.

5.3.1 Stuttering Poisson: A Priori Grounds

The stuttering Poisson shares the memoryless property of demand incidences for all compound Poisson distributions. The geometric distribution of demand sizes is defined only for positive whole numbers, which is in accordance with most demand observed in practice. There is no further a priori justification for the geometric as a distribution of demand sizes. Instead, we must turn to empirical evidence on goodness of fit, which will be reviewed later in this section.

5.3.2 Stuttering Poisson: Ease of Calculation

For the stuttering Poisson, the number of demand incidences per period is Poisson distributed and has a mean of λ, and the demand sizes are geometrically distributed, with parameter ρ. As the mean demand size (per incidence) is $1/\rho$, this gives a mean demand of λ/ρ per period.

The probability of observing zero demand in a unit time period is given by Eq. (5.4).

$$\mathbb{P}(0) = e^{-\lambda} \tag{5.4}$$

This is the same result as for an ordinary (non-compound) Poisson distribution (see Eq. (4.1)). This makes sense because compounding is irrelevant in periods with no demand.

The calculation is straightforward. For example, if $\lambda = 1$ and $\rho = 0.5$, then the probability of zero demand is given by $\mathbb{P}(0) = e^{-1} = 1/e = 0.368$ (to three decimal places). Notice that, if the ρ parameter were to change, it would not affect this calculation.

The general formula for calculating the probability of observing a demand equal to x in a unit time period (where x is a whole number greater than or equal to one) is given by Eq. (5.5).

$$\mathbb{P}(x) = e^{-\lambda} \sum_{j=1}^{x} \frac{(x-1)!}{(j-1)!(x-j)!} \frac{(\lambda\rho)^j}{j!} (1-\rho)^{x-j} \tag{5.5}$$

The rationale behind this formula is given in Technical Note 5.1. It takes a less complicated form for low demand values. The probabilities of demand for $x = 1$ and $x = 2$ are given by Eqs. (5.6).

$$\mathbb{P}(1) = e^{-\lambda} \lambda\rho$$
$$\mathbb{P}(2) = e^{-\lambda} \lambda\rho(1-\rho) + \frac{e^{-\lambda}\lambda^2\rho^2}{2} \tag{5.6}$$

Continuing our example, the probability of demand for one unit is given by: $\mathbb{P}(1) = e^{-1} \times 1 \times 0.5 = 0.368 \times 1 \times 0.5 = 0.184$. For two units, the probability is given

Table 5.1 Poisson ($\lambda = 2$) and stuttering Poisson ($\lambda = 1$ and $\rho = 0.5$) probabilities (prob) and cumulative probabilities (cum prob).

Demand	Poisson prob	Poisson cum prob	Stuttering prob	Stuttering cum prob
0	0.135	0.135	0.368	0.368
1	0.271	0.406	0.184	0.552
2	0.271	0.677	0.138	0.690
3	0.180	0.857	0.100	0.790
4	0.090	0.947	0.070	0.859
5	0.036	0.983	0.048	0.907
6	0.012	0.995	0.032	0.940

by: $\mathbb{P}(2) = (0.368 \times 1 \times 0.5 \times 0.5) + (0.368 \times 1 \times 1 \times 0.5 \times 0.5/2) = 0.092 + 0.046 = 0.138$.

The general expression for the stuttering Poisson, shown in Eq. (5.5), is more complicated than the expression for the Poisson. The formula is quite cumbersome for higher demand values if calculated manually but can be readily programmed.

To illustrate the effect of compounding, we now compare the probabilities and cumulative probabilities of Poisson and stuttering Poisson distributions with the same mean demand of two units per period ($\mu = 2$). In more detail, we compare (i) Poisson demand, based on a mean of two demand incidences per period ($\lambda = 2$) where all the demands are for one unit and (ii) stuttering Poisson demand, with a mean of one demand incidence per period ($\lambda = 1$) but with a mean demand size of two units ($\mu_S = 2$ and $\rho = 0.5$ for the geometric distribution of demand sizes). The detailed comparison is shown in Table 5.1.

In Table 5.1, the stuttering Poisson shows higher probabilities of larger demand values (five and six units) than the Poisson. This yields quite different cumulative probabilities. For example, the final cumulative probability (of demand less than or equal to six) is 0.995 for the Poisson but only 0.940 for the stuttering Poisson.

It is often more convenient to estimate the mean and variance of demand than the λ and ρ parameters of the stuttering Poisson distribution. Estimates of the latter parameters may then be found, using the relationships between the population parameters shown in Eqs. (5.7).

$$\lambda = \frac{2\mu^2}{\sigma^2 + \mu}$$
$$\rho = \frac{2\mu}{\sigma^2 + \mu}$$
(5.7)

Forecasts of the mean (μ) and variance (σ^2) of demand per unit time period give estimates of the λ and ρ parameters, which may be substituted into Eq. (5.5) to give the required probability estimates. Alternatively, a recurrence relationship may be used, relating $\mathbb{P}(x)$ to its two immediate predecessors, $\mathbb{P}(x-1)$ and $\mathbb{P}(x-2)$, for $x \geq 2$, with starting values for $\mathbb{P}(0)$ and $\mathbb{P}(1)$. (For further details, see Nuel (2008) and Özel and İnal (2010).) Both strategies rely on replacing the population means and variances by their forecasted values. In the case of stationary demand, the sample mean and variance may be used. This approach to estimation converges to the correct parameters as demand histories grow longer but may give less accurate and biased results for shorter demand histories. This, in turn, may lead to under- or over-achievement of service targets (Prak 2019). Therefore, in practice, it is important to check its inventory implications, as will be discussed further in Chapter 9.

5.3.3 Stuttering Poisson: Flexibility

The ρ parameter can take any decimal value greater than zero and less than or equal to one. For geometrically distributed demand sizes, this parameter controls both the mean $(\mu_S = 1/\rho)$ and the variance $(\sigma_S^2 = (1 - \rho)/\rho^2)$. Consequently, the variance to mean ratio for demand sizes is $(1 - \rho)/\rho$ and (by applying Eq. (5.2)) the variance to mean ratio for demand is given by Eq. (5.8).

$$\frac{\sigma^2}{\mu} = \frac{2}{\rho} - 1 \tag{5.8}$$

Equation (5.8) shows that the variance to mean ratio is always greater than or equal to one. If all demands are for one unit, then $\rho = 1$ and the stuttering Poisson reduces to the Poisson distribution, and its variance to mean ratio equals one. In all other cases, the ρ parameter is less than one, leading to the variance to mean ratio exceeding one. Therefore, the stuttering Poisson is more flexible than the Poisson in terms of its variance to mean ratio.

The relative variability of demand sizes may also be measured by its coefficient of variation, CV_S, defined as the ratio of the standard deviation to the mean, σ_S/μ_S. This measure has the advantage of being 'scale independent'. To illustrate this concept, we use an example of items that are sold 10 to a pack. If the mean demand size is four packs and the standard deviation is two packs, then the mean demand size is 40 units, and the standard deviation is 20 units. This means that the CV_S value is 0.5, regardless of whether demand is measured in packs or items. The variance values are four if measured in packs and 400 if measured in items. This gives variance to mean ratios of 1 (measured in packs) and 10 (measured in items). These results illustrate that the value of the variance to mean ratio depends on the scale of measurement (packs or items). The coefficient of variation, on the other hand, is scale-independent, as the result is the same for all units of measurement.

The coefficient of variation of demand sizes for a geometric distribution is given by Eq. (5.9).

$$CV_S = \sqrt{1 - \frac{1}{\mu_S}} \tag{5.9}$$

Equation (5.9) shows that the coefficient of variation of the demand sizes is always less than one for the geometric distribution. This is not always a limitation in practice, but it does preclude the stuttering Poisson from representing highly variable demand processes with CV_S values greater than one.

5.3.4 Stuttering Poisson: Goodness of Fit for Demand Sizes

As noted in Chapter 4, there is empirical support for the goodness of fit of Poisson demand incidences, at least as an approximation (e.g. Shale et al. 2008). To test for the goodness of fit of a stuttering Poisson demand distribution, there are two approaches that may be taken: (i) test (separately) for demand incidences being Poisson distributed and demand sizes being geometrically distributed and (ii) test that demand is stuttering Poisson distributed.

The second approach is more decisive, and this type of direct evidence will be reviewed at the end of Section 5.4, when the goodness of fit of the stuttering Poisson will be compared to that of the negative binomial. The first approach is less decisive. As Poisson demand incidences and geometrically distributed demand sizes are assumed in the stuttering Poisson, it is sensible to test these assumptions. However, Poisson demand incidences and geometric demand sizes do not guarantee a stuttering Poisson demand distribution unless demand sizes are also independent and identically distributed, and independent of demand incidences. The evidence to be reviewed in this subsection follows the first approach and tests the geometric distribution of demand sizes (assuming that incidences are Poisson) but does not test the stuttering Poisson demand distribution directly.

Johnston et al. (2003) provided evidence in support of a geometric distribution of demand sizes. Testing that demand sizes are geometrically distributed is not straightforward at the level of an individual SKU because there may be only a small number of non-zero observations when demand is intermittent. However, it is possible to adopt a similar testing strategy to that described for the Poisson distribution in Chapter 4. Firstly, we can examine the relationship between the standard deviation and mean of demand across a range of SKUs. Secondly, we can look at the distribution of demand sizes across a collection of SKUs.

For a geometric distribution, a relationship holds between the standard deviation (σ_S) and the mean (μ_S) of the demand sizes, as shown in Eq. (5.10).

$$\sigma_S = \sqrt{\mu_S(\mu_S - 1)} \tag{5.10}$$

Johnston et al. (2003) pointed out that this relationship enables us to check the geometric distribution of demand sizes over a wide range of SKUs. Their data was at the transactional level, meaning that each order had been recorded, and that 'demand sizes' could be interpreted as 'order sizes'. Using data from a wholesaler of electrical products, they plotted the observed means (horizontal axis) and standard deviations (vertical axis) of demand sizes for 500 SKUs that had between 6 and 12 demand incidences (orders) per year. The data points are shown in Figure 5.2, plotted on a logarithmic scale on both horizontal and vertical axes. The curve given by Eq. (5.10) is also shown, labelled as an 'approximation' to the observed data.

The plot in Figure 5.2 indicates that there is a good fit between the hypothesised curve and the actual data, lending support to a geometric distribution of demand sizes. There is a tendency, though, for the actual standard deviation to be slightly higher than the curve linking the standard deviation to the mean (Eq. (5.10)).

We can also examine the distribution of demand sizes of a collection of SKUs. Johnston et al. (2003) analysed 3500 SKUs, each having between 6 and 12 demand incidences (orders) in a year and average demand sizes between 2.0 and 3.0. The resulting distribution of demand (order) sizes is shown in Figure 5.3.

Figure 5.3 shows a good fit of the observed data to the geometric distribution, but with some overestimation of the frequencies of demand (order) sizes between 11 and 15 and underestimation of frequencies of demand sizes between 46 and 50. Overall, this study

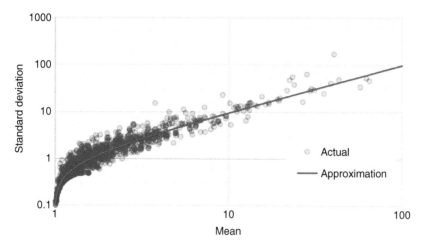

Figure 5.2 Standard deviation and mean of demand sizes. Source: Johnston et al. 2003.

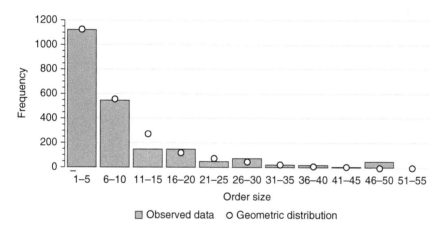

Figure 5.3 Frequency distribution of order sizes. Source: Johnston et al. 2003.

offers some empirical support for the geometric distribution of demand sizes. As we shall see later, there is also more direct empirical evidence showing the goodness of fit of the stuttering Poisson demand distribution.

5.3.5 Summary

As a member of the compound Poisson family of distributions, the stuttering Poisson inherits the memoryless property for demand incidences. Also, its variance can take values greater than the mean. In this sense, it is more flexible than the Poisson, which is always constrained to have its variance equal to the mean. However, the coefficient of variation of the demand sizes must always be less than one, which imposes some limits on the flexibility of the stuttering Poisson.

The distribution is more complicated to calculate than the Poisson, but it depends on only two parameters. The necessary calculations can be programmed reasonably straightforwardly to allow the distribution to be used in practice. There is some evidence in support of the goodness of fit of the Poisson demand incidence distribution, as discussed in Chapter 4. We have just seen that there is empirical evidence in support of a geometric demand (order) size distribution. We have not yet looked at direct evidence of the goodness of fit of the stuttering Poisson. This will be reviewed in Section 5.4.4.

5.4 Negative Binomial Distribution

The stuttering Poisson distribution was not the only early suggestion to represent slow-moving demand. Taylor (1961) proposed the application of the negative binomial distribution (NBD). This distribution is defined in Eq. (5.11) for all non-negative whole-number demands, denoted by x (including zero).

$$\mathbb{P}(x) = \frac{(x + r - 1)!}{x!(r - 1)!} p^r (1 - p)^x \tag{5.11}$$

In some settings, the negative binomial distributed variable, x, may be interpreted as the number of failures before r successes in a series of independent Bernoulli trials, each of which has a probability p of success. This is not a natural interpretation for intermittent demand. However, there are alternative models which do provide an a priori justification for the NBD.

5.4.1 Negative Binomial: A Priori Grounds

There are two distinct ways in which this distribution may arise as a demand distribution:

1. *Compound distribution*: This is based on a Poisson distribution of the number of demand incidences and a logarithmic distribution of demand sizes (Technical Note 5.2).
2. *Mixture distribution*: In this interpretation, demand is Poisson distributed and the mean demand varies over time, following a gamma distribution (Technical Note 5.2).

The first interpretation is consistent with our discussions earlier in this chapter, with a decomposition of demand into demand incidence and demand sizes. We discuss the second interpretation further in Section 5.7, when we consider the implications of the mean demand changing over time.

5.4.2 Negative Binomial: Ease of Calculation

Equation (5.11) is the standard equation for the negative binomial distribution. It is not expressed in a form that is most suitable for demand probability calculations, but may be written in a more convenient form. Let μ be the mean of the demand distribution and z be the variance to mean ratio ($z = \sigma^2/\mu$). Note that these symbols do not have subscripts, as they refer to total demand (over a fixed period of time). Then the demand probabilities can be calculated (Technical Note 5.3) from Eqs. (5.12) (zero demand) and (5.13) (strictly positive whole-number demand values).

$$\mathbb{P}(0) = \left(\frac{1}{z}\right)^{\mu/(z-1)} \qquad (5.12)$$

$$\mathbb{P}(x) = \left(\frac{\frac{\mu}{z-1}+x-1}{x}\right)\left(\frac{z-1}{z}\right)\mathbb{P}(x-1) \qquad (5.13)$$

Equation (5.13) links the probability of each (non-zero) demand value, x, to the probability of its predecessor, $x-1$, in a recursive formula. This makes it easy to implement in a spreadsheet or in a loop in a programming language.

The formulae (5.12) and (5.13) have the virtue that they are expressed solely in terms of the mean (μ) and the variance to mean ratio ($z = \sigma^2/\mu$). So, if we know the mean and variance of demand, then we can calculate the probability of zero demand, $\mathbb{P}(0)$, from Eq. (5.12). For example, if $\sigma^2 = 10$ and $\mu = 4$, then $z = 2.5$, $1/z = 0.4$, $\mu/(z-1) = 4/1.5 = 2.67$ and $\mathbb{P}(0) = 0.4^{2.67} = 0.087$. To calculate $\mathbb{P}(1)$, we can substitute $\mathbb{P}(0) = 0.087$ into the right-hand side of Eq. (5.13). As shown in Table 5.2, $\mathbb{P}(1) = 2.67 \times 0.60 \times 0.087 = 0.139$. Repeating this operation allows calculation of $\mathbb{P}(2)$, and $\mathbb{P}(3)$, and we can keep on going as far as we need with these calculations.

Table 5.2 continues our example by showing the calculation of the negative binomial probabilities in detail. The three central columns correspond to the terms on the right-hand side of Eq. (5.13), and the final column is calculated by multiplying together the three values in these central columns.

In conclusion, Eqs. (5.12) and (5.13) allow negative binomial probabilities to be found. All that is required are values of the mean and variance of demand, and then the probabilities can be calculated.

5.4.3 Negative Binomial: Flexibility

The logarithmic distribution of demand sizes ($S = 1, 2, \ldots$) is given in Eq. (5.14).

$$\mathbb{P}(S) = \frac{-1}{\log(1-p)}\frac{p^S}{S} \qquad (5.14)$$

where log denotes the natural logarithm (to base e).

Table 5.2 Calculation of negative binomial probabilities ($\mu = 4$ and $\sigma^2 = 10$).

Demand (x)	$\left(\frac{\mu}{z-1}+x-1\right)/x$	$(z-1)/z$	$\mathbb{P}(x-1)$	$\mathbb{P}(x)$
0				0.087
1	2.67	0.600	0.087	0.139
2	1.83	0.600	0.139	0.153
3	1.56	0.600	0.153	0.143
4	1.42	0.600	0.143	0.121
5	1.33	0.600	0.121	0.097

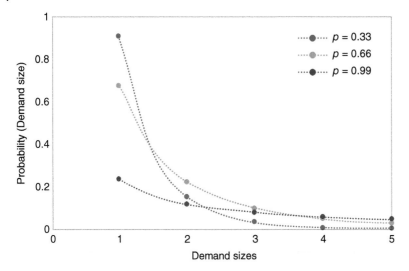

Figure 5.4 Logarithmic distribution ($p = 0.33, 0.66, 0.99$).

The logarithmic distribution, shown in Figure 5.4, has a similar shape to the geometric distribution, shown in Figure 5.1, with the highest probability at one and declining probabilities thereafter.

The distribution is controlled by a single parameter, p (between zero and one). The logarithmic distribution of demand sizes has a coefficient of variation (CV_S) given by Eq. (5.15).

$$CV_S = \frac{\sigma_S}{\mu_S} = \sqrt{-1 - \frac{\log(1-p)}{p}} \tag{5.15}$$

The expression under the square root sign on the right-hand side of Eq. (5.15) is always positive and returns a positive square root for the coefficient of variation. This coefficient of variation can, in fact, take any positive number and is not limited to values less than one. For example, if $p = 0.96$, then $CV_S = 1.53$. This is in contrast to the geometric distribution, whose coefficient of variation cannot be greater than one. Hence, in this sense, the negative binomial (with logarithmic distributed demand sizes) is more flexible than the stuttering Poisson distribution (with geometric distributed demand sizes).

5.4.4 Negative Binomial: Goodness of Fit

We have seen that the stuttering Poisson and negative binomial distributions share similar properties, as they are both based on Poisson demand incidences. The negative binomial is more flexible in terms of the coefficient of variation of demand sizes, but does this translate to a better fit against real data?

Syntetos et al. (2013) undertook a comparison of the Poisson, stuttering Poisson, and negative binomial distributions, using large datasets from the US Defense Logistics Agency, the Royal Air Force (RAF) and the electronics sector. Their results on the goodness of fit of the three distributions for demand per period are summarised in Table 5.3 (see Technical

Table 5.3   Percentages of SKUs with strong fit (demand per period).

Dataset	Number of SKUs	Poisson (%)	Stuttering Poisson (%)	Negative binomial (%)
US Defense	4588	20.1	92.4	87.2
RAF	5000	43.8	99.9	93.2
Electronics	3055	14.2	91.7	95.4

Source: Modified from Syntetos et al. (2013).

Note 5.4 for an explanation of the goodness of fit tests and the meaning of 'strong fit' in Table 5.3).

Table 5.3 shows that the Poisson distribution performs poorly in terms of goodness of fit, especially for the US Defense and electronics datasets. The fit is improved considerably by using either the stuttering Poisson or negative binomial distributions and either of these distributions would be satisfactory for all three datasets.

The stuttering Poisson performs excellently for the RAF dataset. This dataset has the SKUs with the least variance in demand sizes. This is consistent with the earlier observation that the stuttering Poisson is expected to perform better for such cases. Conversely, the negative binomial performs best for the dataset from the electronics sector, which has the highest variance in demand sizes.

A further study on the goodness of fit of these distributions was conducted by Turrini and Meissner (2019). They analysed 4483 SKUs from the renewable energy sector and re-analysed the 5000 SKUs from the RAF that had been studied by Syntetos et al. (2013). The goodness of fit test was undertaken using a new approach which places less weight on the distribution at the left tail and more weight on the right tail of the distribution, to reflect the requirements of inventory systems. Their findings for the RAF dataset agreed with Syntetos et al. (2013), and the findings for the renewables sector also showed both the negative binomial and stuttering Poisson to have good fits, but with the stuttering Poisson having the better fit.

5.4.5   Summary

As a member of the compound Poisson family of distributions, the negative binomial's demand variance can take values greater than the mean. Unlike the stuttering Poisson, its coefficient of variation of demand sizes is not constrained to be always less than one. In this sense, the negative binomial is more flexible than the stuttering Poisson distribution. This is useful for SKUs where there are likely to be some high volume spikes in demand, pushing the coefficient of variation of demand sizes to be higher than one.

Negative binomial probabilities are not difficult to calculate and, in fact, are straightforward to implement in computer software because of the recursive relationship linking the probability of each (non-zero) demand to the probability to its predecessor. Empirical evidence supports its application in real-world situations, making the negative binomial a strong contender for practical applications, alongside the stuttering Poisson.

5.5 Compound Bernoulli Distributions

In Sections 5.2–5.4, we assumed that demand incidences are Poisson distributed. Then, the total demand over a fixed period of time is the sum of the demands from a number of separate demand incidences. This compounding approach can be adapted to other models of demand occurrence and demand incidence. Two alternatives to the compound Poisson that are advocated in the literature are the compound Bernoulli and the compound Erlang distributions. These are discussed in further detail in this section and Section 5.6.

5.5.1 Compound Bernoulli: A Priori Grounds

In Chapter 4, we saw that periods with demand occurrence (or not) could be represented by a Bernoulli distribution. This distribution is memoryless and has just one parameter, namely the probability of demand occurrence.

We can now build on this Bernoulli distribution, by including a distribution for the size of demand during a unit time period ('demand sizes'). These sizes cannot be interpreted as 'order sizes', because there may have been more than one order placed in a period. The distribution of demand sizes can be any distribution with a good fit to the data (e.g. geometric or logarithmic, as discussed in Sections 5.3 and 5.4). Like the compound Poisson, there are two additional requirements for a compound Bernoulli distribution to be memoryless. Firstly, the demand size in the current period should not depend on the demand sizes in previous periods; secondly, the demand size in the current period should not depend on the previous intervals between periods with demand occurrences.

5.5.2 Compound Bernoulli: Ease of Calculation

There are few examples of specific compound Bernoulli distributions being used in practice. Kwan (1991) suggested the log-zero-Poisson distribution. This arises from a Bernoulli demand process and a logarithmic-Poisson distribution of demand sizes. (The logarithmic-Poisson distribution is not the same as the Poisson-logarithmic, which gives the negative binomial distribution.) However, the log-zero-Poisson distribution requires three parameters to be estimated, making it more unwieldy than two-parameter distributions.

5.5.3 Compound Bernoulli: Flexibility

We can examine the flexibility of a compound Bernoulli distribution in terms of its variance to mean ratio, which is given by Eq. (5.16).

$$\frac{\sigma^2}{\mu} = (1 - p)\mu_S + \frac{\sigma_S^2}{\mu_S} \tag{5.16}$$

where p is the probability of demand occurrence in a period, and μ_S and σ_S^2 are the mean and variance of demand size (see Technical Note 5.5 for the derivation of this formula).

Like the compound Poisson distribution, the compound Bernoulli has the flexibility to represent demand patterns where the variance exceeds the mean. The compound Bernoulli has an element of additional flexibility because it can also allow for variance to mean ratios that are less than one. For example, if $p = 0.7$, $\mu_S = 1.5$, and $\sigma_S^2 = 0.25$, then the variance to mean ratio of demand is 0.62.

5.5.4   Compound Bernoulli: Goodness of Fit

As noted in Chapter 4, there is empirical evidence in support of the Bernoulli distribution of demand occurrence. For example, Eaves (2002) found approximately 90% of a large sample of SKUs from the RAF were well fitted by Poisson and Bernoulli demand processes.

Because so few compound Bernoulli distributions have been proposed for intermittent demand forecasting, there is little empirical evidence to review. Kwan (1991) analysed the goodness of fit of the log-zero-Poisson distribution, a member of the family of compound Bernoulli distributions. She examined 85 SKUs, comprising 56 vehicle spare parts and 29 spare parts for steel manufacturing machines.

Kwan's investigation of the log-zero-Poisson offered some encouraging results, with the lead time demand of over 80% of SKUs being well-fitted by this distribution. This data may have been well suited to a compound Bernoulli distribution because 23 of the 85 SKUs had variances less than their means. As noted above, this situation may be better represented by a compound Bernoulli (rather than a compound Poisson) distribution.

5.5.5   Summary

The compound Bernoulli family of distributions has some attractive features. It is based on Bernoulli demand occurrence, which has a theoretical justification as a memoryless distribution. As we shall see in Chapter 6, it was used by Croston (1972) as a basis for intermittent demand forecasting. The compound Bernoulli family is very flexible in terms of variance to mean ratios, allowing for this ratio to be greater than, equal to, or less than one. Unfortunately, there is limited empirical evidence assessing goodness of fit. Because of this, compound Bernoulli distributions are not pursued further in this chapter. However, there is certainly scope for further research on this family of distributions.

5.6   Compound Erlang Distributions

The Poisson distribution represents processes of demand incidence that are memoryless. This property is shared by many intermittent demand items but not all. For example, Larsen and Thorstenson (2008) examined the demand patterns for spare parts in the refrigeration and air conditioning division of the Danfoss Group in Denmark. They found that the demand incidence pattern was often less erratic than assumed by a Poisson process. In this section, we look at an approach to representing patterns of incidence that are not perfectly regular but are less variable than would be expected from a Poisson distribution.

Let us return to the situation when the demand incidences are Poisson. As discussed in Chapter 4, an exponential distribution of demand intervals arises from a Poisson process of demand incidences. If demand incidences are Poisson distributed, with mean λ, then the cumulative distribution of demand intervals is given by Eq. (5.17) (previously shown as Eq. (4.2)).

$$\mathbb{P}(\text{Interval} \leq t) = 1 - e^{-\lambda t} \tag{5.17}$$

The probability density and cumulative distribution of demand intervals are shown in Figure 5.5. The probability density function can be used to specify the probability of a random variable, such as a demand interval, falling within a range of values. The cumulative distribution shows the probability of a random variable being less than or equal to a specified value.

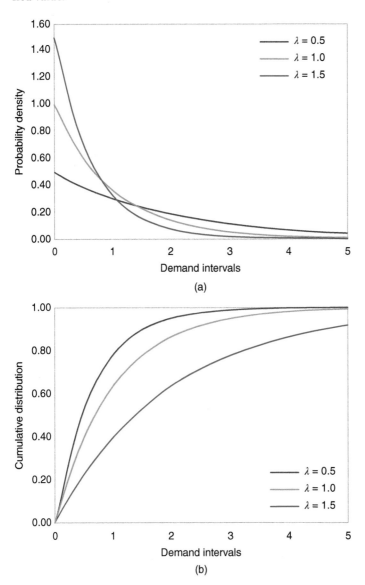

Figure 5.5 Exponential distributions. (a) Probability density; (b) Cumulative distribution function.

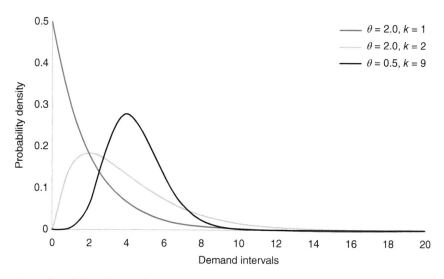

Figure 5.6 Erlang distributions.

From Figure 5.5a, we can see that, for any choice of the mean value (λ) the chance of a demand interval being between two and three is less than the chance of it being between one and two, which is less than the chance of it being between zero and one. From Figure 5.5b, we can read off directly (for each value of λ) the chance of the demand interval being less than that value.

Sometimes, the probability density function of times between incidences of demand does not decline continuously as in Figure 5.5 but, instead, rises to a peak and then declines. Some examples of such distributions are given in Figure 5.6.

Figure 5.6 shows an exponential distribution for $k = 1$ and increasingly symmetrical functions as the k value increases. These distributions are known as Erlang-k distributions, with the exponential as a special case (Erlang-1 distribution). The theta (θ) parameter is known as a scale parameter, and has the effect of stretching or compressing the distribution.

One of the most commonly applied Erlang distributions, apart from the exponential, is the Erlang-2 distribution. Its cumulative distribution is given by Eq. (5.18).

$$\mathbb{P}(\text{Interval} \leq t) = 1 - e^{-\lambda t} - \lambda t e^{-\lambda t} \tag{5.18}$$

In Section 5.6.1, we shall see, from first principles, how this cumulative distribution may arise.

5.6.1 Compound Erlang Distributions: A Priori Grounds

Suppose that a retailer requires a particular SKU from a supplier and the demand on the retailer for this item follows a Poisson distribution. However, the retailer always purchases two of these items and does not place a new order until there is none left. Then, the demand on the retailer follows an 'uncensored Poisson process' but the retailer's purchases follow a 'censored Poisson process'. The word 'censored' is used because every second demand incidence is removed from the time series to give the sequence of purchases.

In this case, the probability that the interval between orders is greater than a given time, t, is found by adding the chance that there is no demand in the time interval up to, and including, time t to the chance that there is one demand in the same interval. Therefore, the cumulative distribution of the interval between orders being less than or equal to the given time, t, is expressed by $\mathbb{P}(\text{Interval} \leq t) = 1 - (\mathbb{P}(0) + \mathbb{P}(1)) = 1 - e^{-\lambda t} - \lambda t e^{-\lambda t}$, which is an Erlang-2 distribution (Eq. (5.18)). Hence, the censored Poisson process provides an a priori justification for the Erlang-2 distribution of demand intervals. Similar arguments, based on ordering after every kth demand observation, may be used to justify an Erlang-k distribution.

An Erlang distribution may be observed even when it does not seem appropriate to represent demand incidence as a censored Poisson process. Smith and Dekker (1997) gave the example of a seal in a pump. Once replaced, it is unlikely that it will fail again within a short period of time. Therefore, it is more likely that the time to the next failure (and ordering of a replacement seal) will follow a pattern such as that shown for an Erlang-k distribution ($k \geq 2$ in Figure 5.6), than for an exponential distribution ($k = 1$).

5.6.2 Compound Erlang Distributions: Ease of Calculation

The compound Erlang is not as straightforward to calculate as the compound Poisson distributions discussed earlier in this chapter. Larsen and Thorstenson (2008) gave general equations for the probability distributions of lead time demand when the demand intervals are Erlang-k distributed (Technical Note 5.6). These equations may be programmed quite straightforwardly but their complexity makes them difficult to explain to anyone other than a technical specialist.

5.6.3 Compound Erlang-2: Flexibility

If the times between incidences are Erlang-2 distributed, then demand incidences themselves follow a condensed Poisson distribution (Chatfield and Goodhardt 1973). The condensed Poisson distribution, for a unit time period, is described in Technical Note 5.7. Its variance to mean ratio is given by Eq. (5.19).

$$\frac{\sigma_N^2}{\mu_N} = \frac{1}{2} + \frac{1}{4\lambda}(1 - e^{-2\lambda}) \tag{5.19}$$

The variance to mean ratio is always greater than a half and less than one, showing that demand incidences are less variable than would be expected from a Poisson distribution. In this sense, the condensed Poisson complements the Poisson distribution.

When condensed Poisson demand incidences are compounded with a demand size distribution, the variance to mean ratio may increase and exceed one, giving the flexibility to address situations where the demand size is highly variable but the demand incidence is more regular than would be expected from the Poisson distribution.

5.6.4 Compound Erlang-2: Goodness of Fit

There is very little evidence available on the goodness of fit of the compound Erlang distribution for intermittent demand. There is some empirical evidence on the Erlang distribution representing time between purchases by individual consumers. Early studies include Herniter (1971), Chatfield and Goodhardt (1973), Jeuland et al. (1980), Dunn et al. (1983), and Gupta (1988). These studies generally support the Erlang as an inter-purchase time distribution for individual consumers, with the Erlang-2 gaining the greatest favour.

Care needs to be taken in extrapolating the results of studies on demand from individual consumers for frequently purchased items (such as instant coffee, baked beans, facial tissue, and laundry detergent) to demand from multiple independent customers for infrequently purchased items (such as spare parts). There is very little evidence available but Kwan (1991) found that the Erlang-2 inter-purchase distribution did not fit the demand intervals of any of the 85 slow-moving parts she analysed. Boylan (1997) found that only approximately 20% of the 230 SKUs analysed were well fitted by the condensed Poisson demand incidence distribution.

5.6.5 Summary

The compound Erlang distributions have a natural a priori justification as a 'censored Poisson process'. In the case of consumer behaviour, there is empirical evidence to support Erlang inter-purchase time distributions.

The condensed Poisson distribution extends the range of variance to mean ratios that may be represented, and so may be considered as a natural complement to the Poisson distribution. The condensed Poisson distribution probabilities are not difficult to calculate. The general compound Erlang-k distribution is more complicated, although there are some special cases that are easier to compute.

When considering demand from multiple independent customers, the a priori case for the Erlang is not so strong. The distribution may still be justified by the observation that failure of a part may be less likely shortly after replacement. Unfortunately, there is little empirical evidence on the goodness of fit of the compound Erlang as a distribution for intermittent demand. The evidence that is available offers only limited support for the distribution. This would indicate that any application of this distribution should be preceded by a thorough examination of real demand data, to ensure that the compound Erlang is appropriate.

5.7 Differing Time Units

Suppose that we have found a distribution that is a good fit for demand over one week periods. Will it also be a good fit for demand over four week periods? Not all the parameters will be the same, but will the distribution be the same?

This question is of practical importance. It will be convenient if we can use the same distribution for demand over any period of time. For example, we may know that demand for all SKUs in a particular product group can be well represented by the Poisson distribution over a single period of time. In that case, it would be beneficial if we can immediately deduce that the Poisson distribution will still apply for demand over the protection interval for all SKUs even if they have different lead times from suppliers, or if these lead times change.

5.7.1 Poisson Distribution

We begin by assuming that demand over a single week is Poisson distributed, with an unchanging mean demand of two units per week over the next four weeks. If the demands over each of the weeks are independent, then the demand over four weeks is also Poisson distributed, with a mean of eight units.

Now suppose that the mean is not fixed at two units per week but changes over time. If it does so, then we have a 'mixture distribution', as mentioned in Section 5.4.1. The distribution of total demand over the whole four week period depends on how the mean is changing over time. If the mean demand is itself gamma distributed (as defined in Technical Note 5.2), then the total demand is negative binomial. In other words, the Poisson distribution of demand over one week has been translated to negative binomial over four weeks.

This discussion provides a warning that we cannot take it for granted that if demand is Poisson distributed over one period of time, then it will also be Poisson distributed over longer periods of time. However, if the changes in the mean demand are small, then the Poisson may still be an adequate approximation of the distribution of demand over the protection interval. In order to be confident of our demand distribution assumptions, we will need to check goodness of fit over the protection interval and not just over single periods of time.

5.7.2 Compound Poisson Distribution

As we saw earlier, even when the Poisson distribution is not a good representation of demand itself, it may still serve as a good distribution of demand incidence, with a separate distribution of demand size. In this case, demand is compound Poisson distributed. How does the compound Poisson, over a single period of time, translate to the whole protection interval?

Firstly, we suppose that the demand is independent over time and the mean rate of demand incidence is not changing. In this case, if demand is compound Poisson distributed over one period, then it is also compound Poisson distributed over several periods. The form of the distribution depends on the distribution of demand sizes. One possibility is that there is a geometric distribution of demand sizes, with the same parameter ρ (the reciprocal of the mean demand size) applying across all periods. Then, demand is stuttering Poisson over several periods. Another possibility is that there is a logarithmic distribution of demand sizes, with the same parameter (p), applying across all periods. Then, demand is negative binomially distributed over several periods.

Secondly, we suppose that the mean demand incidence is changing over time. In this case, the distribution over several periods depends on the mixture distribution. The form of the demand size distribution over several periods depends on the distribution over one period and whether the demand size parameters are changing over time. In general, however, we cannot be assured that a stuttering Poisson will translate to a stuttering Poisson, or a negative binomial will translate to a negative binomial. As with the Poisson distribution, we must check the goodness of fit over the protection intervals and not just over single periods of time.

Table 5.4 Percentages of SKUs with strong fit (lead time demand).

Dataset	Number of SKUs	Poisson distribution (%)	Stuttering Poisson (%)	Negative binomial (%)
RAF	5000	28.9	71.9	59.3
Electronics	3055	11.1	88.9	89.8

Source: Modified from Syntetos et al. (2013).

It is instructive to see some results of goodness of fit tests on real-world data. Returning to the datasets discussed earlier in the chapter, Syntetos et al. (2013) also obtained goodness of fit results for lead time demand, using the same approach as outlined in Technical Note 5.4. Lead times for each SKU were available in the RAF dataset. For the electronics dataset, the SKUs were subject to a common lead time of three periods. No lead time data were available for the US Defense dataset and so this was excluded from the analysis. The findings are summarised in Table 5.4.

In the analysis of goodness of fit for demand per unit time period, the stuttering Poisson and negative binomial had similar results and were both much better than the Poisson. Now, turning to lead time demand, a similar picture emerges for the electronics dataset, so either distribution could be used with confidence there. However, the situation is different for the RAF dataset. The high proportion of SKUs (over 90%) that were well fitted by the two distributions (for unit time periods) has dropped quite markedly. Turrini and Meissner (2019) re-analysed the RAF dataset. They agreed that the fit over lead time was not as good as over a unit time period. They also found that the results were less encouraging when using their modified goodness of fit test, which puts greater emphasis on the upper tail of the distribution, and this was also reflected by their assessment of the inventory implications of using these distributions.

5.7.3 Compound Bernoulli and Compound Erlang Distributions

Over a single period, if demand occurrence is Bernoulli and demand size has its own distribution, then demand is compound Bernoulli distributed. Over more than one period, the situation is slightly more complicated. The simplest case occurs over two periods when demand occurrence in Period 1 is Bernoulli distributed with a certain probability and demand occurrence in Period 2 is Bernoulli distributed with the same probability. In that case, if demand occurrences are independent, then the number of demand occurrences over the two periods is not Bernoulli but binomially distributed. The binomial distribution arises from a Bernoulli demand process naturally, representing the chance of r successes from n 'trials' (see Eq. (4.3)). In our case, each trial has two possible outcomes: demand occurrence and no demand occurrence. The number of trials is the number of periods (two in our example of demand in Period 1 and Period 2). This argument extends to a higher number of periods and, just as a Bernoulli sums to a binomial distribution, so a compound Bernoulli sums to a compound binomial distribution.

The compound Erlang also becomes more complicated as we sum the demand over a number of periods. Some useful expressions for the distribution of demand over lead time have been given by Larsen and Thorstenson (2008). In these cases, as for the compound Poisson, it is necessary to check the goodness of fit over the whole protection interval, and not restrict attention to the distribution of demand over unit time.

5.7.4 Normal Distribution

In the previous discussion, we have seen that distributions such as the stuttering Poisson do not necessarily translate to a stuttering Poisson distribution of demand over the protection interval if the mean demand incidence is changing over time. The distribution may still be approximated by a stuttering Poisson, particularly if the mean incidence is changing slowly over time. Of course, this would need to be checked, as we saw earlier.

We now turn to another way of approximating the distribution of the demand over the protection interval. Rather than using the same distribution that would represent demand over a single period of time, we rely on the normal distribution instead. The normal distribution has often been criticised as a distribution for intermittent demand. To see why this is so, consider the following example, where the line superimposed on the histogram of the frequency data corresponds to the probability density function of the normal distribution (also known as the Gaussian distribution).

In Figure 5.7, the probability density function does not show probabilities directly. Instead, we look at areas under the curve to represent probabilities. In this example, the normal produces a probability density function that does not provide a good fit to the histogram of observed frequencies.

It is clear that the normality assumption can be problematic for intermittent demand items. However, although this is the case when characterising demand per period, the normality assumption may still be useful when looking at demand over longer protection intervals and when demand is not so highly intermittent.

According to the central limit theorem, under certain conditions, the sum of a large number of random variables will be approximately normally distributed. Therefore, although the normal distribution may be a poor approximation to demand over a unit time period, its approximation to the total demand over the protection interval will tend to improve as that

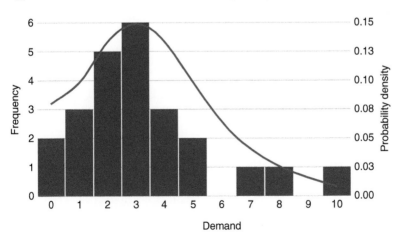

Figure 5.7 Normal distribution (poor approximation).

interval lengthens. This is the a priori justification for the normal distribution to represent demand. There are some arguments against using the normal distribution. The first is that the normal is defined for fractional values that are rarely observed in demand planning. This becomes less problematic as the protection interval lengthens and fractional values become more reasonable approximations to higher demand values. The second argument against the normal is that it is defined for negative values and negative demand values do not make sense. If the left-hand tail of the distribution gives a significant probability of negative values, then an alternative is to use a truncated normal distribution, whereby all values below zero would be disregarded, with appropriate adjustments for the calculation of the remaining probabilities (Thomopoulos 2015).

Let us assume that the protection interval is six months for the SKU whose demand distribution (per month) is shown in Figure 5.7. In Figure 5.8, we show the histogram of the demand distribution over the protection interval and the fit of the normal distribution.

The fit of the normal distribution in Figure 5.8 is a little better than in Figure 5.7, although it is still far from perfect. To use the normal distribution in practice, we need a forecast of the mean and variance over the protection interval. If demand is assumed to be stationary (i.e. neither of these quantities is changing over time), then sample means and variances may be calculated, as shown in Chapter 4. If the mean and variance and changing over time, then the methods to be described in Chapter 6 (mean demand) and Chapter 7 (variance of demand) should be used.

If we have obtained forecasts for the mean demand and the variance over the protection interval, then the chance of demand not exceeding any specified value can be found from a built-in function that converts a standard normal variable to the corresponding (cumulative) probability. This built-in function is available in most spreadsheets and programming languages.

The normal distribution places no constraints on the value of the variance in relation to the mean. However, the distribution is not flexible with regard to its shape. It always takes a symmetric shape, which is one of the reasons that it is less suitable for representing intermittent demand.

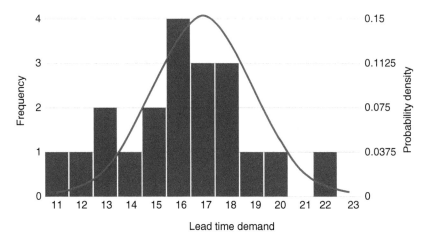

Figure 5.8 Normal distribution (better approximation).

The empirical evidence on the goodness of fit of the normal distribution for intermittent demand over lead time is not encouraging. Eaves (2002) investigated the demand patterns of spare parts for the RAF. He found that the normal was clearly outperformed by the negative binomial, in terms of goodness of fit. Syntetos et al. (2013) agreed with this conclusion, finding that less than 10% of the RAF SKUs had lead time demand with a 'strong fit' to the normal distribution. However, they also found that 42% of the SKUs investigated from the electronics sector did have lead time demand with a 'strong fit' to the normal.

Syntetos and Boylan (2008) analysed 753 SKUs with 12 demand incidences or more over a period of six years. Although the demand was intermittent, it was represented by the normal distribution for lead times of one, five, and nine periods. This research did not analyse goodness of fit, but examined the stock control implications of assuming normally distributed demand. They found that good results were attainable, but did not compare the stock control performance of the normal distribution with any other probability distributions.

5.7.5 Summary

If demand over a unit period of time follows a certain distribution, it is by no means guaranteed that demand over the whole protection interval will follow the same distribution. If the parameters of the distribution (per unit time) do not change over time, and successive demands are independent, then the Poisson, stuttering Poisson, and negative binomial distributions maintain their distributional forms over the protection interval. If the parameters are changing over the protection interval, then this can no longer be guaranteed. The original distributions, which were used for a single unit of time, may still be good approximations over the whole protection interval (with different parameters) but this needs to be checked.

What does this mean from a practical perspective? One of our criteria for a good demand distribution was its flexibility, so that we could cover the whole range of SKUs (and lead times) with a small number of distributions. If we use, say, the negative binomial to represent demand for a particular range of SKUs, then we would prefer not to have to use other distributions depending on the length of the lead time. This indicates that when checking for goodness of fit of a distribution, we should not look just at the fit for demand over unit time, but also at the fit over various typical lengths of the protection interval. In that way, we can select a distribution that performs well over a range of conditions, which will be required in practice. If it is not possible to find such a distribution from the compound Poisson, Bernoulli, or Erlang families, then a normal distribution may be considered instead. The empirical evidence on the goodness of fit of the normal distribution to intermittent demand is not encouraging. More promising results have been obtained when assessing the inventory implications of the application of the normal distribution, although further research is needed to corroborate or challenge these findings.

5.8 Chapter Summary

In summary, we have given most consideration to four specific distributions that may be considered for intermittent demand: (i) Poisson, (ii) stuttering Poisson, (iii) negative binomial, and (iv) normal. For each of these distributions, we have identified the parameters

Table 5.5 Variables to be forecasted for four demand distributions.

Distribution	Parameters	Link to μ, σ^2	To be forecasted
Poisson	λ	$\lambda = \mu$	Mean demand
Stuttering Poisson	λ,ρ	$\lambda = 2\mu^2/(\sigma^2 + \mu)$	Mean demand
		$\rho = 2\mu/(\sigma^2 + \mu)$	Demand variance
Negative binomial	μ,z	$z = \sigma^2/\mu$	Mean demand
			Demand variance
Normal	μ,σ^2	Identical	Mean demand
			Demand variance

that are required to calculate demand probabilities, and have examined their relationship to the mean and variance of demand. These findings are summarised in Table 5.5, which also includes the variables that, if forecasted, will fully specify the demand distribution.

All of the distributions require a forecast of the mean demand. As we shall see in Chapter 6, there are forecasting methods available that will adapt to a mean demand that is evolving over time. For the Poisson, forecasts of the mean demand will suffice. For the other distributions, variance forecasts are also required. This will be the subject of Chapter 7.

Technical Notes

Note 5.1 Form of Stuttering Poisson Distribution

Suppose that demand follows a stuttering Poisson distribution. The probability of observing demand for one unit is found by multiplying the probability of one demand incidence by the probability that the demand size is one, based on the assumption of independence of demand sizes and incidences. The chance of one demand incidence is found from the Poisson distribution (see Chapter 4) and is equal to $\lambda e^{-\lambda}$. The chance of the demand size being one is found from Eq. (5.3) and is equal to ρ. Multiplying these probabilities gives the first of Eqs. (5.6), repeated here as Eq. (5.20).

$$\mathbb{P}(1) = e^{-\lambda}\lambda\rho \tag{5.20}$$

The probability of observing demand for two units (Eqs. (5.6), second equation, repeated here as Eq. (5.21)) is the sum of:

- The probability of one demand incidence ($\lambda e^{-\lambda}$), multiplied by the probability of a demand size of two ($\rho(1 - \rho)$) from the geometric distribution (Eq. (5.3)).
- The probability of two demand incidences ($\lambda^2 e^{-\lambda}/2$) multiplied by the probability of both incidences having a demand size of one (ρ^2).

$$\mathbb{P}(2) = e^{-\lambda}\lambda\rho(1 - \rho) + \frac{e^{-\lambda}\lambda^2\rho^2}{2} \tag{5.21}$$

Table 5.6 'Stars and bars' diagrams.

1 + 3	* |	*	*	*
2 + 2	*	* |	*	*
3 + 1	*	*	* |	*
1 + 1 + 2	* |	* |	*	*
1 + 2 + 1	* |	*	* |	*
2 + 1 + 1	*	* |	* |	*

Calculating the probabilities of higher demand values requires some care. For example, to calculate the probability of demand equalling four units, we need to take into consideration the possibilities of one, two, three, and four demand incidences. We consider the possibility of two and three demand incidences in more detail. For two demand incidences, we should take into account that the demand of four units in total may split into $1 + 3$, $2 + 2$, or $3 + 1$ for the first and second incidences, giving three splits. For three demand incidences, the demand of four units may split into $1 + 1 + 2$, $1 + 2 + 1$, or $2 + 1 + 1$, again giving three splits. These splits may be illustrated using 'stars and bars' diagrams. Let each unit demanded be represented by a star. Then we will place a bar between the stars to represent the splits, as shown in Table 5.6.

If there is just one demand incidence, there is only one case to consider (one demand of four units), and so there are no splits to examine. If there are four demand incidences, then there is only one way that this can occur with a total demand of four, namely $1 + 1 + 1 + 1$. Therefore for a total demand of four units, the number of cases to consider for one, two, three, and four demand incidences are one, three, three, and one, respectively.

To generalise, suppose we have a total demand of x units. Then, we need to take into account $j = 1, 2, \ldots, x$ possible number of demand incidences. To do so, with reference to the 'stars and bars' diagram, we need to find out, for each value of j, the number of ways of arranging $j - 1$ bars in $x - 1$ gaps between the stars. The number of ways the splits can occur is given by $(x - 1)!/(j - 1)!(x - j)!$ (a standard result from combinatorial theory).

The general stuttering Poisson formula takes all of these factors into account. It gives the probability of observing a total demand of x in a unit time period (for any whole number of x greater than or equal to one), as shown by Eq. (5.22), which is a rearrangement of Eq. (5.5).

$$\mathbb{P}(x) = \sum_{j=1}^{x} \frac{(x-1)!}{(j-1)!(x-j)!} \left(e^{-\lambda} \frac{\lambda^j}{j!} \right) \rho^j (1-\rho)^{x-j} \tag{5.22}$$

There are three components of the right-hand side of Eq. (5.22):

1. The first term represents the number of ways in which the demand (x) can split into j incidences $((x-1)!/(j-1)!(x-j)!)$.
2. The middle term $(e^{-\lambda}\lambda^j/j!)$ represents the chance of j demand incidences. This is the standard Poisson formula.
3. The final term $(\rho^j(1-\rho)^{x-j})$ represents the chance, for a total demand of x units and a split into j incidences, of the demand sizes being of the required quantities. For an

individual incidence (which we label as i), the chance that demand size is s_i is given by $p(1 - p)^{s_i - 1}$. The product of these probabilities is $p^j(1 - p)^{x-j}$. The exponent of the second term is found by adding each of the individual terms to give $\sum_{i=1}^{j}(s_i - 1) = x - j$ because the demand sizes at individual incidences (s_i) must sum to the total demand (x).

For any demand (x), the three terms can be multiplied together because (i) the chance of j demand incidences is independent of the way the total demand splits and (ii) the final term is the same no matter how the demand splits, and so can be multiplied by the first term, representing the number of splits.

Finally, the products of the three terms need to be summed for each possible value of j, the number of demand incidences.

Note 5.2 A Priori Models for the Negative Binomial

There are two a priori models for the negative binomial distribution.

Compounding: Suppose that demand incidence is Poisson distributed and demand sizes follow a logarithmic probability mass function, as shown in Eq. (5.23), where log denotes the natural logarithm, to base e.

$$\mathbb{P}(S) = \frac{-1}{\log(1 - p)} \frac{p^S}{S} \qquad (5.23)$$

In this case, demand follows a negative binomial distribution.

Mixing: If the mean demand varies over time, then it will induce greater variance in the demand itself. For example, the mean of a Poisson distribution, λ, may vary over time, following a gamma distribution, $f(\lambda)$, with the probability density function shown in Eq. (5.24) for $\lambda > 0$.

$$f(\lambda) = \frac{\beta^\alpha}{\Gamma(\alpha)} \lambda^{\alpha-1} e^{-\beta\lambda} \qquad (5.24)$$

where $\Gamma(\alpha) = \int_0^\infty \lambda^{\alpha-1} e^{-\lambda} d\lambda$, and is known as the gamma function, α is a shape parameter, and β is an inverse scale parameter. In this case, the demand follows a negative binomial distribution.

Note 5.3 Recursive Form of the Negative Binomial

For a negative binomial distribution, the equivalence of Eq. (5.11) with the Eqs. (5.12) and (5.13) was stated by Prichard and Eagle (1965) and proved by Kwan (1991), whose proof is followed in this technical note.

From Eq. (5.11), the probability of zero demand is given by Eq. (5.25).

$$\mathbb{P}(0) = p^r \qquad (5.25)$$

For a negative binomial distribution, the mean is $\mu = r(1 - p)/p$ and the variance is $\sigma^2 = r(1 - p)/p^2$, yielding the variance to mean ratio in Eq. (5.26).

$$z = \frac{\sigma^2}{\mu} = \frac{1}{p} \qquad (5.26)$$

This yields $z - 1 = (1 - p)/p$ and the result in Eq. (5.27) for $\mu/(z - 1)$.

$$\frac{\mu}{z - 1} = r \tag{5.27}$$

Substituting for p and r in Eq. (5.25) gives Eq. (5.28).

$$\mathbb{P}(0) = \left(\frac{1}{z}\right)^{\mu/(z-1)} \tag{5.28}$$

Equation (5.11) may be re-written recursively, as shown in Eq. (5.29).

$$\mathbb{P}(x) = \frac{(x + r - 1)!}{x!(r - 1)!} p^r (1 - p)^x = \frac{(x + r - 1)}{x}(1 - p)\mathbb{P}(x - 1) \tag{5.29}$$

It is readily established that $r + x - 1 = \mu/(z - 1) + x - 1$ and $1 - p = (z - 1)/z$. By substituting these values into Eq. (5.29), we obtain the recursive relationship shown earlier in the chapter, repeated here as Eq. (5.30).

$$\mathbb{P}(x) = \left(\frac{\frac{\mu}{z-1} + x - 1}{x}\right)\left(\frac{z - 1}{z}\right)\mathbb{P}(x - 1) \tag{5.30}$$

Note 5.4 Kolmogorov–Smirnov Test

To obtain the results in Table 5.3, Syntetos et al. (2013) relied on a different approach to statistical testing of goodness of fit from that used by Kwan (1991), Boylan (1997), and Eaves (2002), who all used chi-square tests. Syntetos et al. (2013) checked the maximum absolute difference between the empirical cumulative demand distribution and each of the theoretical distributions. These differences were then used to determine if the theoretical distributions had a 'strong fit' to the empirical data (using the Kolmogorov–Smirnov test). Expressed more formally, suppose there are n demand observations and they are ordered from the smallest to the largest $(y_1, y_2, \ldots, y_n)$. The Kolmogorov–Smirnov test statistic (D_n) is defined as shown in Eq. (5.31).

$$D_n = \max_{1 \leq i \leq n} \left|F(y_i) - \frac{i}{n}\right| \tag{5.31}$$

where F is the cumulative distribution function according to the particular probability distribution being hypothesised. The test statistic is compared against a critical value, which is a function of the sample size, n, and the specified significance level. If it is found to be larger than the critical value, then the null hypothesis (that the empirical distribution comes from the hypothesised distribution) is rejected. In the results presented in Table 5.3, a significance level of 0.05 has been used to indicate a 'strong fit'. Syntetos et al. (2013) noted that the Kolmogorov–Smirnov test employed in their research is designed for continuous data. When applied to discrete data (as here), the test is conservative: it could result in accepting the null hypothesis of a strong fit at a given critical value when the correct decision would have been to reject the null hypothesis.

Note 5.5 Compound Bernoulli Distribution: Variance to Mean Ratio

Assuming independence of the demand incidence (N) and demand size (S) variables, the expected demand is given by $\mu = \mu_N \mu_S$. In general, the variance of a compound demand variable is given by Eq. (5.32).

$$\sigma^2 = \sigma_N^2 \mu_S^2 + \mu_N \sigma_S^2 \tag{5.32}$$

This is a standard result in probability theory and has also been used to derive the variance of demand over a variable lead time, to be discussed in Chapter 7. It now follows that the variance to mean ratio is given by Eq. (5.33).

$$\frac{\sigma^2}{\mu} = \frac{\sigma_N^2}{\mu_N} \mu_S + \frac{\sigma_S^2}{\mu_S} \tag{5.33}$$

For a Bernoulli process, $\sigma_N^2/\mu_N = 1 - p$. Substituting this expression into Eq. (5.33) gives the variance to mean ratio presented earlier as Eq. (5.16).

Note 5.6 Computation of the Compound Erlang

The chance of observing zero demand over a lead time of L periods ($D_L = 0$) if demand intervals are Erlang-k distributed is given by Eq. (5.34).

$$\mathbb{P}(D_L = 0) = \sum_{i=0}^{k-1} e^{-\lambda L} \frac{(\lambda L)^i}{i!} \tag{5.34}$$

This expression is based on the chance of there being no more than $k - 1$ incidences in the original (uncensored) Poisson process.

Then, for positive values of x, the chance of lead time demand equalling x is given by Eq. (5.35) (Larsen and Thorstenson 2008).

$$\mathbb{P}(D_L = x) = \sum_{m=1}^{x} \mathbb{P}(J^{(m)} = x) \sum_{i=0}^{k-1} e^{-\lambda L} \frac{(\lambda L)^{mk+i}}{(mk + i)!} \tag{5.35}$$

where $J^{(m)} = \sum_{r=1}^{m} J^r$ and $J^1, \ldots, J^m$ represent the demand (customer order) sizes.

In this expression, m represents the number of incidences that could generate a total demand of x units. The minimum number is 1; otherwise there would be no demand. The maximum number is x; otherwise total demand would exceed x. The probability that the total demand (arising from m demand incidences) amounts to x is denoted by $\mathbb{P}(J^{(m)} = x)$. The final term on the right-hand side of Eq. (5.33) represents the chance of there being m demand incidences in the Erlang process. For example, if $k = 2$ and $m = 3$, then these incidences (in the censored process) could arise from six or seven incidences (in the uncensored process).

Note 5.7 Condensed Poisson Distribution

Following the derivation of Chatfield and Goodhardt (1973), if counting of purchases begins at a time independent of the counting of the uncensored process (mean λ), then:

- An even number of events, $2x$, in the uncensored process is certain to give x events in the censored process.
- An odd number of events, $2x + 1$, in the uncensored process is equally likely to give x or $x + 1$ events in the censored process (probability of one half for each possibility).

Therefore, zero events in the censored process could arise from zero events in the uncensored process or (with probability of one half) one event in the uncensored process. Expressing this mathematically gives Eq. (5.36).

$$\mathbb{P}(0) = e^{-\lambda} + \frac{1}{2}\lambda e^{-\lambda} \tag{5.36}$$

A strictly positive number of events, x, in the censored process could arise in three ways: (i) $2x - 1$ events in the uncensored process (with probability one half); (ii) $2x$ events in the uncensored process (with probability one); and (iii) $2x + 1$ events in the uncensored process (with probability one half). Adding the relevant probabilities together gives Eq. (5.37), which holds for $x \geq 1$.

$$\mathbb{P}(x) = \frac{1}{2}\frac{e^{-\lambda}\lambda^{2x-1}}{(2x-1)!} + \frac{e^{-\lambda}\lambda^{2x}}{(2x)!} + \frac{1}{2}\frac{e^{-\lambda}\lambda^{2x+1}}{(2x+1)!} \tag{5.37}$$

By construction, $\lambda/2$ is the mean of the censored demand incidence process. Chatfield and Goodhardt (1973) showed that its variance is $\lambda/4 + (1 - e^{-2\lambda})/8$. This yields the variance to mean ratio given in Eq. (5.19) earlier in the chapter.

6

Forecasting Mean Demand

6.1 Introduction

Identifying a statistical distribution that may adequately represent intermittent demand data, as discussed in the previous chapters, is an important first step for successfully managing inventories. Although it may be reasonable to assume, at least in the short term, that the form of the distribution does not change over time, it would be less reasonable to expect that the mean and variance of the distribution also remain unchanged over time. In practice, these parameters of the demand distribution are not known, and forecasting is concerned with their ongoing estimation. Certain distributions, like the Poisson for example, call for the estimation of one parameter only, namely the mean. For other distributions, such as the negative binomial and the normal, the estimation of the mean demand is not sufficient. Although forecasting the mean demand is often emphasised, estimating the variance is also important for most distributions. In this chapter, we focus on the issue of forecasting mean demand, leaving the forecasting of variance to be covered in Chapter 7.

One crucial issue involved in forecasting of mean demand is the determination of which estimates are relevant to the inventory decisions to be taken. Suppose that the decision is whether to continue stocking the item, or to discontinue re-ordering. In this case, as discussed in Chapter 2, forecasts generally will be made for a whole collection of stock keeping units (SKUs). Whether or not there was demand in the previous period, or number of periods, is not relevant here. Therefore, accuracy of forecasts is required at all points in time.

Now, we turn our attention to the inventory replenishment decision, assuming that reordering has not been discontinued. If the system is one of continuous review, then forecasts made immediately after demand occurrence are the ones that determine stocking requirements. If the system is one of periodic review, then stocking requirements are affected by those forecasts that may initiate an 'issue point'. As explained in Chapter 2, if there are reviews at the end of every period ($R = 1$), then forecasts made at the end of periods containing some demand are those that matter for ordering decisions. For periodic review systems with review every second period or longer ($R \geq 2$), forecasts made at the end of review intervals that have contained some demand are those for which accuracy is required for stock replenishment.

The relevance of this discussion will become evident as the chapter progresses. It is not sufficient for a forecasting method to perform well at all points in time. It is also important that it can perform well when attention is restricted to periods succeeding review intervals in which there has been some demand.

As discussed in Chapter 1, the degree of intermittence of a demand series relates explicitly to the length of the time period (time bucket) over which demand is accumulated and recorded. For example, consider one specific SKU, the demand of which is recorded weekly and demonstrates intermittent behaviour. Would that still be the case if demand were accumulated monthly or quarterly? Perhaps not. Temporal aggregation is the process of aggregating demands from higher-frequency to lower-frequency time buckets – for example, aggregating weekly demands to monthly or quarterly – and using the aggregate time series to generate forecasts.

Another form of aggregation, which emphasises different SKUs rather than different time intervals, is often referred to as cross-sectional aggregation. Instead of aggregating demand over time for a particular SKU, in cross-sectional aggregation, demand is aggregated across SKUs for a specific time period (bucket). It makes sense, for example, to consider the aggregate demand of SKUs that are replenished from the same supplier, to facilitate efficient transportation arrangements. It is also reasonable to consider the aggregate demand of one SKU that is stored across a number of different locations, to facilitate medium term assortment planning. Although demand at the individual SKU (location) level may be intermittent, aggregate demand is less likely to be intermittent. As will be discussed later in this chapter, there are some very desirable features of aggregate demand forecasting and indeed cross-sectional aggregation has been shown, empirically, to be of great value when dealing with fast demand items. Less is known, though, about its value for intermittent demand forecasting.

In the remainder of the chapter, we first examine some assumptions about the structure of demand processes, building on the discussion in Chapters 4 and 5. The links between these processes and different forecasting methods will be reviewed. Two main categories of methods will be considered: (i) methods that do not distinguish between periods with or without demand and (ii) methods that do distinguish between demand and non-demand occurring periods. A critique of these methods of mean demand forecasting will be offered, taking into account their implementation in practice. The value of temporal and cross-sectional aggregation for mean demand forecasting will also be considered. As we noted earlier, estimation of demand variance is an issue left for Chapter 7.

6.2 Demand Assumptions

Before we discuss the performance of various forecasting methods for intermittent demand, we first examine how intermittent demand data is structured. We start with an examination of possible underlying mechanisms that generate the data in the time series. Then we move on to discuss candidate forecasting methods. This will allow us to examine the performance of methods designed for fast-moving demand when applied to intermittent demand. It will also enable us to see how other methods can be developed to reflect the underlying structure of the data.

6.2.1   Elements of Intermittent Demand

In the previous two chapters, we distinguished between two important constituent elements of intermittent demand: (i) the inter-demand intervals, which relate to the probability of demand occurring and (ii) the demand sizes, when demand occurs. The former indicates the degree of intermittence, whereas the latter relates to the behaviour of the positive demands. To recap, memoryless demand intervals may be represented by either the Bernoulli or Poisson process, depending on whether time is treated as discrete or continuous. Demand sizes (when demand occurs) may be represented by such distributions as the logarithmic or the geometric. Compounding the distributions of demand arrivals and demand sizes results in some characterisation of demand per period. For example, the negative binomial distribution arises from Poisson arrivals and logarithmic distributed sizes.

   The previous chapter concluded with an overview of the variables to be forecasted for different demand distributions, including the mean demand. In this chapter, we consider how estimates of the mean inter-demand interval and the mean demand size can inform the forecast of mean demand. As mentioned earlier, it is reasonable to assume that the form of a particular demand distribution will continue to persist into the near future. What is not reasonable to assume is that the parameters of the distribution will remain the same. Thus, the parameters relating to the elements of intermittent demand will need to be forecasted, to give the best prediction of future mean demand.

6.2.2   Demand Models

Every practical forecasting application starts with an examination of the real data available. Assuming no errors in recording the data, and regardless of what that data may look like, this is our raw material. The task then is to introduce a forecasting method, which is a function of past data, that translates them into a forecast, which is 'best' in some way. However, to achieve that, we first need to understand any a priori assumptions being made about the data (for example, that demand occurrences are independent of previous demand occurrences; see Chapter 4). This enables us to conceptualise what is going on beneath the data: what is the possible model that generates the data? One may ask why such knowledge is important, if the only thing needed for practical applications is the method. The answer is really quite simple. Unless we have a model that explains the behaviour of the data and thus of the forecasting method, we are not in a position to improve the performance of the forecasting method or derive insights into why things work the way they do.

   With regard to the demand model then, and as we shall see in Section 6.2.3 of this chapter, one possibility is to assume that the mean demand never changes and any variation in demand is due only to random deviations from the mean. This is known as a demand process with a 'stationary mean'. Another possibility would be to assume that the demand is composed of a mean demand and random fluctuations over time, but with a 'non-stationary mean'. An example is the local level model (Technical Note 6.1), in which the mean is not subject to any systematic movements up or down, but may shift in both directions, over time.

   If we have a stationary mean, the 'best' forecast of the mean demand would be a simple (unweighted) average of all the historical data available. If we have a non-stationary mean, then some other functions will be best (with single exponential smoothing (SES) being the best estimator for the local level model, for example). The issue of what we mean by 'best' is one to which we shall return.

How should we select forecasting methods to be used across a collection of SKUs? There are two approaches to address this very important question:

1. Introduce a classification mechanism that suggests which method should be used when. This is what we do in Chapter 11 when we suggest a way of classifying methods for intermittent demand forecasting.
2. Introduce one method that, although it may not be best under all circumstances, will perform reasonably well in most situations. Such methods are known as 'robust'.

The emphasis of this chapter is on robustness rather than best performance or optimality. The question of what constitutes optimality and how we can utilise optimal methods for forecasting purposes are discussed in detail in Chapter 14.

We start with the modelling assumptions employed by John Croston, and we discuss the implications of these assumptions for intermittent demand forecasting. Croston (1972) assumed a stationary mean demand model, for which the best forecasts are based on averages of all the historical data. However, these forecasts are not robust to any changes in the underlying mean value. Single exponential smoothing (SES) (and simple moving averages, SMA) will be discussed, as alternative methods, because they are known to be more robust estimators. Nevertheless, although SES may perform well for all points in time, we will see that it can suffer from a considerable bias when issue points only are considered. Croston's method was claimed to overcome such bias problems but the method will be shown to suffer from another type of bias. This led to the Syntetos–Boylan Approximation (SBA) which is currently the method in the literature with most empirical evidence in its support.

Before we start with the discussion of the methods outlined above, let us introduce the demand model considered for the purposes of our analysis.

6.2.3 An Intermittent Demand Model

A good start point is the intermittent demand model proposed by Croston (1972). First of all, he assumed that demand is stationary, i.e. the mean demand never changes. This is likely to be true only in the short term. In the longer term, it is possible that the mean may shift to a new level. The method proposed by Croston is robust to such changes but will not be optimal (in the sense of minimising mean square error, MSE; see Chapter 10). The topic of intermittent demand models is still an open research area and will be explored in more depth in Chapter 14.

Croston advocated separating the demand into two components, the inter-demand interval and the size of demand, and forecasting each component separately. He assumed a stationary demand process of the following form:

1. A Bernoulli process of demand occurrence, with constant probability of demand occurrence.
2. Normally distributed demand sizes, with constant mean and variance.

Independence of successive demand intervals follows from the assumption of a Bernoulli process of demand occurrence because the process is memoryless (see Technical Note 4.5). This assumption is often a realistic one and has empirical evidence in its support, as discussed in Chapter 4. A Bernoulli process leads to a geometric distribution of intervals between demand-occurring periods (see Section 4.8.2). As mentioned earlier, the geometric has two quite distinct roles in intermittent demand modelling. It can represent the times between demands if time is treated as 'discrete', as in the Bernoulli model of demand occurrence; it can also represent the sizes of demand, as discussed in Chapter 5.

The second assumption is much less realistic because the normal distribution is rarely appropriate for characterising intermittent demand sizes. However, this assumption was not needed for the forecasting method proposed by Croston, or for the method's modifications to be discussed later in this chapter.

In addition to these two explicit assumptions, Croston made the following implicit assumptions, bringing the total to four:

3. Independence between the demand sizes and the inter-demand intervals (the length of the demand intervals is not related to the magnitude of the demand sizes).
4. Independence of successive demand sizes (a demand size is not related to previous demand sizes).

If Croston's model holds, then demands are independent over time. The i.i.d. assumption is not always valid for intermittent demand, and methods have been developed that do not assume independence of sizes or intervals. Methods based on dependence between demand sizes and intervals are more scarce, although Kourentzes (2013) undertook research on this topic using neural networks, to be reviewed in Chapter 15.

6.2.4 Summary

Demand models are important because they help us to conceptualise the underlying structure of the data and examine in detail the performance of forecasting methods. In this section, a simple model has been outlined, based on assumptions of independence and a mean demand that never changes. These assumptions will be relaxed later.

A distinction has also been made between what is the 'best' forecasting method that can be used under a particular assumed model and a robust forecasting method. A robust method is not necessarily the best under a particular model but performs well under different possible models. Single exponential smoothing (SES) is such a method and it is now discussed in some detail.

6.3 Single Exponential Smoothing (SES)

Single (or simple) exponential smoothing (SES) is very often used in practice to forecast intermittent demand requirements. The method was originally proposed for fast non-trended non-seasonal demands (Brown 1956), but its simplicity has resulted in its wide implementation for slow-moving and intermittent demand items. (In the literature, an SES forecast is sometimes called an exponentially weighted moving average, EWMA.)

6.3.1 SES as an Error-correction Mechanism

The SES forecast produced at the end of period t (estimate of demand in period $t + 1$) is given by Eq. (6.1).

$$\hat{d}_{t+1} = \hat{d}_t + \alpha(d_t - \hat{d}_t) \tag{6.1}$$

SES can be viewed as an error-correction mechanism. The term $d_t - \hat{d}_t$ represents the forecast error, the difference between the current demand and the forecasted demand (forecasted one period ago). This error is 'smoothed' by multiplying by the smoothing constant, alpha (α), which is positive and less than one, and often in the range 0.1–0.3. The method was designed to provide an appropriate response to changes in the demand pattern, and the degree of responsiveness is regulated by the choice of the smoothing constant value.

Suppose, for example, that the forecast produced at the end of the previous time period was for 5 units, and that demand in this current period is for 15 units, resulting in an error (under-forecast) of 10 units. Further suppose that $\alpha = 0.3$. In this case, 0.3 (30%) of the error will be taken into account when producing a forecast for the next time period. So the new forecast will be $5 + (0.3 \times 10) = 8$. (Note that the new forecast is larger than the previous one to reflect the fact that we have previously underestimated the demand. If demand were previously overestimated, with the error being negative, then the new forecast would be smaller than the previous forecast.) However, if $\alpha = 0.1$, then less weight is assigned to the observed error, and thus the method is less responsive to a (potential) change in the demand pattern. The new forecast in that case would be $5 + (0.1 \times 10) = 6$.

So, the higher the α value, the more responsive the system will be to any changes in the underlying mean demand, if such changes are present. Suppose that the mean demand has not changed, and the error arises from demand fluctuating over time. Then a high smoothing constant value will lead to a harmful over-reaction. The lower the smoothing constant value, the less responsive the system will be, as the forecasted mean does not change quickly over time. This is desirable if the mean demand does indeed stay almost the same over time. If the mean demand has changed from the previous period, and the error is the outcome of this change, then a low smoothing constant value will lead to a harmful under-reaction.

In summary, the degree of responsiveness is something that needs to be regulated according to the actual demand pattern. An overstated response to a stable demand pattern (i.e. a high α value when the mean demand varies very little over time) will be as inappropriate as an understated response to a quickly changing demand pattern (i.e. a low α value when the mean demand is changing greatly over time). So, the specification of the smoothing constant values should follow from an examination of the demand patterns. This may take place based on statistical optimisation procedures, discussed later in the chapter, or it may be set on the basis of prior experience on what works well in practice.

6.3.2 SES as a Weighted Average of Previous Observations

The formula for calculating single exponential smoothing forecasts (Eq. (6.1)) can be written in an alternative form (Eq. (6.2)), which is used more commonly in the literature.

$$\hat{d}_{t+1} = \alpha d_t + (1 - \alpha)\hat{d}_t \tag{6.2}$$

This shows that SES may be interpreted as a weighted average of the most recent observation (with weight α) and the previous SES forecast (with weight $1 - \alpha$). Another way of looking at the operation of SES, and understanding its versatile nature, is by considering Eq. (6.2) in more detail. A forecast produced for time $t + 1$ at the end of time t is a function of the demand observed in time t and the forecast produced for time t at the end of time period $t - 1$. But the forecast produced at the end of $t - 1$ was, in exactly the same way, a function of the demand in period $t - 1$ and the forecast produced at the end of $t - 2$, and so on. The forecast for time t, made at the end of period $t - 1$, is given by: $\hat{d}_t = \alpha d_{t-1} + (1 - \alpha)\hat{d}_{t-1}$. Substituting this expression in Eq. (6.2) gives a formula for the SES forecast in terms of the two most recent observations and the forecast made for time $t - 1$ (Eq. (6.3)).

$$\hat{d}_{t+1} = \alpha d_t + (1 - \alpha)(\alpha d_{t-1} + (1 - \alpha)\hat{d}_{t-1}) \tag{6.3}$$

This is a recursive application of Eq. (6.2). Following the exposition by Brown (1959), we have replaced the final term in Eq. (6.2), by an expression for $\hat{d}_t$ which itself comes from Eq. (6.2) lagged by one period. We can now write each term of Eq. (6.3) more explicitly and repeat the recursive method for the final term, which is now $\hat{d}_{t-1}$, as shown in Eqs. (6.4) and (6.5).

$$\hat{d}_{t+1} = \alpha d_t + \alpha(1 - \alpha)d_{t-1} + (1 - \alpha)^2\hat{d}_{t-1} \tag{6.4}$$

$$\hat{d}_{t+1} = \alpha d_t + \alpha(1 - \alpha)d_{t-1} + (1 - \alpha)^2(\alpha d_{t-2} + (1 - \alpha)\hat{d}_{t-2}) \tag{6.5}$$

And we can carry on with this expansion for as many previous terms as we wish, as shown in Eq. (6.6).

$$\hat{d}_{t+1} = \alpha d_t + \alpha(1 - \alpha)d_{t-1} + \alpha(1 - \alpha)^2 d_{t-2} + \alpha(1 - \alpha)^3 d_{t-3} + \cdots \tag{6.6}$$

Equation (6.6) shows the forecast produced for time $t + 1$, at the end of time t, being a function of previous demand observations (in periods $t, t - 1, t - 2, t - 3, \ldots$). In particular, $\hat{d}_{t+1}$ is a weighted average of previous demands with the weights assigned to those demands declining as we go back in time. So, for $\alpha = 0.3$, we assign 0.3 (30%) weight to the most recent demand observation (in time t), $\alpha(1 - \alpha) = 0.3 \times 0.7 = 0.21$ (21%) to the demand in period $t - 1$, $\alpha(1 - \alpha)^2 = 0.147$ (14.7%) to the demand in period $t - 2$, and so on.

Figure 6.1 helps us appreciate the weight given to past observations for different α values. Suppose that we are at the end of the 25th time period (i.e. $t = 25$). Figure 6.1 shows the weights assigned to previous demand observations for α values of 0.3 and 0.1. These figures illustrate an important fact: the weights assigned to previous demand observations decline as we go back in time, and may be approximated by an exponentially declining curve; hence, the name of the method: exponential smoothing.

Higher α values give more weight to very recent observations and give hardly any weight to older observations (e.g. as in Figure 6.1a). Note that the weight assigned to demand observations before Period 11 is (almost) zero. If higher smoothing constant values are employed, then only the more recent observations are useful in estimating current and future mean demand.

Lower α values also result in more recent observations receiving more weight than older observations, but the difference in less marked. Low α values are useful when there is a relatively stable demand pattern and, as such, the more data points we can take into account, the better (e.g. as in Figure 6.1b). For $\alpha = 0.1$, a weight of just under 0.01 is assigned

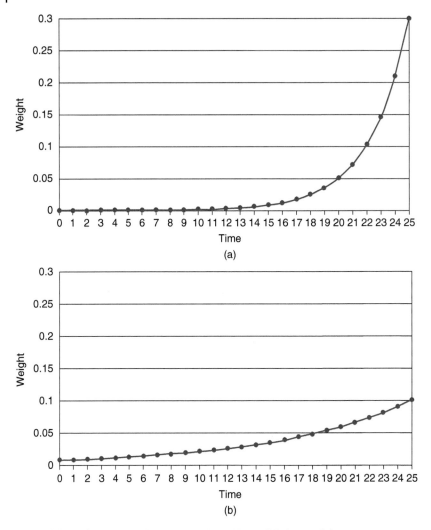

Figure 6.1 Weights of previous observations. (a) $\alpha = 0.3$. (b) $\alpha = 0.1$.

even to the first observation (25 periods ago). If a longer history were available, then older observations (older than 25 periods ago) would be treated as relevant too, by means of being assigned some weights (albeit very small ones) for the calculation of the SES forecast. However, long demand histories are not often available in practice. We return to this issue in Section 6.7.

Finally, let us demonstrate, through an example, how the α value determines the degree of responsiveness of SES to some underlying mean demand change. Suppose that the mean (average) demand for an automotive spare part we hold in stock at a regional warehouse is two units per week. A competitor, who has also been holding stock for that particular spare part, suddenly decides not to stock it any more, unavoidably resulting in an increase of the demand that we face, say to four units per week. In Figure 6.2, we present the response of the SES forecasts to that 'step change' for $\alpha = 0.3$ and for $\alpha = 0.1$. We show in purple the

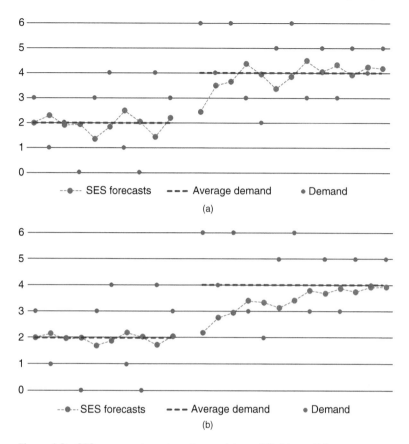

Figure 6.2 SES response to a step-change. (a) $\alpha = 0.3$. (b) $\alpha = 0.1$.

average demand, in blue the demand observations (that first average to two and then to four units), and in red the SES forecasts.

The low weight offered to recent observations for $\alpha = 0.1$ results in a slow response of the method to the step change (Figure 6.2b), and many periods elapse until the forecasts eventually catch up with the change in the underlying mean. When $\alpha = 0.3$, though, SES is more reactive to the underlying change (Figure 6.2a) and the forecasts reflect the new situation more rapidly.

6.3.3 Practical Considerations

At this point, having already discussed the operation of the method, an important practical concern should be addressed. To produce a new SES forecast, the forecast from the previous time period is needed. This leads to the observation that, to start using SES, an initial forecast is required. The forecasting procedure is typically initialised (at time $t = 0$) with the mean (straight average) of the demand data available at the point of introducing the method. So, if for monthly data, 10 months' worth of demand history is available and we wish to employ SES, then the very first forecast can be set to be the straight average of the 10 monthly demand observations available.

For the extreme case of $\alpha = 0$, never used in practice, each new forecast simply equals the one produced in the previous time period, a process that results in the very first (initial) forecast being used without ever being changed. Given that the initial forecast is a straight average, this (theoretically) implies a stationary mean model. At the other extreme, when $\alpha = 1$, we have a naive forecast (i.e. the last actual observation becomes the forecast for the next time period). In this case, the demand pattern is such that only the very last demand observation contains any information that is valuable towards the production of the new forecast. As previously discussed, the α value is often specified on the basis of prior experience. Alternatively, it may be determined based on statistical optimisation procedures. The same applies to the choice of initial forecasts. We return to this issue in Section 6.7.

6.3.4 Summary

Single exponential smoothing is a robust method that has been very successfully employed in the vast majority of real-world inventory forecasting applications since its introduction in the 1950s. The method has not been designed for intermittent demand but nevertheless it can perform well for such items, when all points in time are considered. For issue points only, though, the method is biased high, as we shall see in Section 6.4, and thus it cannot be recommended for general application. This issue is explained in detail presently.

Before we close this section, we should mention that the simple moving average (SMA) is another robust forecasting method that shares many of the benefits of SES, both for intermittent and non-intermittent demand, and is particularly easy to apply. However, details regarding this method's application are presented as a technical note to ensure an uninterrupted discussion of the key developments in intermittent (mean) demand forecasting (Technical Note 6.2).

6.4 Croston's Critique of SES

Croston (1972) examined the application of SES to intermittent demand. He found that if we isolate the forecasts that are made after a demand occurs (i.e. the forecasts produced at the end of demand occurring periods), then they are too high on average ('biased'). Of course, it is to be expected that they will sometimes be too high and sometimes too low, but it would be desirable if the forecasts could be correct on average ('unbiased'). Here, 'bias' is understood in the statistical sense, meaning a systematic tendency to forecast too high, or too low, on average. It may have nothing to do with human biases. In fact, this is the case here: a bias arises from a statistical forecasting technique that may be fully automated in computer software. Forecast biases may also arise from human biases, when demand planners amend statistical forecasts. This is a separate issue, and we postpone discussion of it until Chapter 10.

6.4.1 Bias After Demand Occurring Periods

Croston (1972) showed that SES is biased after a demand occurring period. These are the periods that may generate 'issue points' if stock is reviewed at the end of every period

($R = 1$). He also quantified the expected value of the bias of SES for these periods, assuming stationary demand. The expected value is the long-run average that we would expect from theory and is denoted by the symbol $\mathbb{E}$. The expected value of demand in the next period, denoted by $\mathbb{E}(d_{t+1})$, is, quite naturally, the expected demand size divided by the expected demand interval. It is shown in Eqs. (6.7), together with the expected value of the SES forecast, which is denoted by $\mathbb{E}(\hat{d}_{t+1})$.

$$\mathbb{E}(d_{t+1}) = \frac{\mu_S}{\mu_I}$$

$$\mathbb{E}(\hat{d}_{t+1}) = \frac{\mu_S}{\mu_I}(1 + \alpha(\mu_I - 1)) \tag{6.7}$$

where μ_S is the expected demand size (when demand occurs), and μ_I is the expected length of demand intervals. An alternative, more precise, notation is to write the expectation of the SES forecast in Eq. (6.7) as $\mathbb{E}(\hat{d}_{t+1}|d_t > 0)$, which makes explicit the conditioning on the previous demand being non-zero. (No such conditioning is required for demand itself, as it is assumed to be independent and identically distributed, according to Croston's model.) Updating of forecasts every period is standard for a periodic review system when $R = 1$.

If SES were unbiased, then the expected value of the forecast would be μ_S/μ_I. Equation (6.7) shows that the expected bias, expressed as a percentage of the mean demand is $100\alpha(\mu_I - 1)$. As this quantity is always strictly positive for intermittent demand, we can see that SES forecasts are biased high after demand occurrence.

In Figure 6.3, we may see why the method is biased after demand occurring periods (issue points for $R = 1$, denoted by yellow filled circles). A forecast produced at the end of a demand occurring period for the next time period (issue point forecast) tends to be higher than those succeeding it. Unless demand occurs in the following time period, the forecast decreases and it continues to decrease in every subsequent period with no demand, not increasing again until the next demand occurs. The average demand per period in the example shown in Figure 6.3 is approximately 0.52, and so is the average SES forecast for

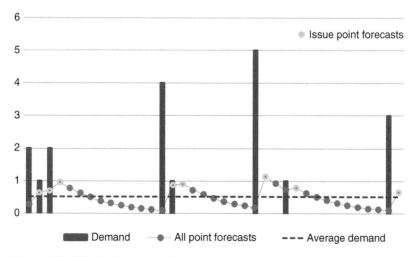

Figure 6.3 SES bias for issue points only ($R = 1$).

all points in time (i.e. the forecasts are unbiased). However, the average of the 'issue points only' SES forecasts is 0.82.

The SES forecast is higher than the true mean demand by about 58%, after an issue point, and this difference can be important in practice. Admittedly, 0.82 does not appear to be much larger than 0.52 – especially if in someone's mind these forecasts need to be rounded up to one. However, the mean demand forecasts are not rounded up (or down) to an integer number because the mean demand may be fractional. In our example, if demand is assumed to be Poisson distributed, and the cycle service level (CSL) target is 90%, then an OUT level of one unit suffices if the mean demand is forecasted to be 0.52, but an OUT level of two units is required if the forecasted mean demand is 0.82.

6.4.2 Magnitude of Bias After Demand Occurring Periods

The magnitude of SES's bias after an issue point, for $R = 1$, depends on the smoothing constant value and the average inter-demand interval. The bias increases as a function of both of these factors. In Table 6.1, the magnitude of the bias is expressed as a percentage of average demand for some typical combinations of smoothing constant (α) values and degrees of intermittence (probability of demand occurrence).

Table 6.1 shows that SES has little bias when demand is only slightly intermittent (e.g. 90% chance of demand occurrences). This makes sense, as the method is unbiased when the demand is not intermittent at all (100% of periods contain demand occurrences). However, the problem of forecast bias becomes more severe as the data becomes more highly intermittent. When the chance of demand occurrence is only 10%, and the smoothing constant value is equal to 0.2, SES can be heavily biased (by 180% of the average demand). This matters, from an inventory perspective, as it can result in over-stocking.

6.4.3 Bias After Review Intervals with Demands

Croston's critique of SES is encapsulated in Eqs. (6.7), which show the bias of SES after a demand occurring period, and is calculated in Table 6.1. For periodic review systems, Table 6.1 is relevant when the review interval is of one period ($R = 1$). In Technical Note 6.3, we show that the bias of SES reduces as the review interval lengthens, and a general bias expression is given, which applies for any (positive whole-number) review interval. This technical note also contains a tabulation of bias percentages for a range of review intervals, for $\alpha = 0.2$. The results show that, for a review interval of 10 periods, the bias is very small, unless the demand is highly intermittent. Of course, increasing the review interval is not

Table 6.1 SES bias (issue points only, $R = 1$) as a percentage of average demand.

α	Probability of demand occurrence				
	10%	30%	50%	70%	90%
0.1	90%	23%	10%	4%	1%
0.2	180%	47%	20%	9%	2%

usually recommended. Although it reduces the bias of SES, it does so at the cost of increased inventories to cover a lengthened protection interval.

6.4.4 Summary

Single exponential smoothing is biased high when we isolate the forecasts made at issue points only. This bias can be quantified and is highest for $R = 1$, and declines for longer review intervals. The existence of the bias implies that another method is needed that avoids this problem. Croston (1972) proposed such a method, which is discussed in detail in Section 6.5.

6.5 Croston's Method

To address the bias problem associated with the application of SES for intermittent demand, Croston proposed an alternative method that builds demand estimates from the constituent elements of demand sizes and inter-demand intervals.

6.5.1 Method Specification

According to Croston's method, separate exponential smoothing estimates are made of (i) the average size of the demand (when demand occurs) and (ii) the average interval between demand occurrences. These estimates are updated after demand occurs, using the same smoothing constant value for sizes and intervals. If no demand occurs, the estimates remain the same.

Let $\widehat{\mu}_{S,t+1}$ be the forecast of the mean demand size for period $t + 1$ (made at the end of period t, during which time some demand has occurred). We also let $\widehat{\mu}_{I,t+1}$ be the corresponding forecast of the mean demand interval. Then Croston's method (Croston 1972), for updating forecasts after demand occurs, is given by Eqs. (6.8).

$$\widehat{\mu}_{S,t+1} = \alpha S_t + (1 - \alpha)\widehat{\mu}_{S,t}$$

$$\widehat{\mu}_{I,t+1} = \alpha I_t + (1 - \alpha)\widehat{\mu}_{I,t} \tag{6.8}$$

$$\widehat{d}_{t+1} = \widehat{\mu}_{t+1} = \frac{\widehat{\mu}_{S,t+1}}{\widehat{\mu}_{I,t+1}}$$

In these equations, S_t denotes the demand size in period t; note that $S_t > 0$, as demand has occurred in period t. Also, I_t denotes the most recent demand interval, the time that elapsed from the previous demand-occurring period to the latest (at time t).

Note that $\widehat{d}_{t+1}$ is the forecast of mean demand not only for the next time period $(t + 1)$ but also for each period over the protection interval $(t + 1, \ldots, t + R + L)$ or, indeed, for any future time period. This is also the case for all other methods discussed in this chapter. As we assume that demand is independent and mean demand is not subject to systematic variation such as trend or seasonality, the forecast of mean demand produced at the end of time t will be the same for any future time period.

6.5.2 Method Application

Croston's method is implemented in many software packages. The following example illustrates the application of the method, updating estimates using Eqs. (6.8). Consider an intermittent demand series consisting of eight observations, as shown in Table 6.2.

This series can be decomposed into two other series: demand sizes (when demand occurs) and inter-demand intervals (Table 6.3). The length of those series will equal the number of demand occurrences (four in this case).

Concerning the inter-demand interval series, please note that (i) we start counting immediately after a demand occurrence and we assume that there was demand in time period zero (immediately preceding our first observation) and (ii) counting includes the demand occurring period (e.g. the last inter-demand interval is recorded as four rather than three).

SES is applied separately to each series to estimate the mean demand size and mean inter-demand interval. In both cases, the forecasts can be updated only when a new demand occurs. Unless a demand occurs, no new demand size or inter-demand interval information is available and thus no new forecasts can be produced.

Suppose, for example, that we wish to start using Croston's method and the demand data presented above is available. In line with previous discussions on the initialisation of SES (see Section 6.3), the initial inter-demand interval forecast, for Period 9, will be taken to be the average of the historical inter-demand intervals (1, 2, 1, and 4), which is equal to two periods ($\hat{\mu}_{I,9} = 2$). Similarly, the initial demand size forecast will be taken to be the average of the previously recorded demand sizes (4, 2, 5, and 1), which is equal to 3 units ($\hat{\mu}_{S,9} = 3$). The initial mean demand forecast will be $\hat{\mu}_9 = 1.5$ units per period, which is the average of all the demand observations available (4, 0, 2, 5, 0, 0, 0, and 1).

In terms of the implementation of Croston's method, let us now assume that the smoothing constant value (used for both the inter-demand intervals and the demand sizes) is set to 0.2 and that the demand realised in Periods 9 and 10 is for 6 and 0 units, respectively, as shown in Table 6.4.

Table 6.2 Intermittent demand series (first eight periods).

Time period	1	2	3	4	5	6	7	8
Demand	4	0	2	5	0	0	0	1

Table 6.3 Series of demand sizes and demand intervals.

Demand sizes	4	2	5	1
Demand intervals	1	2	1	4

Table 6.4 Intermittent demand series (first 10 periods).

Time period	1	2	3	4	5	6	7	8	9	10
Demand	4	0	2	5	0	0	0	1	6	0

In that case, the demand size and inter-demand interval forecasts for Period 10 (produced at the end of Period 9) are given by Eqs. (6.9).

$$\hat{\mu}_{S,10} = 0.2S_9 + 0.8\hat{\mu}_{S,9} = (0.2 \times 6) + (0.8 \times 3) = 3.6$$

$$\hat{\mu}_{I,10} = 0.2I_9 + 0.8\hat{\mu}_{I,9} = (0.2 \times 1) + (0.8 \times 2) = 1.8$$

(6.9)

The actual inter-demand interval (I_9) was recorded as 1 to reflect the consecutive demand occurrences (from Period 8 to Period 9). Croston's forecast of demand in Period 10 (produced at the end of Period 9) would be: $\hat{d}_{10} = \hat{\mu}_{S,10}/\hat{\mu}_{I,10} = 3.6/1.8 = 2$.

At the end of Period 10, when there has been no demand at all, neither the inter-demand interval nor the demand size forecast will be updated, and Croston's forecast (at the end of Period 10) for Period 11 will remain unchanged (i.e. 2). Therefore, $\hat{\mu}_{S,11} = \hat{\mu}_{S,10} = 3.6$, $\hat{\mu}_{I,11} = \hat{\mu}_{I,10} = 1.8$ and $\hat{d}_{11} = \hat{d}_{10} = 2$.

Both the demand size and inter-demand interval forecasts produced with SES are unbiased (under Croston's demand model assumptions). This means that the expected values of the forecasts are equal to the expected values of what is being forecasted. Expressed mathematically, $\mathbb{E}(\hat{\mu}_{S,t+1}) = \mu_S$ and $\mathbb{E}(\hat{\mu}_{I,t+1}) = \mu_I$.

According to Croston (1972), the expected estimate of demand per period in that case would be given by Eq. (6.10).

$$\mathbb{E}(\hat{d}_{t+1}) = \mathbb{E}\left(\frac{\hat{\mu}_{S,t+1}}{\hat{\mu}_{I,t+1}}\right) = \frac{\mathbb{E}(\hat{\mu}_{S,t+1})}{\mathbb{E}(\hat{\mu}_{I,t+1})} = \frac{\mu_S}{\mu_I} = \mu$$

(6.10)

In that case, the method would be unbiased. This result is not correct, as we shall see in Section 6.6.

An advantage of Croston's method is that when demand occurs in every period, the method is identical to SES. Thus, it can be used not only for intermittent demand items but for the rest of the SKUs as well. Croston's estimator is widely used in practice; the method is available in demand planning modules of component based enterprise and manufacturing solutions (e.g. Industrial and Financial Systems) and in integrated real-time sales and operations planning processes (e.g. SAP Advanced Planning and Optimization).

Schultz (1987) proposed a modification to Croston's method, suggesting that a different smoothing constant value should be used in order to update the inter-demand interval and the size of demand, when demand occurs. It has been shown that accuracy improvements are possible by using two parameters instead of one (Kourentzes 2014), although the benefits may be quite modest. However, this modification to Croston's method has not been widely adopted in practice. It is not discussed further in this chapter, except for an important qualification that needs to be made when presenting the SBA method in Section 6.7. We return to this issue in Chapter 12, when discussing a variant of Croston's method that has been developed with the issue of obsolescence in mind.

6.5.3 Summary

Croston's method was proposed to overcome the bias problem of SES. When demand is not intermittent, the method collapses to SES. Croston's method was claimed to be unbiased and was regarded until recently as the state of the art in intermittent demand forecasting.

6.6 Critique of Croston's Method

Syntetos and Boylan (2001) demonstrated the biased nature of Croston's estimator and showed that there is scope for improving the accuracy of its forecast of mean demand. In this section, the source of the bias is explained and quantified.

6.6.1 Bias of Size-interval Approaches

Let us consider a very simple example to demonstrate the bias associated with Croston's method. Let us also use a variant of its operation by not considering SES. In this variant, we will continue to use a size-interval ratio but will use the naive method instead of SES to forecast the mean demand size and the mean demand interval. The naive method takes the last actual observation as the next forecast. It is not recommended for practical applications but it makes the explanation more transparent and reveals the source of the bias problem.

Consider the sequence of demand observations shown in Table 6.5. As discussed in Section 6.5, suppose that we start counting (observing demand) immediately after the first demand occurrence, the size of which is not known and is denoted by X.

In this example, both of the demand sizes are one, giving an average demand size of one unit. The naive forecasts after each demand occurrence would also be one, and so the average forecast is one, matching the average demand size. There is no bias problem here.

The first inter-demand interval is two periods, and the second is four periods. Thus, the average inter-demand interval is three periods, and the probability of demand occurrence is 0.333 (to three decimal places). In our variant of Croston's method, the first forecast of the mean demand interval is two periods, and the second forecast is four periods because the naive method is being used. When these forecasts are used in the denominators of the size-interval ratios, the relevant (reciprocal) values are 1/2 and 1/4. The average of these reciprocal values is $(0.50 + 0.25)/2 = 0.375$, somewhat higher than 0.333. Consequently, by using a size-interval ratio approach, we believe that demand occurs more often than it actually does. We tend to overestimate the probability of demand occurrence and, thus, we tend to overestimate mean demand.

6.6.2 Inversion Bias

In more technical terms, the bias, as illustrated above, stems from the fact that the expected value of the reciprocal of a random variable is not, in general, equal to the reciprocal of its expected value. Returning now to Croston's method, rather than a variant of it, we know that Eq. (6.11) holds, assuming that demand sizes and intervals are independent (as discussed in Section 6.2).

$$\mathbb{E}\left(\frac{\widehat{\mu}_{S,t+1}}{\widehat{\mu}_{I,t+1}}\right) = \mathbb{E}(\widehat{\mu}_{S,t+1})\mathbb{E}\left(\frac{1}{\widehat{\mu}_{I,t+1}}\right) \qquad (6.11)$$

Table 6.5 Intermittent series (after demand occurrence in period zero).

Time period	0	1	2	3	4	5	6
Demand	X	0	1	0	0	0	1

But the inequality labelled as (6.12) expresses an important result for random variables.

$$\mathbb{E}\left(\frac{1}{\hat{\mu}_{I,t+1}}\right) \neq \frac{1}{\mathbb{E}(\hat{\mu}_{I,t+1})} \tag{6.12}$$

The reasons for the inequality (6.12) were illustrated in the previous example. The inequality does not apply when the demand intervals are deterministic and are always equal to a constant value. However, in that case, the mean inter-demand interval does not need to be forecasted. Because the timing of the next demand occurrence is assumed to be known, all that would need to be forecasted is the mean demand size, when demand occurs.

Therefore, Croston's size-interval ratio approach is statistically biased. Using the reciprocal of the smoothed inter-demand interval to estimate the probability of demand occurrence leads to an inflated estimate of that probability. This is often called the 'inversion bias'. The occurrence of this bias will be realised regardless of the estimation procedure being used (e.g. single exponential smoothing or simple moving averages) and regardless of how demands are assumed to arrive (Bernoulli or Poisson). Both issues are discussed in more detail in Section 6.7. In addition, the bias occurs, in the same magnitude, for both all points in time and issue points only.

6.6.3   Quantification of Bias

Under the assumptions considered so far in this chapter, the bias associated with Croston's method can be approximated, for all smoothing constant values, by Eq. (6.13).

$$\text{Bias} \approx \frac{\alpha}{2-\alpha}\mu_S\frac{\mu_I - 1}{\mu_I^2} \tag{6.13}$$

A more detailed explanation of the bias expression is given in Technical Note 6.4. The approximate bias can be conveniently expressed as a proportion of the average demand ($\mu = \mu_S/\mu_I$), as shown in Eq. (6.14).

$$\frac{\text{Bias}}{\mu} \approx \frac{\alpha}{2-\alpha}\left(1 - \frac{1}{\mu_I}\right) \tag{6.14}$$

In Table 6.6, we use Eq. (6.14) to show the approximate percentage bias for a range of realistic combinations of the smoothing constant value (α) and the probability of demand occurrence.

Although the biases shown in Table 6.6 are not as great as for SES, they can still be significant, particularly for sparse data with only a 10% chance of a period showing any demand.

Table 6.6   Croston's bias as a percentage of average demand.

α	Probability of demand occurrence				
	10%	30%	50%	70%	90%
0.1	5%	4%	3%	2%	1%
0.2	10%	8%	6%	3%	1%

In Section 6.7, an adaptation to Croston's method is discussed that deflates the estimator and reduces its bias.

6.6.4 Summary

Croston's method successfully addresses one source of bias ('issue point bias') but, unfortunately, introduces another source of bias ('inversion bias'). This bias grows as data becomes more sparse and as the smoothing constant increases, and can lead to inflated stock levels. It would be desirable to keep the features of Croston's method that avoid the issue point bias but also to address the problem of inversion bias. This was the motivation for the development of the method described in Section 6.7.

6.7 Syntetos–Boylan Approximation

Syntetos and Boylan (2005) proposed an approximately unbiased estimator, shown in Eq. (6.15), which is a forecast of the mean demand for period $t + 1$, and subsequent periods.

$$\widehat{d}_{t+1} = \left(1 - \frac{\alpha}{2}\right) \frac{\widehat{\mu}_{S,t+1}}{\widehat{\mu}_{I,t+1}} \tag{6.15}$$

where the notation is the same as before. If separate smoothing constants are used for sizes and intervals, then α refers to the smoothing constant for demand intervals.

This method provides a good approximation of the mean demand per period, especially for the cases of low α values and large inter-demand intervals. This estimator is known in the literature as the SBA method (after Syntetos-Boylan Approximation) and has a small negative bias, which is $-(\alpha/2)(\mu_S/\mu_I^2)$ (Technical Note 6.5). It replaces an earlier Croston adaptation by Syntetos and Boylan (2001) (Technical Note 6.6). Some other Croston variants have also been discussed in the literature (Teunter and Sani 2009b; Teunter et al. 2011) but SBA is the only adaptation to Croston's method with considerable empirical evidence in its support. The method has been assessed on 18 750 SKUs from the Royal Air Force (RAF) and found to outperform Croston's estimator (Eaves and Kingsman 2004). In addition, evidence in support of this method's utility has been provided by Gutierrez et al. (2008), Van Wingerden et al. (2014), and Nikolopoulos et al. (2016).

6.7.1 Practical Application

In terms of the method's application in practice, an initial SES forecast is required both for the demand sizes and inter-demand intervals, in the same way as Croston's method. As discussed in Section 6.5, both demand size and inter-demand interval forecasts are typically initialised with a straight average of the respective data available at the point of introducing the methods, but can also be optimised. This implies that to apply Croston and SBA, at least two positive demand observations are required; otherwise, an average cannot be computed.

As noted earlier, Schultz (1987) suggested applying Croston's method with different smoothing constant values for the demand sizes and inter-demand intervals (see Section 6.5). For systems that already rely upon such an application and wish to move to the use of SBA, or for companies that are embarking on intermittent demand forecasting and wish to experiment with the implications of Schultz's suggestion, please recall that the smoothing constant value used in Eq. (6.15) is the smoothing constant for the inter-demand intervals.

6.7.2 Framework for Correction Factors

At this point, we need to emphasise again that all the work presented so far is based upon the assumption of a Bernoulli demand arrival process and SES estimates of sizes and intervals. Alternatively, demand may be assumed to arrive according to a Poisson process, as discussed in Chapter 4. It is also possible to adapt Croston's method so that sizes and intervals are updated based on an simple moving average (SMA) procedure instead of SES (see Technical Note 6.2).

Boylan and Syntetos (2003), Shale et al. (2006), and Syntetos et al. (2015b) presented correction factors to overcome the bias associated with Croston's approach under a Poisson demand arrival process and/or estimation of demand sizes and intervals using an SMA. The correction factors are summarized in Table 6.7 (where k is the length of the Simple Moving Average and α is the smoothing constant for SES).

The bias correction factors in Table 6.7 are all approximate, except for the SMA correction factor of Shale et al. (2006) for Poisson demand incidences $((k-1)/k)$, which is exact. As the length of the moving average increases, the Bernoulli and Poisson correction factors for SMA become ever closer to one another.

6.7.3 Initialisation and Optimisation

Now we return to some earlier discussions on the initialisation and optimisation of forecasting methods. These issues are often ignored in intermittent demand forecasting, but they may be crucial in determining a method's performance. Let us first consider the sensitivity of the methods to (poor) initialisation. We do so by examining the application of SES in some more detail.

SES is a weighted average forecasting method, as shown by Eq. (6.6), which may also be written as: $\hat{d}_{t+1} = \sum_{i=0}^{\infty} \alpha(1-\alpha)^i d_{t-i}$. The sum of the weights assigned to previous demand observations should equal one, i.e. $\sum_{i=0}^{\infty} \alpha(1-\alpha)^i = 1$. However, in practice, we always have a finite number of observations, and the finite sum will not equal one, and may not do so even approximately, depending on (i) the smoothing constant value α and (ii) the length of the demand history.

Table 6.7 Bias correction factors.

Estimation method	Incidence process	
	Bernoulli	Poisson
Single exponential smoothing	$1 - \dfrac{\alpha}{2}$	$1 - \dfrac{\alpha}{2}$
Simple moving average	$\dfrac{k}{k+1}$	$\dfrac{k-1}{k}$

For very high α values, weights will be 'exhausted' within not too many historical demand observations. For $\alpha = 0.8$, for example, six demand observations will be (practically) sufficient for producing a new forecast. So, a short demand history is not necessarily an issue. However, the typical range of smoothing constant values employed in practice, especially for intermittent demand series, is between 0.05 and 0.2 (Syntetos and Boylan 2005). Should that be the case, long demand histories would be needed to apply SES. Alternatively, and as sometimes occurs in practice, the forecast updating equation described above is appropriately amended to reflect the fact that a finite number of observations is available for forecasting purposes, as shown in Eq. (6.16).

$$\widehat{d}_{t+1} = \sum_{i=0}^{t-1} \alpha(1 - \alpha)^i d_{t-i} + (1 - \alpha)^t \widehat{d}_0 \qquad (6.16)$$

where $\widehat{d}_0$ is the initial forecast.

As previously discussed, $\widehat{d}_0$ may be set to be the (straight) average of all available information; it may also be set to be equal to the very last demand observation (naive forecast). The latter sometimes reflects a choice, but typically would be a necessity (in the presence of only one demand observation). Alternatively, optimisation of $\widehat{d}_0$ is possible, as discussed later.

The weight of $(1 - \alpha)^t$ given to the initial forecast ensures that the weights add up to 1. However, for a low α value, the initial forecast has a high weight, unless we have a long demand history. This means that the method is not robust to poor initial forecasts, such as those often resulting from the naive approach. Therefore, of course, Croston and SBA are also not robust to poor initialisation.

Once the SES forecast is initialised, the value of the smoothing constant needs to be determined to enable the application of the method. As previously discussed, the α value is sometimes determined judgementally (based on experience). Alternatively, statistical optimisation of the α value may take place by means of minimising some appropriate forecast error metric (see discussion in Chapter 9). The Mean Square Error, in particular, is most commonly used for this purpose because it has some desirable statistical properties (see Chapter 10).

Assuming sufficient data is available, the data history (sample) is divided into two parts: (i) a part (subsample) of the data that is used for forecast initialisation purposes and (ii) another part (subsample) that is used for optimisation purposes. Once an initial SES forecast is available (by means of using the initialisation subsample), then forecasts can be produced over time for any given smoothing constant value (over the optimisation subsample) and the resulting forecast errors can be recorded over time and summarised in some appropriate way. The one-step-ahead MSE, for example, is the straight average of the resulting one-step-ahead squared errors. (Forecast errors are squared and then the straight average of those squared errors is calculated.) The α value that minimises the MSE is known as the optimal α value. It is natural to use this value for future one-step-ahead forecasts; it is often also used for forecasts over longer horizons. This process is visualised in Figure 6.4.

An alternative approach, advocated by Kourentzes (2014), is to optimise parameters by minimising the squared (or absolute) difference between the forecast and the average demand over the optimisation subsample, known as the mean squared rate (MSR). Similar measures, based on differences from the average demand, were introduced by Prestwich et al. (2014a) for forecast evaluation, rather than parameter optimisation. Kourentzes' optimisation approach is based on the idea of using demand rates over time to calculate

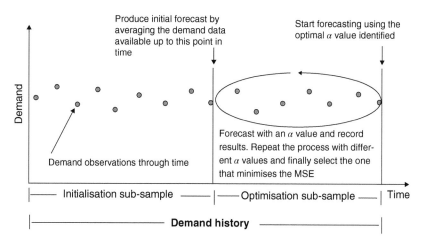

Figure 6.4 Forecast initialisation and optimisation.

the error, rather than realised demand. Empirical experiments, including Croston and SBA methods, found that this approach produced more stable intermittent demand forecasts, with less tendency to identify high smoothing parameters.

The 'search' for the optimal α value may take place in the entire range of $[0, 1]$, or it may be constrained to some other range that is known to work well in practice. That would typically be $[0.1, 0.3]$ for fast demand and $[0.05, 0.2]$ for intermittent demand. Petropoulos et al. (2013) found that optimising the smoothing parameter of SBA (to minimise in-sample MSE) over a range from 0.05 to 0.20 produced a significant reduction in bias.

A parameter search may be conducted in a continuous fashion (i.e. looking at any possible α value) or in steps of some 'reasonable' magnitude (e.g. 0.01). As discussed above, the process described in Figure 6.4 depends on sufficient demand history being available to consider both an initialisation and optimisation subsample. What may be regarded as sufficient varies, of course, depending on the context. For intermittent demand, for example, a long demand history is not necessarily of any value if it contains very few (or no) positive demand observations. Neither an initialisation resulting in a zero forecast nor optimisation in a subsample that contains no positive demand information would be particularly helpful. There is very little published in the academic literature on this subject. In that respect, and as previously noted, managerial knowledge may play an important role in determining the α value when the demand data available is limited, permitting only initialisation to take place. Alternatively, optimisation may take place, cross-sectionally, to allocate the same smoothing constant across a number of SKUs that are known to exhibit, or are expected to exhibit, similar demand behaviour.

For both Croston's method and SBA, statistical optimisation takes place in a similar fashion to that discussed above. Once an initial forecast is available, either the common (for demand sizes and inter-demand intervals) α value that minimises the MSE can be determined or a joint search can be performed for the (different) smoothing constant values that should be used for the demand sizes and inter-demand intervals.

Kourentzes (2014) found that significant gains in accuracy and inventory performance were possible by optimising the initial values of Croston and SBA methods, based on analysis of the same dataset of automotive spare parts investigated by Syntetos and Boylan (2005). So, a joint search for optimal smoothing constants and initial values can be conducted. For further discussion on optimisation related issues for intermittent demand, interested readers are referred to Kourentzes (2014).

6.7.4 Summary

Croston's method has been amended, to account for its bias, under both Bernoulli and Poisson demand arrival processes, and estimation of demand sizes and intervals based on single exponential smoothing and simple moving averages. The resulting methods are as easy to apply as Croston's original method.

An overlooked issue in intermittent demand forecasting is the initialisation and optimisation of smoothing methods. Initial forecasts do matter, especially for shorter demand histories and more heavily intermittent SKUs. They may be set based on an averaging technique or optimised per series. Smoothing constant values may be determined in three ways: (i) fixed values may be considered based on experience; (ii) the values may be optimised per series (specific SKU); and (iii) the values may be optimised across series. Smoothing constants and initial forecasts should be chosen with care, as they have important implications for forecasting.

6.8 Aggregation for Intermittent Demand

So far, we have emphasised single series, single period approaches to mean demand forecasting. We have considered the treatment of one SKU at a time, and the generation of point forecasts by utilising demand information recorded in some predetermined (single) periods of time. We now extend the discussion to some interesting possibilities enabled by the practice of aggregation.

As discussed in Section 6.1 of this chapter, we can distinguish between two types of aggregation for demand forecasting: temporal and cross-sectional. Both forms of aggregation are relevant to demand forecasting in general but are particularly appealing for intermittent series because of the paucity of non-zero observations.

6.8.1 Temporal Aggregation

Forecasting by temporal aggregation is the process of aggregating demands from higher frequency to lower frequency time buckets – for example aggregating weekly data to quarterly – and using the aggregate time series to generate forecasts. Assuming that we are not willing to change the time periods in which demand is recorded (or, alternatively, the relevant IT infrastructure does not offer such opportunities), the aggregate forecasts usually need to be disaggregated back to the original higher frequency time buckets. There is an exception to this rule. We discuss, later in this section, that if the time bucket is set to be equal to the protection interval, then no disaggregation is required.

For intermittent demand, this approach may be very useful because temporally aggregated demand data may resemble the behaviour of fast demand series more closely, and thus be much easier to forecast. (It is, in general, true that fast demand series are easier to forecast than intermittent series.) For example, weekly intermittent demand may not be intermittent when aggregated to quarterly time buckets, thereby enabling the application of methods that have been designed for fast demand data (e.g. SES). The disaggregated forecasts may have greater accuracy than the forecasts produced by methods for slow demand (e.g. Croston) applied directly to the weekly data.

However, and despite its intuitive appeal, the benefits of temporal aggregation are not well understood by managers and relevant applications are not typically supported by forecasting software – in contrast with cross-sectional aggregation, which is supported by inventory and supply chain software packages.

There are two forms of temporal aggregation: non-overlapping and overlapping. The first divides the historical information into consecutive non-overlapping blocks of equal length. In overlapping aggregation, the blocks are also of equal lengths but, at each period, the oldest observation is dropped and the newest is included. In this case, the data are actually moving subtotals of demand history. Non-overlapping aggregation results in a considerable reduction of the number of periods, for example from 21 daily demands to 3 weekly demands. Calendar adjustments may sometimes be required when aggregating daily or weekly data into monthly, in which case the blocks will not have the exact same length (e.g. monthly blocks will consist of 28, 29, 30, or 31 days). Practitioners have expressed concerns over the natural loss of information associated with temporal aggregation. However, this concern is most pertinent for shorter demand histories (and non-overlapping aggregation). Should longer demand series be available, the loss of information resulting from aggregation needs to be considered in contrast with the potentially improved forecast accuracy associated with the transformed (aggregated) series.

Although this area has attracted considerable attention in the forecasting literature in general (see, e.g. Rostami-Tabar et al. 2013, 2014), relevant theory has not been as well developed for the case of intermittence (see Chapter 13 for a discussion on the research which has been conducted). The same is true in terms of empirical studies. The first contribution in the area of intermittent demand is the study by Nikolopoulos et al. (2011). The researchers conducted an empirical evaluation of temporal aggregation for intermittent demand forecasting, by emphasising non-overlapping aggregation and comparisons at the disaggregate level (original time periods). The experimentation framework was called an 'aggregate disaggregate intermittent demand approach' (ADIDA) to forecasting. Disaggregation of the aggregate forecasts into the original time periods was conducted by employing equal weights (e.g. a quarterly forecast is disaggregated into three monthly forecasts by simply dividing by three). Other disaggregation mechanisms may be more appropriate depending on the nature of the original series, but this is not further discussed here. Figure 6.5 shows a graphical illustration of ADIDA, for monthly demand data aggregated to quarters.

The ADIDA approach works in three stages. First, demand data are aggregated into non-overlapping quarterly time buckets. Second, forecasting takes place at the aggregate level. The framework is not constrained to the application or consideration of specific forecast methods. In Figure 6.5, and for simplicity, the naive method is used: the very last actual demand observation is the forecast for the next time period (the next quarter in this case). Third, the aggregate forecast is disaggregated to the original time buckets (based on equal weights in this particular case).

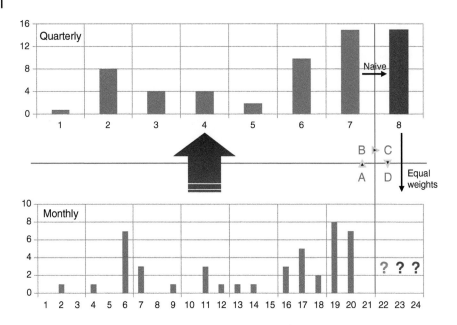

KEY: A: Original data (months) – 24 periods of history; B: Aggregate data (quarters); C: A quarterly forecast is produced; D: The quarterly forecast is broken down to three equal monthly forecasts.

Figure 6.5 ADIDA forecasting framework. Source: Nikolopoulos et al. (2011). © 2011, Taylor & Francis.

An important variation of the framework discussed above, is one where the aggregate time bucket is conveniently set to match the decision-making process that forecasting serves. In the context of inventory forecasting, forecasts are required over the protection interval. If we were to set the aggregate time bucket equal to the lead time plus review interval (for a periodic inventory policy), disaggregation is not needed. In the example discussed above, if the protection interval equals three months, then the forecast produced at the temporally aggregated series is what is needed for inventory purposes, and no forecasts are required for the original series. An obvious constraint to such an approach is that different SKUs are associated with different lead times, and thus the determination of different time buckets is needed across a stock base. However, there is certainly merit in considering such an approach further.

The main outcome of the study by Nikolopoulos et al. (2011) was two fold:

- The ADIDA process may lead to substantial improvements in a single method's application. SBA, for example, applied at the aggregate series level may produce better results than its application at the original time series. Thus, ADIDA may be perceived as a self-improvement mechanism for any forecasting method.
- Setting the aggregation level equal to the protection interval is a very promising approach to inventory forecasting.

Another approach to temporal aggregation was proposed by Kourentzes and Athanasopoulos (2020). Using this approach, a monthly series, for example, is also considered as aggregated bi-monthly, quarterly, half-yearly, and yearly series. These series may be forecasted using methods designed for intermittent data or by exponential smoothing methods designed for non-intermittent data, with the latter including the scope for modelling trend and seasonality. The approach can be used with various intermittence thresholds, which determine whether to use a method designed for intermittent or non-intermittent data. Forecasts are obtained at each level of the temporal hierarchy and are adjusted to ensure that they are reconciled, using a process of 'structural scaling' (Athanasopoulos et al. 2017). This reconciliation process ensures that, for example, weekly forecasts sum correctly to the quarterly forecasts, and the quarterly forecasts sum to the yearly forecasts. In addition to ensuring temporal consistency of forecasts, the process allows features identified at higher levels of aggregation, such as seasonality, to influence forecasts at lower levels of aggregation.

The importance of temporal aggregation for intermittent demand forecasting is reasonably evident at the time of writing. Although there has been some good recent progress, more remains to be done both in terms of theory development and empirical studies in this area.

6.8.2 Cross-sectional Aggregation

Cross-sectional (or 'contemporaneous') aggregation is the practice of aggregating demand for a specific time period across a number of SKUs, and using this aggregate data to produce forecasts. This is an intuitively appealing approach when forecasts are required at some 'group' level, and suitable algorithms have long been incorporated in the standard functionality of supply chain software packages. Consider, for example, a number of items, all of which are replenished from the same supplier. Then, it seems natural to aggregate their demand, and produce forecasts at the aggregate level, in order to facilitate efficient transportation arrangements. Similarly, more efficient warehousing provisions may be achieved as a result of an aggregate forecast that refers to a group of items that collectively occupy a certain part of a warehouse.

An alternative way of generating aggregate forecasts is the following: single period forecasts produced at the individual SKU level are added up (across all relevant SKUs) in order to reach the aggregate (group) forecast of interest. The argument for opting for such an approach is that information available on an individual SKU basis is not being lost due to aggregation, and thus more accurate forecasts can be potentially achieved. This is an important argument. Think of a non-intermittent demand SKU, associated with a very long series and relatively low variability. It will not be difficult to identify the model that reflects the underlying demand structure of that series, and to select a forecast method that is optimal in some sense. If we were to aggregate demand though, this rich individual series related information would be potentially lost, due to aggregation. Thus, it is possibly preferable to first produce forecasts at the individual series level and then aggregate those forecasts, rather than first aggregate demand and then produce a forecast at the aggregate level. (We say 'possibly', because, at the time of writing, there is no consensus in the literature as to which approach should generically perform best. Rather, comparative performance is subject to the characteristics of the individual series, and consequently the characteristics of the resulting aggregate series.)

Consider now a group of, say, three very short intermittent demand series (SKUs), each associated with only one positive demand observation. Assume also that all three SKUs are replenished from the same supplier and have the same lead time, and thus an aggregate forecast is needed to facilitate their collective delivery arrangements. The little information available precludes the application of Croston or SBA at the individual SKU level (let alone having some certainty as to what the underlying demand model may be), since the data is not sufficient to allow for the methods' initialisation in any of the individual series (see Section 6.7). In this case, aggregation of demand across all three SKUs would enable the application of Croston or SBA (assuming that positive demand has not occurred in the exact same period for all SKUs, in which case we would still end up with only one [aggregate] positive demand observation). In this example, aggregate forecasts can be achieved only by means of using aggregate demand data.

Further, and assuming a larger group of intermittent demand SKUs (say 10), demand aggregation may eventually lead to a time series that is not intermittent at all, thereby enabling the application of methods that have been designed for non-intermittent demand items. This could include methods addressing trend in demand such as Holt's method or damped Holt's method. There has been some research on forecasting intermittent demand with trend, without recourse to aggregation. Altay et al. (2008) proposed an adaptation to the modification of Holt's exponential smoothing, introduced by Wright (1986) for data with missing values. They compared their 'Wright modified Holt' (WMH) method with SBA on 4225 aircraft service parts, of which 594 parts indicated a significant trend for non-zero demand. The results show SBA with lower inventories but WMH with higher service levels; there were somewhat mixed results for the total inventory costs. To date, there has been no empirical comparison between WMH and cross-sectional aggregation methods.

It is possible that there may be benefits associated with cross-sectional aggregation for individual SKU forecasting purposes. It is not unreasonable to anticipate that forecasting at the aggregate level followed by a disaggregation of the forecast to individual SKU requirements could perform better than extrapolating demand at the individual series level. The fact of the matter, though, is that this is merely speculation, owing to the unfortunate lack of research and empirical work in this area. The value of cross-sectional aggregation for demand forecasting purposes has been demonstrated in academic studies (Technical Note 6.7), but this work emphasises non-intermittent demand items only. Despite the intuitive appeal of cross-sectional aggregation in an intermittent demand context, very little is actually known about its effectiveness at the time of writing.

6.8.3 Summary

Temporal aggregation relies upon the assumption that forecasting at lower frequency time buckets results in improved forecast performance. This depends not only on the nature of the series but also on the mechanism employed when disaggregating the forecasts. Any accuracy improvement after aggregation may be reduced (or eliminated) by the subsequent loss of accuracy after disaggregation. Interestingly, the problem of disaggregation may, very conveniently, become redundant, if the aggregation level is chosen to reflect the context in which forecasting takes place. For inventory replenishment, setting the aggregation level to be equal to the protection interval means that disaggregation is not needed.

Cross-sectional aggregation is another intuitively appealing approach to forecasting intermittent demand. However, and although it has, in theory, great potential for improving forecasts, at the time of writing there is relatively little known or understood about its benefits when implemented in practice.

The consideration of single or multiple SKUs (and their corresponding demand series) as well as single or multiple time periods, for forecasting purposes, leads to the following progression in terms of possible combinations.

1. *Single SKU (series), single period approaches*: This constitutes the primary focus of this book.
2. *Single SKU (series), multiple period approaches*: Approaches such as ADIDA and temporal hierarchies may be particularly helpful in an intermittent demand context.
3. *Multiple SKUs (series), single period approaches*: There is merit in further considering, both empirically and theoretically, the value of cross-sectional aggregation for intermittent demand forecasting.
4. *Multiple SKUs (series), multiple period approaches*: Combined temporal and cross-sectional approaches are currently the focus of academic forecasting research, though the emphasis, as with cross-sectional aggregation, is on fast rather than intermittent demand items.

In Section 6.9, we review the empirical evidence available in the area of intermittent demand forecasting. We start by reviewing evidence on the application of single SKU, single period approaches, followed by some evidence available on the performance of single SKU, multiple period approaches. To date, there is a lack of empirical evidence on the application of multiple SKU-single period and multiple SKU-multiple period approaches.

6.9 Empirical Studies

Empirical evidence on the performance of forecasting methods for intermittent demand series has grown over recent decades but is still not extensive.

6.9.1 Single Series, Single Period Approaches

Willemain et al. (1994) compared SES and Croston's method on both theoretically generated data and empirical intermittent demand data (54 series). They concluded that Croston's method is robustly superior to exponential smoothing and can provide tangible benefits to stockists dealing with intermittent demand. An important feature of their research, however, was that industrial results showed very modest benefits as compared with the simulation results.

Sani and Kingsman (1997) compared the performance (service level and inventory costs) of various empirical and theoretically proposed stock control policies for low demand items as well as that of various forecasting methods (SMA, SES, Croston) on 30 service parts. Their results indicated (i) the very good overall performance of SMA and (ii) stock control policies that have been developed in conjunction with specific distributional assumptions (e.g. compound Poisson) perform particularly well.

Willemain et al. (2004) assessed the forecast accuracy of SES and Croston's method (both in conjunction with a hypothesised normal distribution) and their non-parametric (bootstrap) approach (see Chapter 13) on 28 000 service inventory items. They concluded that the bootstrap method was the most accurate forecasting method and that Croston's method had no significant advantage over SES. As will be discussed in Chapter 13, some reservations have been expressed regarding the study's methodology (see, also, Syntetos et al. 2015a). Nevertheless, the bootstrapping approach is intuitively appealing for very lumpy demand items. More empirical studies are needed to substantiate its forecast accuracy in comparison with other methods.

Syntetos and Boylan (2005) conducted an empirical investigation to compare the forecast accuracy of SMA, SES, Croston's method, and the SBA. The forecast accuracy of these methods was tested, using a wide range of forecast accuracy metrics, on 3000 service parts from the automotive industry. The results demonstrated quite conclusively the superior forecasting performance of the SBA method.

In a later project, Syntetos and Boylan (2006) assessed the empirical stock control implications of the same estimators on the same 3000 SKUs. The results demonstrated that the increased forecast accuracy achieved by using the SBA method (previously known as the 'approximation method') translated to better stock control performance (service level achieved and stock volume differences). A similar finding was reported in an earlier research project conducted by Eaves and Kingsman (2004). They compared the empirical stock control performance (implied stock holdings given a specified service level) of the above estimators on 18 750 service parts from the RAF (United Kingdom). They concluded that 'the best forecasting method for a spare parts inventory is deemed to be the approximation [SBA] method', (p. 436).

At the time of writing, the SBA constitutes the benchmark against which other (new) proposed methodologies in the area of intermittent demand forecasting are assessed. It has been found repeatedly to account for considerable empirical inventory forecasting improvements (e.g. Gutierrez et al. 2008; Van Wingerden et al. 2014; Nikolopoulos et al. 2016).

6.9.2 Single Series, Multiple Period Approaches

We close this section with some empirical evidence that has been offered in the literature on the value of (non-overlapping) temporal aggregation for intermittent demand forecasting. Nikolopoulos et al. (2011) demonstrated the forecast accuracy gains resulting from the implementation of ADIDA on 5000 SKUs (spare parts) from the RAF (United Kingdom). In a later project, Babai et al. (2012) assessed, on the same data, ADIDA's empirical stock control implications. They showed that forecast accuracy improvements translate to superior stock control performance (as judged by the trade-offs between service levels and inventory investments).

Kourentzes and Athanasopoulos (2020) evaluated a temporal hierarchy approach to the same 5000 series from the RAF. They used the Teunter-Syntetos-Babai (TSB) method (to be discussed in Chapter 12) for data deemed as intermittent and exponential smoothing (using the exponential smoothing state space model (ETS) formulation, Hyndman et al. 2008) for data deemed as non-intermittent. They found small accuracy improvements over the TSB benchmark for mean demand forecasts, based on the root MSE, but more noticeable reductions in forecast bias, using a measure based on the mean error. (These error measures will be discussed in more detail in Chapter 9.)

Temporal aggregation is known to be applied widely in practical military settings (associated with very sparse data), the after-sales industry (service parts) and elsewhere. Less is known, though, about the implications and comparative benefits achieved in some of these settings. More studies are needed to expand the empirical knowledge base in the area of intermittent demand forecasting by temporal aggregation.

6.9.3 Summary

The number of empirical studies in the area of intermittent demand forecasting has increased in recent years, and an empirical knowledge base has started to emerge in this area. However, there is a need to expand this knowledge base, critically appraise the practical implications of employing various methodologies and offer insights into managerial issues that arise from using different forecasting methods. SBA is, at the time of writing this book, the method with most empirical evidence in its support, both in terms of forecast accuracy and inventory implications. Beyond single period/single SKU forecast methods, there is also some evidence to suggest that temporal aggregation can result in forecast accuracy improvements for intermittent demand.

6.10 Chapter Summary

Forecasting of mean demand is a task that is explicitly linked to the inventory decisions that it informs. For stock/non-stock decisions, forecasts at any point in time are relevant, and so forecast accuracy should be evaluated over all points in time.

For replenishment decisions, a distinction needs to be drawn between continuous review and periodic review systems. For continuous review systems, only those forecasts made immediately after demand occurrence may generate an issue point. For periodic review systems, if stock is reviewed every period, then forecasts generated at the end of demand occurring periods are relevant to ordering decisions and, consequently, their accuracy should be assessed. If the review interval is longer, then forecast accuracy should be assessed only at the end of those review intervals in which there has been some demand.

It has been found that single exponential smoothing (SES) is unbiased when considering all points in time. However, it has an issue point bias when evaluated after demand occurring periods only (review interval of one period, $R = 1$) and, to a lesser degree, at the end of longer review intervals which are constrained to contain non-zero demand ($R \geq 2$).

The problem of issue point bias motivated, back in the early 1970s, the development of Croston's method. Croston's forecasting method was claimed to be unbiased (under all inventory review cases), but the method was shown to suffer from another type of bias (inversion bias) leading to the development of the Syntetos-Boylan Approximation, which has been found to perform well in empirical tests, and is straightforward to implement in practice.

In this chapter, some introductory discussion was also offered on the issue of modelling for intermittent demand forecasting and why models are important. A detailed discussion on this issue follows in Chapter 14. Further, the distinction between a theoretically 'best' and a practically robust forecasting method was introduced, and this discussion is also extended in Chapter 14, when optimal (theoretically 'best') forecasting methods are discussed.

Finally, temporal and cross-sectional aggregation approaches to intermittent demand forecasting were considered. The importance and potential value of the former for improving intermittent demand forecasting practices are reasonably evident, at the time of writing. Less is known or understood about the value of the latter. Cross-sectional aggregation is a promising approach for intermittent demand, whose value will become evident as empirical evidence is collected.

Technical Notes

Note 6.1 Stationary Mean and Local Level Models

Under the local level model assumption, the mean demand level is not stationary but rather it varies stochastically through time (Hyndman et al. 2008; Durbin and Koopman 2012). This model is often referred to as the local constant mean model; the mean demand is not constant for the whole demand history but rather only locally, for some part of the demand history. The analytical form of the model is a subject that has been debated in the academic literature, but is not further pursued here. Figure 6.6 illustrates the difference between a stationary mean model and a local level model.

Note 6.2 Simple Moving Averages

The simple moving average (SMA) is a very popular method in industry, owing to its robustness and ease of implementation. The SMA forecast produced at the end of period t (estimate of demand in period $t + 1$) is given in Eq. (6.17).

$$\hat{d}_{t+1} = \frac{1}{k}\sum_{j=0}^{k-1} d_{t-j} \tag{6.17}$$

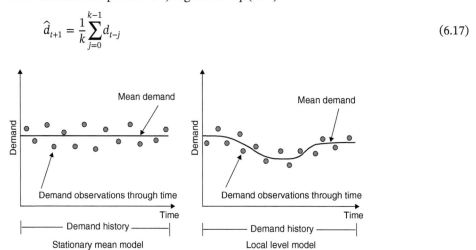

Figure 6.6 Comparison of model forms.

where k is the moving average length. This is a straight (unweighted) average of the last k demand observations. In every new time period, the oldest demand observation is dropped and the newest is included in the moving average to update the forecast.

SMA has its own underlying models, which are rather different to those for SES, whether expressed in autoregressive or state space form (Svetunkov and Petropoulos 2018). Under a stationary mean model assumption, SMA is unbiased, though not the best estimator unless averaging takes place over all the observations available in the demand history.

SMA is appropriate for a locally constant mean (Johnston et al. 1999a). The k value may be decided based on managerial knowledge or statistical optimisation. It has been reported that, for monthly data, it is typically set somewhere between 3 and 12 points, and, for weekly revisions, between 8 and 24 points (Johnston et al. 1999b). The value of k should reflect the underlying demand pattern. A low moving average length should be used when the underlying mean demand is changing rapidly, allowing for a quick response to such a change (just as SES does with a high α). On the contrary, a high value of k is used when the mean demand is changing slowly (similarly to SES with a low α value).

SMA is a popular estimator in practice when dealing with intermittent demand items and it has been shown, through empirical studies, to be a difficult benchmark to beat (Sani and Kingsman 1997; Syntetos 2001; Eaves and Kingsman 2004) both in terms of forecast accuracy and inventory implications of the forecasts. The method is unbiased if we consider all points in time; however, it does suffer from an issue points bias, just like SES, which eventually leads to overstocking.

Rather than applying SMA directly to intermittent demand, it may be applied to the demand intervals and demand sizes (when demand occurs) separately. Then, a ratio of these SMA forecasts may be used as a forecast of mean demand. This ratio suffers from 'inversion bias', which may be corrected using an appropriate bias correction factor (see Table 6.7).

Note 6.3 SES Bias: End of Review Intervals with Demand

The general expression for the expected value of an SES forecast at the end of review intervals (of length R) containing some demand is given by Eq. (6.18).

$$\mathbb{E}(\hat{d}_{t+1}|D_R > 0) = \frac{\mu_S}{\mu_I}\left(\frac{1-(1-\alpha)^R}{1-(1-1/\mu_I)^R} + (1-\alpha)^R\right) \tag{6.18}$$

Table 6.8 Bias of SES ($\alpha = 0.2$) as a percentage of average demand conditional on demand during the review interval.

Review interval	Probability of demand occurrence				
	10%	30%	50%	70%	90%
1	180.0%	46.7%	20.0%	8.6%	2.2%
2	153.5%	34.6%	12.0%	3.6%	0.4%
3	131.3%	25.5%	7.0%	1.4%	0.0%
5	96.9%	13.6%	2.2%	0.2%	0.0%
10	47.8%	2.6%	0.1%	0.0%	0.0%

for $0 < \alpha \leq 1$, $\mu_I \geq 1$ and where $D_R = d_t + \cdots + d_{t-R+1}$ is the total demand in the most recent review interval. This is a new result and holds generally for any (strictly positive) whole-number length of review interval. A special case of Eq. (6.18) was given earlier as Eq. (6.7), established by Croston (1972), which applies when stock is reviewed at the end of every period ($R = 1$).

It also follows from Eq. (6.18) that $\mathbb{E}(\hat{d}_{t+1}|D_R > 0) \to \mu_S/\mu_I$ as $R \to \infty$, for $\mu_I \geq 1$ (i.e. all possible mean inter-demand intervals) and $0 < \alpha \leq 1$. (For $\alpha = 0$, never used in practice, the expected value is equal to μ_S/μ_I only if the initial forecast is set to this value.) Hence, SES is asymptotically unbiased as a function of the length of the review interval.

The expression in (6.18) arises from Eq. (6.19), which is obtained in the same way as Eq. (6.4).

$$\hat{d}_{t+1} = \alpha d_t + \alpha(1-\alpha)d_{t-1} + \cdots + \alpha(1-\alpha)^{R-1}d_{t-R+1} + (1-\alpha)^R\hat{d}_{t-R+1} \tag{6.19}$$

The term $\hat{d}_{t-R+1}$ represents the last forecast to be made before the start of the most recent review interval. Because this forecast is not conditioned on demand occurrence during the previous review interval, it has expected value, $\mathbb{E}(\hat{d}_{t-R+1}) = \mu_S/\mu_I$.

The demands $d_t, \ldots, d_{t-R+1}$ are conditional on at least one of them being positive or, equivalently, conditional on not all of them being zero. This yields the conditional mean value for d_{t-j} for $j = 0, \ldots, R-1$ shown in Eq. (6.20).

$$\mathbb{E}(d_{t-j}) = \frac{\mu_S}{\mu_I}\left(\frac{1}{1-(1-1/\mu_I)^R}\right) \tag{6.20}$$

Substituting the expected values for $\hat{d}_{t-R+1}$ and d_{t-j} for $j = 0, \ldots, R-1$ in Eq. (6.19) gives the expected values for SES forecasts, conditional on demand occurrence during the review interval, as shown in Eq. (6.18).

The bias implications of Eq. (6.18) are illustrated in Table 6.8, for a smoothing constant of $\alpha = 0.2$ and a range of review intervals and probabilities of demand occurrence.

Note 6.4 Approximate Bias of Croston's Method

In this note, we quantify the bias of Croston's method, following Syntetos and Boylan (2005). Let the exponentially smoothed demand size forecast be $x_1 = \hat{\mu}_{S,t+1}$ and suppose this estimator is unbiased, $\mathbb{E}(x_1) = \mu_S$. Let the exponentially smoothed inter-demand interval forecast be $x_2 = \hat{\mu}_{I,t+1}$ and suppose it is also unbiased, $\mathbb{E}(x_2) = \mu_I$.

Applying Taylor's theorem to a function $g(x_1, x_2)$ yields the series given in Eq. (6.21), under certain conditions on the function g, where terms are shown up to second-order.

$$g(x_1, x_2) = g(\mu_S, \mu_I) + \frac{\partial g(\mu_S, \mu_I)}{\partial x_1}(x_1 - \mu_S) + \frac{\partial g(\mu_S, \mu_I)}{\partial x_2}(x_2 - \mu_I)$$

$$+ \frac{1}{2}\frac{\partial^2 g(\mu_S, \mu_I)}{\partial x_1^2}(x_1 - \mu_S)^2 + \frac{\partial^2 g(\mu_S, \mu_I)}{\partial x_1 \partial x_2}(x_1 - \mu_S)(x_2 - \mu_I) \tag{6.21}$$

$$+ \frac{1}{2}\frac{\partial^2 g(\mu_S, \mu_I)}{\partial x_2^2}(x_2 - \mu_I)^2 + \cdots$$

Suppose $g(x_1, x_2) = x_1/x_2$. Taking expectations of both sides of Eq. (6.21), and assuming independence of the smoothed estimates of sizes and intervals (which follows from independence of sizes and intervals), gives the expression in Eq. (6.22).

$$\mathbb{E}\left(\frac{x_1}{x_2}\right) = \frac{\mu_S}{\mu_I} + \frac{\mu_S}{\mu_I^3}\mathrm{Var}(x_2) + \cdots \tag{6.22}$$

This result follows because the expectations of $(x_1 - \mu_S)$, $(x_2 - \mu_I)$, and their product, are all zero, and the second (partial) derivative of x_1/x_2 with respect to x_1 is zero.

In this case, x_2 is an exponentially smoothed forecast of independent inter-demand intervals; therefore, $\mathrm{Var}(x_2) = (\alpha/(2-\alpha))\sigma_I^2$ (with smoothing constant α). Because the intervals are geometrically distributed with variance $\sigma_I^2 = \mu_I(\mu_I - 1)$, Eq. (6.22) can be re-expressed as the approximation in (6.23).

$$\mathbb{E}\left(\frac{\hat{\mu}_{S,t+1}}{\hat{\mu}_{I,t+1}}\right) \approx \frac{\mu_S}{\mu_I} + \frac{\alpha}{2-\alpha}\mu_S\frac{\mu_I - 1}{\mu_I^2} \tag{6.23}$$

This shows that the inversion bias from Croston's method may be approximated by the final term in (6.23), namely $[\alpha\mu_S(\mu_I - 1)]/[(2-\alpha)\mu_I^2]$. Syntetos (2001) showed, by means of experimentation on simulated data, that for $\alpha \le 0.2$, the difference between this approximate bias and the simulated bias lies within a 99% confidence interval of $\pm 0.2\%$ of the mean simulated demand.

Note 6.5 SBA is Approximately Unbiased

The expected value of the Syntetos-Boylan Approximation (SBA) follows directly from the (approximate) Eq. (6.23) in the previous technical note, and is expressed in Eq. (6.24) (which is also an approximation).

$$\mathbb{E}\left(\left(1-\frac{\alpha}{2}\right)\frac{\hat{\mu}_{S,t+1}}{\hat{\mu}_{I,t+1}}\right) \approx \frac{\mu_S}{\mu_I} - \frac{\alpha}{2}\frac{\mu_S}{\mu_I} + \frac{\alpha}{2}\mu_S\frac{\mu_I - 1}{\mu_I^2} = \frac{\mu_S}{\mu_I} - \frac{\alpha}{2}\frac{\mu_S}{\mu_I^2} \tag{6.24}$$

SBA has a (negative) bias term proportional to $1/\mu_I^2$, whereas Croston has a (positive) bias term proportional to $1/\mu_I$. Because $\mu_I > 1$ for intermittent demand, the bias of SBA diminishes more rapidly than Croston as the inter-demand interval lengthens.

Note 6.6 Revised Croston's Method

In an early study, Syntetos and Boylan (2001) proposed a different adaptation to Croston's method, known as the 'Revised Croston's method'. In this adapted method, demand size estimates are updated using exponential smoothing, just as in Croston's method. This estimate is then divided by an exponentially smoothed estimate of the quantity $I_t c^{I_t - 1}$, where c is a tuning parameter, and updates occur immediately after a demand occurrence at time t, with I_t denoting the latest demand interval. As the value of the tuning parameter, c, increases, the bias of this estimator decreases, becoming asymptotically unbiased (as $c \to \infty$). However, this estimator has greater variance than Croston and SBA and, for that reason, is no longer recommended.

Note 6.7 Cross-sectional Aggregation

Beyond the production of aggregate demand forecasts, another, often overlooked, advantage of cross-sectional aggregation is that it offers an opportunity to approximate individual series characteristics that are not visible at the individual series level. The emphasis here is not on producing group forecasts, but rather individual SKU forecasts. It is often the case that, due to high variability and/or the shortness of the time series, certain characteristics that we suspect are present in the individual series (such as seasonality) cannot be easily retrieved from the information available to us.

Assume for example that we know of a group of items that share similar seasonal profiles, but due to the shortness of data or the very high variability of the individual series, these profiles may not be clearly identified at the individual SKU level. (The assumption that the SKUs under concern form a 'homogeneous' group, i.e. one that all its constituent items indeed share the characteristic of interest, is a key one in this process.) Aggregating demand across SKUs may facilitate the identification of such characteristics, knowledge of which can then be used at the individual level. That is, important characteristics may be revealed at the aggregate level and then used at the individual level, whereas it would not be possible to directly identify them if we were to consider one SKU at the time.

Chen and Boylan (2007, 2008) discussed the practice of cross-sectional aggregation for seasonal (non-intermittent) demand forecasting, and showed forecast performance improvements related to such approaches on real data. Boylan et al. (2014) extended this work by focusing on how the groups of SKUs may be decided. It is important to note that all related work in this area has emphasised fast demand items. Although some benefits are expected when cross-sectional aggregation practices are considered for intermittent demand items, such benefits have not yet been demonstrated.

7

Forecasting the Variance of Demand and Forecast Error

7.1 Introduction

In Chapter 4, we saw that if demand is Poisson, then its distribution is completely characterised by its mean. In Chapter 5, we found that the negative binomial and the normal distributions are not fully characterised by the mean alone, but are completely specified by the mean and variance.

We have already seen, in Chapter 6, how the mean value may be forecasted for intermittent demand series. In this chapter, we turn our attention to forecasting the variance of demand and the variance of forecast error. In inventory management, such forecasts are needed not only over a single period of time but over the whole protection interval.

Throughout the chapter, we assume that the demand variance is unknown. We begin our discussion by assuming that the mean demand is known. This is not a realistic assumption, but it allows us to conduct a careful analysis of how the variance of demand per unit time can be translated to the variance of demand over the protection interval. We then proceed to the more realistic case where the mean is forecasted, and there is a need to estimate the variance of forecast error rather than the variance of demand. In Section 7.4, we analyse the case of variable lead times. Finally, we draw together the main conclusions of the chapter.

7.2 Mean Known, Variance Unknown

In this section, we analyse the hypothetical situation where the mean is known but the variance is not and must be forecasted.

Suppose that the mean demand over the forthcoming protection interval is known, although the demand over this period is unknown. If this were true, then there would be no need for a formula to generate a forecast of the mean demand. Instead, we could simply use the known mean value as the forecast. This would be exact as a forecast of the mean demand, but it would be inexact as a forecast of the demand itself because of the variability in demand about the mean value.

Intermittent Demand Forecasting: Context, Methods and Applications, First Edition.
John E. Boylan and Aris A. Syntetos.
© 2021 John Wiley & Sons Ltd. Published 2021 by John Wiley & Sons Ltd.
Companion Website: www.wiley.com/go/boylansyntetos/intermittentdemandforecasting

7.2.1   Mean Demand Unchanging Through Time

The 'sample variance' of a number of demand observations is calculated according to the following method, if the mean is known and not changing through time.

1. The difference between each observation and the (known) mean is found.
2. Each difference is squared.
3. The squared differences are totalled and divided by the number of observations (t).

This is expressed in Eq. (7.1), which shows the forecast of demand variance for time $t + 1$, produced at the end of time t (denoted as $\hat{\sigma}^2_{1,t+1}$, which includes the subscript 1 to emphasise that we are referring to the estimate of the unknown variance of demand per single period).

$$\hat{\sigma}^2_{1,t+1} = \frac{1}{t}\sum_{j=0}^{t-1}(d_{t-j} - \mu)^2 \tag{7.1}$$

In Eq. (7.1), μ is the known mean demand (per period). This result can be used directly in order-up-to level calculations only if the protection interval ($R + L$) is equal to one period. In a periodic review system, if we review the inventory position every period, then $R = 1$, and so the only way that we can have $R + L = 1$ is if the lead time (L) is zero. This means that orders are satisfied instantaneously. Obviously, this is highly unusual. We generally need to calculate the variance of demand when the protection interval includes a non-zero lead time. How this should be done is an important issue and is the focus of the remainder of this section. It will be picked up again later in the chapter when we move to the more realistic scenario of unknown mean demand.

7.2.2   Relating Variance Over One Period to Variance Over the Protection Interval

The variance of demand over the protection interval, σ^2_{R+L}, for independent and identically distributed (i.i.d.) demand, is linked to demand variance over a single period, σ^2_1, by Eq. (7.2).

$$\sigma^2_{R+L} = (R + L)\sigma^2_1 \tag{7.2}$$

This relationship depends on the 'independent' and 'identically distributed' assumptions, defined in Chapter 3 and summarised below.

- *Independent* means that the demand probabilities in one period do not depend on the demands in previous periods. This assumption is often made for intermittent demand.
- *Identically distributed* means that the probabilities are not changing over time. This will be ensured if the form of the demand distribution (e.g. negative binomial) and the distribution's parameters (e.g. mean and variance) do not change over time.

When demand is not i.i.d., then Eq. (7.2) does not hold. Johnston and Harrison (1986) dropped the i.i.d. assumptions and supposed, instead, that demand follows a 'local level model' (Technical Note 6.1). In this situation, in which the mean demand shifts over time, there is a different formula linking the variance of demand over the protection interval to the variance of demand over a unit period of time (see Technical Note 7.1 for further details).

When the i.i.d. assumption does hold, and the mean demand is known, but the variance is unknown, then the forecasted variance of demand over the protection interval, commencing at time $t+1$, is linked to the forecasted variance of demand over the unit time period $(t+1)$, as shown in Eq. (7.3).

$$\hat{\sigma}_{R+L,t+1}^2 = (R+L)\hat{\sigma}_{1,t+1}^2 \tag{7.3}$$

In this case, when the mean demand is known, Eq. (7.3) also yields an estimate of the variance of the forecast error over the protection interval. The variance of demand and variance of forecast error are the same because no forecasting, in the usual sense, is required. The forecast is simply taken to the true mean demand, assumed to be known. As we shall see later, when the mean demand is unknown, and must be forecasted, the variances of demand and forecast error are no longer the same.

7.2.3 Summary

If the mean and variance of demand, per unit time period, are known, and demand is i.i.d., then Eq. (7.2) provides a convenient formula for the variance of demand over the protection interval. This formula is correct only if demands are independent and identically distributed. The formula for i.i.d. demands translates to a similar form (Eq. (7.3)) when the variance is assumed to be unknown but the mean is still supposed to be known. However, this no longer holds when both mean and variance of demand, per unit time period, are unknown. An alternative approach to estimating the variance of forecast error over the protection interval will be introduced in Section 7.3.4 to address this more realistic situation. The approach avoids assumptions of independent and identically distributed demand, or of a local level model.

7.3 Mean Unknown, Variance Unknown

In this section, we turn to the situation where both the mean and variance are unknown. This is what we always encounter in practice. In this situation, the variance of forecast error and the variance of demand are different whereas, if the mean demand is known, then they are the same.

In Section 7.2, we assumed that the mean demand is known and not changing through time. In this case, the k-step-ahead forecast error is given by $e_{t+k} = d_{t+k} - \mu$ where, as before, μ denotes the (known) mean demand for a single period. Because this mean demand is assumed to be known and unchanging, the forecast error and the demand differ only by a known constant value (μ). This fixed quantity introduces no additional variability and, consequently, the variance of forecast error is the same as the variance of demand.

Now we suppose that the mean demand is not known but must be forecasted. In this situation, assuming that the mean demand is unchanging but unknown, the k-step-ahead forecast error is given by $e_{t+k} = d_{t+k} - \hat{\mu}_{t+k|t}$, where $\hat{\mu}_{t+k|t}$ is the k-step-ahead forecasted mean demand (over a single period of time), using all the demand history up to, and including, time t.

In this situation, the variances of forecast errors and demand are not the same because the constant mean demand (μ) has been replaced by the forecasted mean demand ($\hat{\mu}_{t+k|t}$) which changes through time. Even though the true (but unknown) mean demand is unchanging, more information is becoming available after the end of every time period, and the forecasted mean demand is being updated accordingly. Because the mean demand is not assumed to be known, we can no longer rely on using the variance of demand as a proxy for the variance of forecast error. Rather, we must estimate the variance of forecast error directly.

7.3.1 Mean and Variance Unchanging Through Time

Having moved to the more realistic assumption of the mean and variance both being unknown, we now proceed in two stages, assuming these values to be constant over time in this subsection, and then allowing them to vary over time in Section 7.3.2. In almost all organisational settings, variation of the mean and/or the variance is the norm. As before, the less realistic assumption acts as a stepping-stone to the more realistic case.

Suppose that the forecasting method and the mean and variance of demand are not changing through time. Then, a natural estimate of the variance of forecast error, for a horizon of a single period, is given by Eq. (7.4).

$$\hat{s}^2_{1,t+1} = \frac{1}{t-1} \sum_{j=0}^{t-1} (e_{t-j} - \bar{e})^2 \qquad (7.4)$$

Notice the change in notation. We now use $\hat{s}^2_{1,t+1}$ to denote our estimate of (one-step-ahead) forecast error variance, to distinguish it from $\hat{\sigma}^2_{1,t+1}$, our estimate of demand variance for a single period. The term $e_{t-j} = d_{t-j} - \hat{d}_{t-j}$ is the observed forecast error, where the forecast for time $t-j$ (made one period prior to this) is subtracted from the actual demand at time $t-j$. The division by $t-1$ instead of by t (as in Eq. (7.1)) is to ensure an unbiased estimator when the mean is unknown. (If we use a denominator of t, then the estimator has a bias, which decreases towards zero as the length of history (t) increases.)

The term $\bar{e}$ is the sample mean of the observed (one-step-ahead) forecast errors. This average should be close to zero if the forecast method is unbiased. So, if our forecasting method gives approximately unbiased forecasts, as advocated in Chapter 6, then Eq. (7.4) can be simplified by approximating the mean of the errors to be zero, giving the expression in Eq. (7.5).

$$\hat{s}^2_{1,t+1} \approx \frac{1}{t-1} \sum_{j=0}^{t-1} e^2_{t-j} = \frac{1}{t-1} \sum_{j=0}^{t-1} (d_{t-j} - \hat{d}_{t-j})^2 \qquad (7.5)$$

Equation (7.5) is a good approximation to the variance of forecast errors provided that the forecasts remain unbiased. Even if a forecasting method is well chosen, it is unwise to assume that its forecasts will always remain unbiased. For example, the Syntetos–Boylan approximation can become biased if there is a persistent downward trend in demand sizes. For this reason, it is important to monitor forecast errors to ensure that forecasts remain unbiased. Methods for monitoring forecast bias will be discussed in Chapter 9.

7.3.2 Mean or Variance Changing Through Time

We now move to the more realistic situation where there may be changes in the mean or variance of demand over time. In this situation, there may be a tendency for forecast errors to become more volatile over time, or less volatile. Simply averaging over all squared errors, as in Eq. (7.5), would underestimate the future variance if errors are becoming more variable, and overestimate it if errors are becoming less variable. An alternative approach is needed.

This problem has long been recognised by inventory management experts. An early solution, proposed by Brown (1959), was rather indirect. The variance is based on squared errors, but Brown based his method on absolute errors, to gain an estimate of the mean absolute error, also known as the mean absolute deviation (MAD), of one-step-ahead forecast errors, as shown in Eq. (7.6).

$$\widehat{\text{MAD}}_{1,t+1} = \omega|d_t - \hat{d}_t| + (1 - \omega)\widehat{\text{MAD}}_{1,t} \qquad (7.6)$$

where ω is a smoothing constant between zero and one: the higher the value of ω, the more responsive is the updated MAD to large absolute errors. The expression $\widehat{\text{MAD}}_{1,t+1}$ represents the estimate of the one-step-ahead MAD of forecast error, for time $t + 1$, made at the end of period t.

This MAD estimate can be converted to an estimate of the standard deviation of forecast errors by multiplying by 1.25 for normally distributed errors. (The ratio of the standard deviation to the MAD, for a normal distribution, is $\sqrt{\pi/2}$, which is approximately equal to 1.25.) By squaring the estimate of the standard deviation, we obtain an estimate of the variance of forecast errors.

It can be seen that Eq. (7.6) is an application of single exponential smoothing (SES). In Chapter 6, SES was applied to the actual demand values, to give a forecast of mean demand. Here, it is used to give a forecast of the mean absolute deviation of forecast errors.

The main practical advantages of using absolute errors, rather than squared errors, were to simplify the calculations and to avoid the storage of large numbers. These were issues of some importance in the 1950s. Over the 1960s and 1970s, the processing and storage capabilities of computing technology rapidly improved, and Brown (1982) recommended the direct approach of using exponential smoothing on the squared errors instead. This was supported by Bretschneider (1986) who found that smoothing squared errors gives more precise estimates of the forecast variance, even if there are some outlying observations. To adopt the squared error approach, the latest estimate of the mean square error (MSE) of forecasts made one-step-ahead ($\text{MSE}_{1,t+1}$) is used as our estimate of the variance of one-step-ahead forecast errors ($s_{1,t+1}^2$), as shown in Eq. (7.7).

$$\hat{s}_{1,t+1}^2 = \widehat{\text{MSE}}_{1,t+1} = \omega(d_t - \hat{d}_t)^2 + (1 - \omega)\widehat{\text{MSE}}_{1,t} \qquad (7.7)$$

In Eq. (7.7), $\hat{s}_{1,t+1}^2$, the forecast of the (one-step-ahead) error variance, made at the end of time t, is related to the same quantity estimated at the end of the previous period through exponential smoothing, with smoothing parameter ω (between zero and one). The updating of the one-step-ahead variance of forecast error is illustrated in Table 7.1, with results rounded to the second decimal place in the final four columns.

Table 7.1 Updating of mean and variance using SES.

Period	Actual demand	Forecast demand	Forecast error	Squared error	Smoothed variance
1	1	*1.00*	0.00	0.00	*1.00*
2	0	1.00	−1.00	1.00	0.90
3	0	0.80	−0.80	0.64	0.91
4	1	0.64	0.36	0.13	0.88
5	0	0.71	−0.71	0.51	0.81
6	5	0.57	4.43	19.63	0.78
7	0	1.46	−1.46	2.12	2.66
8	0	1.16	−1.16	1.36	2.61
9	1	0.93	0.07	0.00	2.48
10	5	0.95	4.05	16.44	2.24
11	0	1.76	−1.76	3.08	3.66
12	0	1.40	−1.40	1.97	3.60

In Table 7.1, the first two columns contain the data we have available. The third column shows the one-step-ahead forecasts, using single exponential smoothing (SES) with a smoothing constant of 0.2. For example, the last figure in the third column (1.40) is the forecast for Period 12, made at the end of Period 11. SES forecasts are initialised at 1.00 in Period 1, highlighted in italics. In Chapter 6, we saw that other methods may be better than SES but the method has been used in this example for simplicity and to allow the main focus to be on forecast error variance.

The fourth column shows the one-step-ahead forecast error and the fifth column shows its square. Then, the final column is based on the smoothing of squared forecast errors specified in Eq. (7.7). The squared forecast errors are initialised at 1.00 in Period 1, highlighted in italics, and a smoothing constant of 0.1 has been used. Methods for setting initial values and smoothing constants are discussed later in this chapter, in Section 7.3.5.

Now if we look more closely at the forecasts of the one-step-ahead forecast error variance in the final column, we can see that it seems to go through two stages:

1. Values less than 1.0 in Periods 2–6.
2. Values over 2.2 in Periods 7–12, after the observation of a demand of five units in Period 6 (and a further observation of five units in Period 10).

This shows how the smoothing method (Eq. (7.5)) is allowing the smoothed variance to increase in response to the larger forecast errors in Periods 6 and 10, which have arisen because of the unusually high demand values in these periods.

7.3.3 Relating Variance Over One Period to Variance Over the Protection Interval

Now that we have a method of forecasting the variance of one-step-ahead errors, we may ask how to extend our approach to forecasting the variance of forecast errors over the whole protection interval. The discussion in Section 7.2, which related to known mean demands, should make us wary of using the equivalent 'scaling formula' to Eq. (7.3) when the mean demand is unknown and needs to be forecasted: $\hat{s}^2_{R+L} = (R + L)\hat{s}^2_1$ (dropping the time subscripts).

If demand is not independent and identically distributed (i.i.d.), then the problems of using this formula, identified for known means, carry over to unknown means. Moreover, even if demand is i.i.d., the formula is still inappropriate when the mean demand must be forecasted. This was highlighted by Prak et al. (2017) who have offered a detailed explanation of the problem, summarised below.

Let us suppose that demand is independent and identically distributed. Therefore, we are returning to the situation where the mean demand is unknown but not changing over time. Forecasts for the next $R + L$ periods are calculated by single exponential smoothing. SES assumes no trend or seasonality, and so the forecast for two periods ahead is the same as the forecast for one period ahead. Similarly, the remaining forecasts (for all periods in the protection interval) are all equal to the one-step-ahead forecast, and all forecasts are assumed to be unbiased. In these circumstances, Prak et al. (2017) remarked that the variance of forecast error over the protection interval is given by Eq. (7.8), where the variance of forecast errors relates to the forthcoming protection interval (from $t + 1$ to $t + R + L$).

$$s^2_{R+L} = \text{Var}\left(\sum_{j=1}^{R+L} e_{t+j}\right) = (R + L)\sigma^2_1 + (R + L)^2 \text{Var}(\widehat{d}_{t+1}) \tag{7.8}$$

This formula was also given by Strijbosch et al. (2000) and Syntetos et al. (2005). It shows the variance of forecast errors, rather than its estimate, as the formula involves terms on the right-hand side that require estimation. In Eq. (7.8), σ^2_1 represents the variance of demand over a single period. As demand is assumed to be i.i.d., this is multiplied by $R + L$ to give the variance over the protection interval. The term $\text{Var}(\widehat{d}_{t+1})$ is the variance of the one-step-ahead forecast. Note that the forecast variance is not multiplied by $R + L$ but by $(R + L)^2$ (see Technical Note 7.2 for an explanation).

For a protection interval of just one period, we have $s^2_1 = \sigma^2_1 + \text{Var}(\widehat{d}_{t+1})$. Now suppose that this expression were simply multiplied by the length of the protection interval, $R + L$, as often occurs in practice. This would give a 'scaling formula' of: $s^2_{R+L} = (R + L)\sigma^2_1 + (R + L)\text{Var}(\widehat{d}_{t+1})$. There is an important difference between Eq. (7.8) and the scaling formula: the protection interval of $R + L$ is squared in the final term of Eq. (7.8) but not in the scaling formula. Therefore, Eq. (7.8) will yield larger values than the scaling approach, whenever the protection interval is longer than one period. The difference becomes more marked as the protection interval lengthens or the forecasts become more variable. The same issue arises if we operationalise the formula by replacing σ^2_1 and $\text{Var}(\widehat{d}_{t+1})$ by their estimates to give $\hat{s}^2_{R+L}$.

Closer inspection of the scaling formula shows why it is correct if demand is independent and identically distributed and the mean demand is known, but incorrect if the mean demand is unknown. If an unchanging mean is assumed to be known, then the forecast is simply the known value, and so is also unchanging. In this case, $\text{Var}(\widehat{d}_{t+1}) = 0$ and the scaling formula gives exactly the same result as Eq. (7.8), namely $(R + L)\sigma^2_1$. On the other hand, if the mean demand is unknown, then the forecast changes as new data becomes available. Therefore, there is a positive variance of forecasts.

One approach that addresses the problem has been advocated by Silver et al. (2017). Expressing the scaling relationship in terms of standard deviations gives the formula

$\hat{s}_{R+L} = (R+L)^{0.5}\hat{s}_1$. As this relationship is not correct when the mean is unknown, we may consider a different relationship, of the form $\hat{s}_{R+L} = (R+L)^c\hat{s}_1$. In this formula, the parameter c is not known and must be estimated empirically, using regression, based on the data available. There is a lack of published empirical evaluations on the effectiveness of this approach, although Silver et al. (2017) reported satisfactory performance in their experience of inventory systems.

7.3.4 Direct Approach to Estimating Variance of Forecast Error Over the Protection Interval

To estimate forecast error variance over the protection interval, it would be desirable to be responsive to changes in variance, for example by smoothing, but to avoid using the scaling approach because of the reasons explained above.

Syntetos and Boylan (2006) proposed direct estimation of the variance of forecast errors over the protection interval. Using this method, there is no need to estimate a relationship between $\hat{s}_{R+L}$ and $\hat{s}_1$. This is because we use the smoothing formula in Eq. (7.9) to update directly our estimate of forecast error variance, $\hat{s}^2_{R+L,t+1}$, for time $t+1$.

$$\hat{s}^2_{R+L,t+1} = \widehat{\mathrm{MSE}}_{R+L,t+1} = \omega\left(\sum_{j=t-R-L+1}^{t}(d_j - \hat{d}_j)\right)^2 + (1-\omega)\widehat{\mathrm{MSE}}_{R+L,t} \tag{7.9}$$

This is a similar approach to the exponential smoothing equation for one-step-ahead squared errors (Eq. (7.7)). It differs in two important respects:

1. The forecasts $(\hat{d}_j)$ are no longer all one-step-ahead forecasts. Suppose the last observed demand was at $t = 12$ and $R + L = 2$. Then the summation in the first expression on the right-hand side of Eq. (7.9) runs from $t = 11$ to $t = 12$. The forecasts are those made at the end of Period 10. So, $\hat{d}_{11}$ is the one-step-ahead forecast and $\hat{d}_{12}$ is the two-step-ahead forecast. (These are sometimes written as $\hat{d}_{11|10}$ and $\hat{d}_{12|10}$ to stress that the forecasts were made at the end of Period 10.)
2. Correspondingly, the forecast errors are not restricted to one-step-ahead forecast errors. Continuing the previous example, the one-step-ahead forecast error $(d_{11} - \hat{d}_{11|10})$ is added to the two-step-ahead forecast error $(d_{12} - \hat{d}_{12|10})$ to give the total error over the protection interval (of two periods). This is the same as the difference between the total demand $d_{11} + d_{12}$ and the total forecast $(\hat{d}_{11|10} + \hat{d}_{12|10})$ which is the forecast error over the whole protection interval of two periods.

The move away from one-step-ahead forecasts gets around the problems of using relationships between $\hat{s}_{R+L}$ and $\hat{s}_1$ and avoids assumptions of independence of forecast errors over periods during the protection interval. It also addresses problems that may arise if the variance of one-step-ahead forecast errors differs from the variances of forecast errors over longer horizons. This should not occur if demand is i.i.d. but is often observed in practice, when real data deviate from the i.i.d. assumption. We would not be surprised, for example, if 10-step-ahead forecast errors were more variable than one-step-ahead forecast errors. By focussing directly on the forecast error of total demand over the protection interval, we do not need to make an assumption of constant forecast error variance over the forecast horizon.

Table 7.2   Updating of variance over protection interval: scaled and direct.

Period	Demand	Scaled variance	Forecast (R+L=4)	Forecast error	Squared error	Direct variance
1	1					
2	0					
3	0					
4	1	3.53	4.00	−2.00	4.00	3.53
5	0	3.23	4.00	−3.00	9.00	3.58
6	5	3.11	3.20	2.80	7.84	4.12
7	0	10.65	2.56	3.44	11.83	4.49
8	0	10.43	2.85	2.15	4.63	5.23
9	1	9.93	2.28	3.72	13.85	5.17
10	5	8.94	5.82	0.18	0.03	6.04
11	0	14.62	4.66	1.34	1.80	5.44
12	0	14.39	3.73	2.27	5.17	5.07

The 'direct estimation' approach is illustrated in an example, shown in Table 7.2, which compares the 'scaling' formula ($\hat{s}^2_{R+L} = (R+L)\hat{s}^2_1$) with the 'direct' formula (Eq. (7.9)). The protection interval is of four periods.

In Table 7.2, the first two columns contain the same data as in Table 7.1. The third column shows the scaled variance. This is calculated by taking the smoothed variance in the final column of Table 7.1 and multiplying it by four (the length of the protection interval).

The fourth column contains the forecasts over the whole protection interval ($R + L = 4$). The forecast for demand over Periods 1–4 is taken to be the first one-step-ahead forecast (1.00, see Table 7.1) multiplied by four. The next column contains the error of that forecast (for the first forecast of 4.00, the error is $(1 + 0 + 0 + 1) − 4 = −2$). The sixth column contains its square. The direct approach of Eq. (7.9) has been used in the final column, with an initial estimate of 3.53 and smoothing constant of 0.1. (The initial value has been set to be equal to that for the scaled variance, for ease of comparison.) Just as for the scaled approach, the direct approach gives an estimate of variance of forecast errors over the whole protection interval.

The forecasts of the variance of forecast errors may now be compared. In this example, the scaled approach produces higher forecasts than the direct approach in the final column. This is because rolling four-period totals of demand have lower variance than the variance over one period (scaled by four). Other examples can be given where the opposite is true.

Syntetos and Boylan (2008) analysed 753 stock keeping units (SKUs) from the Royal Air Force and showed that the direct approach helped towards reaching service level targets. Using this approach requires setting different forecasting horizons (equal to $R + L$) if protection intervals differ between SKUs. This is in contrast to the traditional approach which requires the same forecasting horizon (of one period) for all SKUs.

7.3.5 Implementing the Direct Approach to Estimating Variance Over the Protection Interval

As with all forms of exponential smoothing, there are two practical issues that must be addressed for successful implementation of the direct approach to estimating variances over the protection interval. These issues are initialisation of estimates and choice of smoothing parameters.

A simple way to initialise the MSE estimate is to use the sum of the first $R + L$ observations, at the end of period $R + L$ as the forecast for the next $R + L$ observations, and to calculate their squared difference.

This method of initialisation can work well with intermittent demand that is non-lumpy. However, it can be sensitive to outlying observations, which may occur with lumpy demand. Such outliers can lead to a simple initialisation of the MSE to be set at an unreasonably high value, and it may take a long time for the smoothing updates to bring the MSE estimate down to more realistic levels, particularly with low smoothing parameters. Another approach to initialisation is to use a 'backcasting method'. In this approach, we reverse the time series and estimate the initial MSE on the reversed time series. This approach is described in fuller detail in Technical Note 7.3.

The implementation of MSE updates, using Eq. (7.9), usually relies on lower smoothing constants, such as $\omega = 0.1$ or $\omega = 0.2$, to avoid an over-reaction to any individual large errors that may arise. The smoothing constant is often fixed without any evaluation of its implications. An alternative approach requires the evaluation of the inventory holdings and service levels that would be achieved with different smoothing constants for the error variance, and selection of the smoothing constant value that leads to the best results. The approach can be extended to an evaluation of both smoothing constants and initial values.

If there is an insufficient length of demand history to implement the direct approach, then alternatives are available. Brown (1959) suggested fitting a 'power law' relationship across a family of SKUs. This would be of the form $\hat{\sigma}^2_{R+L} = \alpha \hat{\mu}^\beta_{R+L}$, where α and β are parameters that are estimated using regression. Once this equation has been established, mean demand estimates for each SKU (which tend to be more reliable than variance estimates for short histories) can be used to obtain demand variance estimates for each SKU. These serve as proxies for estimates of variances of forecast errors. Alternatively, a 'quadratic law' of the form $\hat{\sigma}^2_{R+L} = \alpha \hat{\mu}_{R+L} + \beta \hat{\mu}^2_{R+L}$ may be used (Stevens 1974; Boylan and Johnston 1996). 'Laws' of this type are no more than approximate relationships, but they allow variance estimation for each SKU when it would not otherwise be feasible.

7.3.6 Summary

In this section, we have seen that the variance of one-step-ahead forecast errors may be estimated dynamically by using exponential smoothing on the mean square errors. This approach depends on having unbiased forecasts and, so, forecast bias should be monitored on an ongoing basis.

It has been found that a scaling formula relating variance of forecast errors over the protection interval to a single period is problematic even if demands are independent and identically distributed. An alternative approach has been suggested, which is based on extending exponential smoothing of mean square errors to the whole protection interval.

7.4 Lead Time Variability

In the previous discussions, it has been assumed that the review interval (R) and the lead time (L) are not subject to any variation. In the case of the review interval, this seems reasonable. This interval is under the control of the organisation, which may choose to review the inventory position daily, weekly, monthly, or at some other frequency. There is no inventory benefit in introducing unnecessary variability. In fact, the opposite is true: higher stocks will be needed to maintain service levels if the review interval becomes variable. Waller et al. (2008) showed that the resulting increase in variability in demand over the protection interval may be propagated upstream to suppliers, leading to further inflation in stock requirements. These authors did point to potential transportation cost savings through higher truckload utilisation, which may result from varying the review interval. However, these need to be weighed against the higher inventory costs throughout the supply chain. In practice, the review interval is almost always held fixed.

The assumption of a fixed lead time is not always realistic. Some variations may be known in advance. For example, there may be planned shutdowns of manufacturing plants. In that case, the lead time needs to be adjusted accordingly in the inventory system, to allow for the temporary additional delay, and then reset when the plant reopens. Because this variation is foreseen, there is no additional complexity in modelling. The same models can be used, but with adjusted lead time parameters.

Other variations in lead times are not known in advance. Suppliers may be confident that they will meet the standard fixed lead time target, but fail to do so, for a variety of reasons. This introduces additional variability into the process which cannot be addressed by a temporary adjustment because the variation is not foreseen. So far in this chapter, this additional variability has not been taken into account.

7.4.1 Consequences of Recognising Lead Time Variance

It should be recognised that taking unforeseen lead time variability into account may be more realistic but will result in higher forecast error variance estimates than not doing so. This will mean that order-up-to levels and average inventory holdings will also rise. Managers may feel that it is not acceptable for their own organisation to be obliged to hold higher inventories because of the unreliable delivery performance of their suppliers. Nevertheless, if they do not do this, then service levels will suffer until supplier delivery lead times become more consistent.

If the variance of forecast error over the protection interval is estimated more realistically, taking lead time variability into account, then these estimates can be applied in two different ways.

The estimates can be used to calculate the inventory holdings required to hit service level targets while delivery performance remains at the same level. The estimates of lead time variance may be adjusted as supplier performance improves (or worsens) and lead time variability is reduced (or increased).

The estimates can be used to compare the inventory holdings required to hit service level targets with and without lead time variability. The difference in inventories is the basis for estimating the additional costs incurred by lead time variability, and to inform negotiations with suppliers on penalties for late deliveries. It can also act as a 'wake-up call' and a spur to better supplier performance.

There are three ways in which lead time variability may be taken into account in determining order-up-to levels:

1. Estimating the variance of forecast errors over the protection interval, and using this as an input to an appropriate probability distribution.
2. Using an empirical distribution of lead times, bypassing the need to estimate the variance of lead times.
3. Using a bootstrapping approach, resampling not only from previous observed demands but also from previous lead times.

The first approach is widely advocated, and will be discussed further in this chapter. The second approach will be covered in Section 8.6. The bootstrapping approach will be addressed in Chapter 13.

7.4.2 Variance of Demand Over a Variable Lead Time (Known Mean Demand)

There is a general result in probability theory for the variance of the sum of a variable amount of independent and identically distributed random variables. The significance of this result for demand forecasting was first recognised by Clark (1957) who applied it to the variance of demand over a variable lead time. Assuming that the review interval (R) is fixed, we can allow for the variability of the lead time in Eq. (7.10).

$$\sigma_{R+L}^2 = (R + \mathbb{E}(L))\,\sigma_1^2 + \text{Var}(L)\mu_1^2 \tag{7.10}$$

In Eq. (7.10), the mean and variance of the lead time are represented by $\mathbb{E}(L)$ and $\text{Var}(L)$, respectively. The other notation is unchanged.

Equation (7.10) assumes that both the mean demand per period (μ_1) and the variance of demand per period (σ_1^2) are known. The result also assumes that demand is independent and identically distributed (i.i.d.). Snyder et al. (2004) gave a formula for the variance of demand over a variable lead time for a non-i.i.d. demand process for which single exponential smoothing is the optimal method.

Equation (7.10) shows that the variance of demand over the protection interval diminishes as the variance in lead time ($\text{Var}(L)$) reduces, and reaches $(R + L)\sigma_1^2$ when there is no variability in the lead times, and $\mathbb{E}(L)$ may be replaced by the fixed lead time, L. Conversely, the variance of demand over the protection interval rises as the variance in lead time increases. This can be a problem in organisations with complex supply chains, where there can be considerable variation in lead time. Bagchi et al. (1986) gave an example of an item from the inventory of the US Air Force Logistics Command, where the lead time had a mean of 379 days and a standard deviation of 64 days. This lead time variability increased the standard deviation of demand over lead time from approximately 20 units (no variability in lead time) to approximately 70 units (with variability in lead time), raising required inventory levels significantly.

7.4.3 Variance of Demand Over a Variable Lead Time (Unknown Mean Demand)

Now we may proceed to analyse the situation when the mean demand is unknown and must be forecasted. In this case, the total of the forecast errors over the protection interval may be written as in Eq. (7.11).

$$\sum_{j=1}^{R+L} e_{t+j} = \sum_{j=1}^{R+L} d_{t+j} - (R + \mathbb{E}(L))\hat{d}_{t+1} \tag{7.11}$$

On the right-hand side of Eq. (7.11), the sum of demands and the forecast over the protection interval merit some further explanation. The sum of demands can be calculated only after the lead time has transpired and, therefore, L is known. The forecast, on the other hand, must be made before the lead time has transpired. It assumes that the review interval (R) is fixed and known, but the lead time (L) is variable, and the next lead time is not known in advance. So, our best forecast is to take the one-step-ahead forecast $\hat{d}_{t+1}$ and multiply it by the expected length of the protection interval.

In this case, the variance of the total forecast error over the protection interval is given by Eq. (7.12).

$$\text{Var}\left(\sum_{j=1}^{R+L} e_{t+j}\right) = (R + \mathbb{E}(L))\,\sigma_1^2 + \text{Var}(L)\mu_1^2 + (R + \mathbb{E}(L))^2 \text{Var}(\hat{d}_{t+1}) \tag{7.12}$$

Equation (7.8) is a special case of Eq. (7.12). It holds when there is no variability in lead time (Var(L) = 0, and $\mathbb{E}(L)$ may be replaced by L).

To use Eq. (7.12), which assumes the review interval to be fixed and known, would require estimates of the mean and variance of the lead time. Getting reliable estimates of the quantities $\mathbb{E}(L)$ and Var(L) may be difficult. If there have been relatively few orders made for a particular SKU, then it is hard to estimate the variance of lead time with any degree of accuracy. One way of getting round this problem is to assume that the mean and variance of lead time vary by supplier but not by the SKUs provided by each supplier. This then enables more orders to be analysed, yielding more accurate estimates of $\mathbb{E}(L)$ and Var(L), provided it is safe to assume that these values are the same, or nearly the same, for all the SKUs in a supplier's range. If this can be done, the estimated mean and variance of demand (per unit time period) would need to replace the variables μ_1 and σ_1^2 in Eq. (7.12) to make it operational.

It would be desirable to use a simpler formulation than Eq. (7.12), which is somewhat cumbersome. Unfortunately, the direct estimation approach (Eq. (7.9)) cannot be used here because the protection interval is not fixed.

7.4.4 Distribution of Demand Over a Variable Lead Time

If we have estimated the mean and variance of demand over the variable protection interval, then we must ask what distribution should be used. In Section 5.7, it was pointed out that if demand is Poisson, stuttering Poisson, or negative binomially distributed for a single period of time, then these distributions may also be used for the whole protection interval if the parameters do not change over time. However, this assumed a fixed lead time. When the lead time varies, then it can no longer be guaranteed that the distribution will remain unchanged.

Table 7.3 summarises the distributions of demand over lead time, given various distributions of demand over unit time, if the lead time is gamma distributed.

The gamma distribution was defined in Chapter 5 (Technical Note 5.2). It is a continuous distribution, defined only for non-negative values and is flexible with regard to its shape. It has been recommended as a demand distribution (Burgin 1975; Snyder 1984) and has been implemented in manually operated systems (Burgin and Wild 1967) and stock control software (Johnston 1980; Janssen 2010). In Table 7.3, it is used as a lead time distribution. A number of researchers have based their analyses on gamma distributed lead times. Burgin (1972) discussed the case of (non-intermittent) normally distributed demand and gamma lead times. Dunsmuir and Snyder (1989) established properties of intermittent demand distributions with Bernoulli demand occurrences, general demand size distributions, and gamma distributed lead times. Johansen and Thorstenson (1993) analysed (s, Q) inventory systems, with Poisson demand and gamma lead times. Segerstedt (1994) derived inventory rules for a periodic review system with intermittent demand, based on demand intervals, demand sizes, and lead times all being gamma distributed.

Table 7.3 shows that if demand per unit time period is normal or Poisson, then demand over a variable lead time can be characterised by two-parameter distributions (gamma, negative binomial). However, if demand per unit time period is stuttering Poisson or negative binomial, then more complex three-parameter distributions are required. (For a technical discussion of the issues involved, see Park 2007.) Although these distributions have been suggested in the academic literature, there is a lack of empirical evidence in their support. A further complication arises from the addition of the demand during the review interval to the demand during the lead time. For example, this may involve adding a stuttering Poisson (over the review interval) to a geometric Poisson gamma (over lead time). These

Table 7.3 Distributions of demand over gamma distributed lead times.

Demand distribution per unit time	Demand distribution during lead time	Source
Normal	Gamma approximation	Ord and Bagchi (1983)
Poisson	Negative binomial	Hadley and Whitin (1963)
Stuttering Poisson	Geometric Poisson gamma	Bagchi (1987)[a]
Negative binomial	Logarithmic Poisson gamma	Nahmias and Demmy (1982)

a) Based on Bagchi (1983), presented at the American Institute of Decision Sciences.
Source: Adapted from Bagchi et al. (1986).

considerations make it difficult to recommend the use of more complex distributions in practice. In these situations, it may be better to adopt either the second or third approaches listed in Section 7.4.1.

7.4.5 Summary

It has been proposed that consideration of lead time variability may be helpful in two ways: evaluation of the cost of lead time variability and operational calculation of inventory requirements.

Formulae have been given for the variance of demand and forecast error over a variable lead time. These estimates may be used in the cases when demand per unit time period is normal or Poisson distributed. However, when demand is stuttering Poisson or negative binomial, estimates of mean and variance are insufficient because the resulting distributions are characterised by three parameters. In these cases, alternative approaches, based on empirical distributions of lead time may be more appropriate.

7.5 Chapter Summary

In this chapter, we have seen that there are three distinct but related concepts that are relevant to demand variance in an inventory management context:

- Variance of demand.
- Variance of forecast error.
- Mean square error.

The variance of demand is a property of the demand itself and is not dependent on the choice of forecasting method. It would be relevant for determining inventory requirements when the mean demand is assumed to be known, and so the only variability arises from the demand itself. Although this is not realistic, it enables us to look at the relationship between (i) demand variance over a single period and (ii) demand variance over the whole protection interval. It was found that the standard approach, of multiplying (i) by the length of the protection interval to give (ii), is correct (for known mean demand) only if demand is independent and identically distributed.

It is more realistic to assume that both the mean and the variance of demand are unknown and must be estimated. In this case, it is the variance of forecast errors that is required for inventory management, rather than the variance of demand itself. Of course, the variance of forecast errors depends on the choice of forecasting method. This variance over the whole protection interval is often estimated by multiplying the variance over a single period by the length of the protection interval. However, we saw that this simple rule is problematic when the mean demand is unknown. Even if demand is independent and identically distributed, the variance of forecast errors cannot be found using this rule. Therefore, it is not recommended for practical application.

If our forecasts are unbiased, then the variance of forecast error is the same as the mean square error. This gives us the opportunity to estimate the variance of forecast errors by smoothing the squared errors. This may be done for a single period or for the whole protection interval. For the whole interval, we simply compare the forecasted demand with the actual demand over the protection interval to give the forecast errors. This approach avoids the difficulties inherent in translating variance over a single period to variance over the whole protection interval.

If the lead time is variable, smoothing over the whole protection interval is no longer feasible, as the lead time is not fixed. Variance formulae may be applied. However, the resultant distribution of demand becomes complicated if demand per period is stuttering Poisson or negative binomially distributed. In these cases, alternative approaches may be preferred.

For fixed lead times, we have reliable methods to forecast both the mean demand and the variance of forecast error over the protection interval. These will be essential inputs to the inventory formulae discussed in Chapter 8.

Technical Notes

Note 7.1 Variance of Demand Over the Protection Interval

Suppose demand at time t, denoted by d_t, is not independent and identically distributed but follows a 'local level model' of the multiple source of error (MSOE) form, as shown in Eqs. (7.13).

$$d_t = \mu_t + \epsilon_t$$
$$\mu_t = \mu_{t-1} + \eta_t$$

(7.13)

In this model, μ_t denotes the underlying mean demand at time t. The noise terms, ϵ_t and η_t, are assumed to (i) have zero means and constant variances ($\text{Var}(\epsilon_t) = V$, $\text{Var}(\eta_t) = W$); (ii) be independent and identically distributed; and (iii) be independent of one another.

Johnston and Harrison (1986) gave the correct formula for the variance of demand over a fixed period of time, if demand follows a MSOE model. This is shown in Eq. (7.14), where the fixed period of time is taken to be the protection interval.

$$\sigma^2_{R+L} = (R+L) \left(1 + \frac{\alpha(R+L-1)(1 + \alpha(2R + 2L - 1))}{6} \right) \sigma^2_1$$

(7.14)

In Eq. (7.14), $R + L$ is the protection interval and $\alpha = r(\sqrt{1 + 4/r} - 1)/2$, where $r = W/V$. This α value is the optimal smoothing constant for single exponential smoothing (SES). When operated with this smoothing constant, SES is the minimum mean square error forecasting method for the MSOE form of the local level model shown in Eqs. (7.13). Under a single source of error form of the local level model (for which SES is still the optimal forecasting method), the same formula applies (see Snyder et al. 1999, for further details). Johnston and Harrison (1986) extended their findings to a linear growth model, for which Holt's exponential smoothing method is optimal. Later, Snyder et al. (2004) extended their earlier work to include models for which other forms of exponential smoothing (e.g. trend corrected, additive seasonal) are the optimal methods.

Note 7.2 Variance of Forecast Errors Over the Protection Interval

In this note, we suppose that demand, d_t, is independent and identically distributed and the forecast, $\hat{d}_{t+1}$, of demand at time $t + 1$, is updated using single exponential smoothing

(SES). Then, the forecast error over the protection interval (from $t + 1$ to $t + R + L$) can be decomposed as shown in Eq. (7.15).

$$\sum_{j=1}^{R+L} e_{t+j} = \sum_{j=1}^{R+L} ((d_{t+j} - \mu) + (\mu - \widehat{d}_{t+j})) \tag{7.15}$$

For SES, or any method that produces a constant forecast for each period over the protection interval, $\widehat{d}_{t+1} = \widehat{d}_{t+2} = \cdots = \widehat{d}_{t+R+L}$. Then, Eq. (7.15) can be written as Eq. (7.16).

$$\sum_{j=1}^{R+L} e_{t+j} = \sum_{j=1}^{R+L} (d_{t+j} - \mu) + (R + L)(\mu - \widehat{d}_{t+1}) \tag{7.16}$$

To calculate the variance of the forecast error over the protection interval, we now need to recognise that (i) the variance of the first term on the right-hand side of Eq. (7.16) is $(R + L)\mathrm{Var}(d_t) = (R + L)\sigma_1^2$; (ii) the variance of the second term is $(R + L)^2 \mathrm{Var}(\widehat{d}_{t+1})$, assuming unbiased forecasts; and (iii) the covariance between the two terms is zero because of the assumption that the demand process is independent and the forecast, $\widehat{d}_{t+1}$ is a function of demand values only up to and including time t. Taking all these three points into account yields Eq. (7.8).

Note 7.3 Backcasting for Initial MSE Estimation

In the backcasting approach, the time series is reversed so, for example, a sequence $(y_1, y_2, \ldots, y_{23}, y_{24})$ becomes $(y_{24}, y_{23}, \ldots, y_2, y_1)$ with the last element of the reversed time series being the oldest observation. A forecasting method is applied to this reversed series to give a 'forecast' (in reality, a 'backcast') for the protection interval immediately preceding the first period.

The mean square error (MSE) estimate for the reversed time series is initialised using a simple approach, such as using the first squared error over the protection interval. This estimate can then be continually updated, on the reversed series, using Eq. (7.9), finally giving an estimate of the MSE for the protection interval immediately preceding the first period. This is then used as the initial estimate of the MSE for forecasting the original (non-reversed) timeseries.

8

Inventory Settings

8.1 Introduction

In Chapter 2, we reviewed a number of inventory rules that may be used to manage the stock of intermittent demand items. We paid particular attention to the periodic review (R, s, S) and (R, S) policies. In both policies, the inventory position is reviewed every R periods, and enough stock is ordered to raise it to the order-up-to (OUT) level (S) (also known as the OUT level). The difference between the two policies lies in the condition for triggering an order. In the (R, s, S) system, the condition is that the inventory position falls at or below the order point, s, whereas in the (R, S) system, the condition is that the inventory position falls below the OUT level, S. We noted that an (R, S) system is often used in practice, for intermittent demand items, based on its simplicity and robustness.

The (R, S) system requires the determination of the review interval (R) and OUT level (S) for each individual stock keeping unit (SKU). In practice, though, the review interval is usually set to be the same for all SKUs or for whole classes of SKUs, for reasons discussed in Chapter 2. The setting of the review interval varies according to industry sector. In grocery retail, this may be daily or twice daily, whereas automotive spare parts may be reviewed weekly or monthly.

The OUT level (S) needs to be determined separately for each individual SKU, to take into account its demand uncertainty. The setting of the OUT level depends on both the form of the demand distribution and on its parameters. In this chapter, we start by analysing normally distributed demand. Although this distribution has limitations for intermittent demand modelling, it gives the clearest illustration of some issues that affect all of the distributions discussed in this chapter. Then we move on to intermittent demand that is characterised by the Poisson distribution. This raises some new issues, which also affect compound Poisson distributions, discussed in the following sections. Up to this point in the chapter, lead times are assumed to be constant. The case of variable lead times is then analysed, and a pragmatic solution is recommended.

Intermittent Demand Forecasting: Context, Methods and Applications, First Edition.
John E. Boylan and Aris A. Syntetos.
© 2021 John Wiley & Sons Ltd. Published 2021 by John Wiley & Sons Ltd.
Companion Website: www.wiley.com/go/boylansyntetos/intermittentdemandforecasting

8.2 Normal Demand

Meeting service level targets depends on recognising the nature and level of demand uncertainty over the protection interval. This was discussed in detail in Chapters 4 and 5, where we focused on three types of distributions to represent demand variability, namely the normal, Poisson, and compound Poisson distributions (stuttering Poisson and negative binomial).

In this section, we concentrate on 'normal demand'. This is demand that may be characterised by the normal distribution. In Chapter 5, it was acknowledged that the normal distribution is often a poor fit to the pattern of slow-moving demand per period and so, ironically, is not 'normal' for them in the usual sense of the word. However, the normal distribution may be a better approximation to the pattern of demand over the whole protection interval if this is of long duration and if demand, per unit time period, is not highly intermittent.

8.2.1 Order-up-to Levels for Four Scenarios

The normal distribution is characterised by its mean and its standard deviation. To fully appreciate how these two parameters relate to the determination of OUT levels, we take a sequential approach, looking at the following four scenarios:

1. Mean demand known, standard deviation known.
2. Mean demand unknown, standard deviation known.
3. Mean demand known, standard deviation unknown.
4. Mean demand unknown, standard deviation unknown.

The first three scenarios are not directly relevant to real-life situations because the mean and standard deviation of demand are always unknown and must be forecasted. Nevertheless, these unrealistic scenarios will help to clarify some important concepts, and will serve as useful building blocks in calculating OUT levels for the final realistic scenario.

8.2.2 Scenario 1: Mean and Standard Deviation Known

In Scenario 1, the OUT level of an (R, S) system depends on the mean and standard deviation of demand over the protection interval $(R + L)$. These quantities are denoted by μ_{R+L} and σ_{R+L}.

If μ_{R+L} and σ_{R+L} are both known, and we are working to a cycle service level (CSL) target of 95%, then the standard OUT level (S) calculation is given by Eq. (8.1).

$$S = \mu_{R+L} + 1.645\sigma_{R+L} \tag{8.1}$$

The value of 1.645 in Eq. (8.1) is an example of a safety factor. Although the future mean and standard deviation are assumed to be known, we are not supposing that we know the future demand itself. This uncertainty in future demand is represented in Figure 8.1, which shows 95% of the area under the curve (in lighter shading) to correspond to values less than or equal to 1.645, and 5% (in darker shading) to values greater than 1.645. In this diagram, the standard normal distribution is shown, for which the mean is zero and the standard

Figure 8.1 Standard normal distribution.

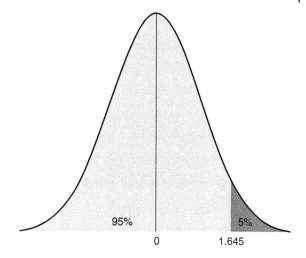

95%   0   5%   1.645

Table 8.1 Safety factors for CSL targets, normal demand.

CSL target (%)	Safety factor
90.0	1.282
92.5	1.440
95.0	1.645
97.5	1.960

deviation is one. A similar diagram can be drawn, replacing zero by μ_{R+L} and 1.645 by $1.645\sigma_{R+L}$, in which the proportions of lighter and darker shading would be unaltered.

Setting the OUT level according to Eq. (8.1) will guarantee that a 95% CSL target will be met. For a general CSL target, not restricted to 95%, the formula is as follows:

$$S = \mu_{R+L} + c_1\sigma_{R+L} \tag{8.2}$$

where c_1 denotes the safety factor.

The setting of the safety factor depends on the target CSL. The safety factor would be exactly the same for the CSL$^+$ measure, introduced in Chapter 3, which counts only those review intervals with some demand. There is no difference between the CSL and CSL$^+$ measures in this case because normally distributed demand is assumed to be non-intermittent over the protection interval even if it is intermittent over a single period. Some common safety factors are listed in Table 8.1.

If demand is normally distributed and the mean and standard deviation of demand are known, and the OUT level is set according to Eq. (8.2) using a safety factor of $c_1 = 1.96$, then we can be assured that 97.5% of replenishment cycles will have no stockouts. By reducing the safety factor to 1.645, the assurance drops to 95% of replenishment cycles, and so on.

The CSL is a measure of the probability of there being a stockout but gives no indication of the quantity unfulfilled or how this relates to the total quantity demanded, as discussed in

Table 8.2 Safety factors for fill rate (FR) targets, normal demand.

FR target (%)	Coefficient of variation (CV_{R+L})				
	0.50	0.75	1.00	1.25	1.50
90.0	0.493	0.741	0.902	1.021	1.115
92.5	0.671	0.902	1.055	1.167	1.256
95.0	0.902	1.115	1.256	1.360	1.443
97.5	1.256	1.443	1.569	1.663	1.738

Source: Strijbosch and Moors (2005). © 2005, Elsevier.

Chapter 3. The unit fill rate, on the other hand, measures the proportion of units demanded that are immediately satisfied from stock. If our fill rate target is 95%, this means that we want at least 95% of units demanded to be fulfilled immediately from stock. A formula for determining the OUT level is given in Eq. (8.3). It is of the same form as Eq. (8.2), but with a different safety factor (Strijbosch and Moors 2005); see Technical Note 8.1 for further explanation.

$$S = \mu_{R+L} + c_2\sigma_{R+L} \tag{8.3}$$

Equation (8.3) relates to the usual fill rate calculation, rather than the amended fill rate calculation (Zhang and Zhang 2007) discussed in Chapter 3 (Technical Note 3.1). Although the fill rate calculation still requires some adaptation when demand is normal, the correction is not as substantial as for erratic or lumpy demand.

The setting of the safety factor c_2, for fill rate targets, is not as straightforward as for c_1, for CSL targets. It depends not only on the target fill rate but also on the coefficient of variation (CV) of demand. As mentioned in Chapter 5, the CV is calculated as the ratio of the standard deviation to the mean. For periodic review systems, the value of c_2 depends on the CV of demand over the protection interval $(R + L)$ denoted by CV_{R+L}, which is calculated as shown in Eq. (8.4).

$$CV_{R+L} = \frac{\sigma_{R+L}}{\mu_{R+L}} \tag{8.4}$$

Examples of safety factors for fill rate systems, with normally distributed demand, are given in Table 8.2.

In conclusion, if demand is normally distributed with known mean and standard deviation, then an exact OUT level can be calculated. If this is fractional, and demand is always for whole number quantities, then rounding up to the next whole number will guarantee meeting CSL or fill rate targets if appropriate safety factors are used.

8.2.3 Scenario 2: Mean Demand Unknown Standard Deviation Known

The formula for the OUT level for CSL systems (Eq. (8.2)) is presented in many textbooks and may be regarded as 'standard'. It is correct if the mean and standard deviation are known. However, it is highly unrealistic to assume that these quantities are known. After all, there would be no point in trying to forecast the mean demand if it were known! We will now proceed by assuming that the standard deviation of demand is known but the mean demand is not and needs to be forecasted. It is still unrealistic to suppose the standard deviation to be known but this assumption will isolate the effect of forecasting the mean demand on the OUT level.

As the mean demand is unknown, we need a forecast of it over the protection interval $(R + L)$, which we denote by $\hat{\mu}_{R+L}$. This may be obtained by using one of the methods discussed in Chapter 6, such as Croston's method or the Syntetos–Boylan Approximation (SBA). In Eq. (8.2), for CSL systems, it would be natural to replace the mean demand over the protection interval (previously assumed to be known) by the forecast of this mean demand value, as shown in Eq. (8.5).

$$S = \hat{\mu}_{R+L} + c_1 \sigma_{R+L} \tag{8.5}$$

In Eq. (8.5), the standard deviation of demand over the protection interval, σ_{R+L}, does not have a 'hat' symbol because it is assumed to be known and so does not need to be forecasted.

This new OUT level (S) will not always be accurate, as sometimes the value will be too low (when there is an under-forecast) and sometimes too high (when there is an over-forecast). This may lead to situations when the target CSL will be underachieved or overachieved. It would be advisable, nevertheless, for an OUT level equation to provide OUT levels that will result in attaining the target CSL on average over many replenishment cycles.

It is generally desirable to identify forecasting methods that are unbiased. In Chapter 6, we saw that some forecasting methods, including Croston's method, are biased, whereas the SBA is approximately unbiased. Suppose that our forecasting method is exactly unbiased. This can be difficult to achieve for forecasts immediately after issue points, but the assumption will serve to make an important point. Two questions arise in relation to Eq. (8.5) when it includes an unbiased forecast:

1. Does Eq. (8.5) provide an unbiased estimate of the OUT level?
2. Does Eq. (8.5) result in attainment of the target CSL on average?

The answer to the first question is 'yes' if the forecasting method is unbiased. The answer to the second question is generally 'no' even if the forecasting method is unbiased (Strijbosch et al. 1997). This is counter-intuitive and merits further discussion. The answer to the first question is not a surprise. If our forecasts are correct on average, and we know the standard deviation of demand, then it follows that the estimate of the OUT level is also correct on average. So, why do we not, on average, achieve the desired target CSL? To see why, consider the diagram in Figure 8.2.

In Figure 8.2, the wider normal curve represents the distribution of demand over the protection interval, with a mean of μ_{R+L}, abbreviated to μ in the figure. We suppose that $\mu_{R+L} = 12.16$ and that the standard deviation of demand is given by $\sigma_{R+L} = 4$. The narrower curve, on the right of the diagram, represents the distribution of the OUT levels generated by different forecasts of mean demand. The forecasts are assumed to be unbiased and normally distributed. Then the OUT level estimates are also normally distributed, as shown on the right of the diagram. Equation (8.6) (mean demand known) gives an OUT level of 20 units for a CSL target of 97.5%.

$$S = 12.16 + (1.96 \times 4) = 20 \tag{8.6}$$

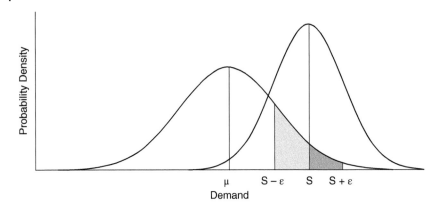

Figure 8.2 Normally distributed demand and OUT levels. Source: Janssen et al. (2009).

Table 8.3 Asymmetric effect of under- and over-forecasting.

$\hat{\mu}_{R+L}$	σ_{R+L}	OUT level	CSL (%)
10.16	4	18	92.8
12.16	4	20	97.5
14.16	4	22	99.3

Equation (8.7) (mean demand unknown) gives a result that depends on the forecast of the mean demand over the protection interval, $\hat{\mu}_{R+L}$.

$$S = \hat{\mu}_{R+L} + (1.96 \times 4) = \hat{\mu}_{R+L} + 7.84 \qquad (8.7)$$

If the mean demand were known, then Eq. (8.6) would give a 97.5% CSL, as required. In the more realistic situation of the mean demand being unknown, Eq. (8.7) will give a 97.5% CSL when we get our forecast exactly right ($\hat{\mu}_{R+L} = 12.16$) but will give a CSL higher than 97.5% when the forecast is greater than 12.16 and a CSL lower than 97.5% when the forecast is less than 12.16.

From our previous discussion in response to Question 1, we know that the average value of S will be 20, as the forecast is unbiased. Because the normal distribution is symmetric, it is equally likely that Eq. (8.7) will give OUT levels between $20 - \epsilon$ and 20 as it will give OUT levels between 20 and $20 + \epsilon$, for any value of ϵ. Take the example of $\epsilon = 2$. This corresponds to under- and over-forecasts by two units and OUT levels of 18 and 22, respectively. The effect on the CSL is given in Table 8.3 (with further details in Technical Note 8.2).

Table 8.3 shows that, although the OUT levels themselves are equally distanced from the correct OUT level (20 units), their effect is not. The added CSL by having an OUT level of 22 (instead of 20) is given by 99.3% − 97.5% = 1.8%. This is illustrated by the darker shaded area in Figure 8.2. The loss in CSL by having an OUT level of 18 (instead of 20) is 97.5% − 92.8% = 4.7%. This is illustrated by the lighter shaded area in Figure 8.2. It is clear that the loss (4.7%) outweighs the gain (1.8%), and the same would be true for any other comparison of OUT levels equally spaced from the central value of 20. Overall, we can expect an under-achievement of the average CSL against the target of 97.5%. A similar underachievement effect will be observed for other realistic CSL targets.

This explains why the answer to Question 2 is 'no' although the answer to Question 1 is 'yes'. Even if the forecasts (and hence the OUT levels) may be symmetrically distributed, their effect is asymmetric. Under-forecasting has a stronger effect on CSLs than over-forecasting. Therefore, unbiased forecasts lead to an overall underperformance according to the CSL measure.

Strijbosch and Moors (2005) examined the effect of unbiased forecasts on the fill rate measure, and arrived at similar conclusions: for normally distributed demand, unbiased forecasts lead to an overall underperformance according to the fill rate measure.

It may be asked why unbiased forecasts are needed if they result in service level underperformance. The reason is that there is no systematic way of resolving the issue by producing biased forecasts. To address the problem of underperformance in CSLs (and fill rates) for normally distributed demand, it is not the unbiased forecast that should be changed but the safety factor. We return to this resolution when examining Scenario 4. This is the realistic case for which adjustments to the safety factor will need to be made in practice.

8.2.4 Scenario 3: Mean Demand Known Standard Deviation Unknown

Let us return temporarily to Scenario 1, when both the mean and standard deviation of demand are assumed to be known. The two equations for determining the OUT levels (one for CSL, and one for fill rate) may be written more concisely as one equation, as shown in Eq. (8.8).

$$S = \mu_{R+L} + c_\beta \sigma_{R+L} \tag{8.8}$$

In Eq. (8.8), $c_\beta = c_1$ for a CSL driven system and $c_\beta = c_2$ for a fill rate driven system. This equation refers to the case when the mean and standard deviation of demand are both supposed to be known. In Scenario 3, it is assumed that the mean demand is known, but the standard deviation of demand is unknown. Then, we have Eq. (8.9).

$$S = \mu_{R+L} + c_\beta \widehat{\sigma}_{R+L} \tag{8.9}$$

In the right hand sides of Eqs. (8.8) and (8.9), the second components ($c_\beta \sigma_{R+L}$ and $c_\beta \widehat{\sigma}_{R+L}$) allow for variation of demand (over the protection interval) about the known mean level (μ_{R+L}). They are usually known as the 'safety stock' components of inventory holdings. The degree of variation, as represented by the standard deviation, is assumed to be known in Eq. (8.8) but requiring estimation in Eq. (8.9). In the latter scenario, the standard deviation of demand is the same as the standard deviation of forecast error. This is because the mean demand and the forecast are the same (μ_{R+L}) and so any differences between actual observations and the mean are identical to the differences between actuals and forecasts. In the next scenario, the standard deviations of demand and forecast error are no longer identical. Corrected safety factors are presented for this fourth scenario (rather than for the second and third scenarios) because this is the situation we always face in practice.

8.2.5 Scenario 4: Mean and Standard Deviation Unknown

We now turn to the realistic case in which both the mean and standard deviation need to be estimated. In this case, OUT levels are given by Eq. (8.10).

$$S = \hat{\mu}_{R+L} + c_\beta \hat{s}_{R+L} \qquad (8.10)$$

Comparing Eq. (8.10) to Eq. (8.9), we can see that the mean demand over the protection interval is no longer known but must be forecasted. The other change is from the estimate of the standard deviation of demand ($\hat{\sigma}_{R+L}$) to the estimate of the standard deviation of forecast errors ($\hat{s}_{R+L}$). The reasons for this change were explained in Chapter 7. To recap, in Eq. (8.10), the mean demand is not known and we must rely on the forecasted mean demand ($\hat{\mu}_{R+L}$). In this case, then, any variation must be measured about the forecast value. The differences between the actual demand (over the protection interval, $R + L$) and the forecasted demand (over the same time period) are, by definition, forecast errors. So, instead of estimating the standard deviation of demand, we focus instead on the standard deviation of forecast errors.

Our estimate of the OUT level using Eq. (8.10) (mean unknown, standard deviation unknown) suffers from the same problem as Eq. (8.5) (mean unknown, standard deviation known). In both cases, the mean demand is unknown and must be forecasted. As we saw earlier, this results in an overall underachievement of CSLs.

Strijbosch and Moors (2005) quantified the underachievement for a CSL system. They assumed that both the mean demand and mean absolute deviation of forecast errors were being forecasted using single exponential smoothing. The forecasted standard deviation of forecast errors was estimated by multiplying the forecasted mean absolute deviation of forecast errors by 1.25, which is appropriate for a normal distribution (see Chapter 7).

The researchers found that the effect on performance for low target CSLs and low smoothing constants was very small. However, the effect becomes more pronounced as the target CSL increases or the smoothing constants rise, with shortfalls that become more significant. Strijbosch and Moors (2005) also quantified the effect on fill rates, and found similar results: a small underperformance against target, but one that grows with increasing target fill rates and smoothing constants (and also grows with an increasing CV of demand).

How can this underperformance be addressed? For lower service targets, such as 85.0%, the effect may be so small as to require no action. For higher service targets, one approach is to 'scale up' the estimate of the standard deviation, by quantities greater than the standard safety factors. This would mean replacing the OUT level formula by Eq. (8.11).

$$S = \hat{\mu}_{R+L} + r_\beta \hat{s}_{R+L} \qquad (8.11)$$

Equation (8.11) differs from Eq. (8.10) in that the standard safety factors (c_1 and c_2) have been replaced by adjusted safety factors (r_1 and r_2). The new factors, r_1 and r_2, take into account service level underperformance for CSL and fill rate systems, respectively. Table 8.4 shows the standard safety factors alongside the adjusted safety factors (Strijbosch and Moors 2005) for a CSL system and for a range of smoothing constants for the mean absolute deviation of forecast errors (ω) and a fixed smoothing constant for mean demand ($\alpha = 0.15$).

Table 8.4 shows that the differences between the standard safety factors and the adjusted safety factors are generally quite small. The greatest differences occur for the highest CSL

Table 8.4   Adjusted safety factors for cycle service levels.

CSL target (%)	Standard factors	Adjusted factors		
		$\alpha = 0.15$ $\omega = 0.03$	$\alpha = 0.15$ $\omega = 0.06$	$\alpha = 0.15$ $\omega = 0.09$
90.0	1.282	1.284	1.290	1.301
92.5	1.440	1.450	1.466	1.477
95.0	1.645	1.671	1.686	1.716
97.5	1.960	2.006	2.044	2.092

Source: Adapted from Strijbosch and Moors (2005).

target and the highest smoothing parameters. For a target CSL of 97.5% and a smoothing constant (for mean absolute deviations of forecast errors) of 0.09, the safety factor rises from 1.960 to 2.092. These adjusted safety factors are based on normally distributed demand for CSL systems. Strijbosch and Moors (2005) also calculated adjusted safety factors for fill rate systems (see Technical Note 8.3).

8.2.6   Summary

For normally distributed demand, we have seen that unbiased estimation of the OUT level does not guarantee achievement of the CSL target on average. Generally, for realistic CSL targets, the average achieved CSL will be lower than the target because of the asymmetric effect of over- and underestimation of the OUT level. It is possible to adjust the safety factors to address this problem, which affects both CSLs and fill rates. We have noted previously that the normal distribution is not the usual choice for intermittent demand. However, the issue of the asymmetric effect of over- and under-estimation also affects other demand distributions, including the Poisson, to which we now turn.

8.3   Poisson Demand

In this section, we address the calculation of the OUT level when demand is Poisson distributed. We move on to compound Poisson distributions in Section 8.4.

To clarify the exposition, we first deal with the unrealistic situation of the mean demand being known. If this were the case, we would know the entire Poisson distribution, thus simplifying the problem. Then, we move on to the more realistic case of the mean demand being unknown and having to be forecasted.

8.3.1   Cycle Service Level System when the Mean Demand is Known

The determination of the OUT level depends on the service level measure employed, with different calculations needed for the CSL (P_1) and fill rate (P_2) measures. In this subsection, we restrict our attention to the CSL.

Table 8.5 Cycle service level for Poisson demand $((R+L)\lambda = 3\lambda = 1.2)$.

Demand	Probability	CSL	CSL$^+$
0	0.301	0.301	
1	0.361	0.663	0.365
2	0.217	0.879	0.731
3	0.087	0.966	0.916
4	0.026	0.992	0.979

Suppose that the demand over one week is independent and identically Poisson distributed with a known mean demand of 0.4 units. If the review interval is one week and the lead time is two weeks, then the protection interval is three weeks, and demand over this interval is Poisson distributed, with a mean demand of 1.2 units. The probabilities of demand, shown in Table 8.5, are calculated as described in Chapter 4. The CSL values are given directly by the cumulative probabilities, as they represent the chance that demand over the protection interval does not exceed these values. In Chapter 3, we discussed a modified measure, denoted CSL$^+$, which restricts attention to those review intervals in which there has been some demand. The CSL$^+$ values, for different OUT levels, can be calculated using the procedure described in Technical Note 8.4. The results for mean demand of 1.2 units (over three weeks) are given in Table 8.5.

The third column of Table 8.5 shows that if we require a CSL of at least 90%, then an OUT level of three units is required. This yields a CSL of 96.6%, which is quite some way in excess of the target of 90%. The final column of the table shows that, for an OUT level of three units, a CSL$^+$ value of 91.6% will be attained. This is less than the CSL value of 96.6% for the same OUT level, but still exceeds a target value of 90% by 1.6%.

This example illustrates a more general phenomenon for discrete demand distributions. If the mean demand is known, then the target CSL or CSL$^+$ will be exceeded by setting the OUT level at the minimum value (three in this example) to ensure that the target is met. The only exception to the rule is if the target is hit exactly, which happens very rarely in practice.

8.3.2 Fill Rate System when the Mean Demand is Known

We now turn our attention to the fill rate measure. The fill rate may be calculated using Eq. (8.12) (Sobel 2004) for a unit-time review interval ($R = 1$), which is expressed slightly differently to the formula in Chapter 3:

$$FR(S) = 1 - \frac{\mathbb{E}\left(d_{L+1} - (S - D_L)^+\right)^+}{\mu} \tag{8.12}$$

where, as before, S is the OUT level, D_L denotes the demand over lead time, d_{L+1} is the demand in the single period immediately after the lead time, μ is the mean demand per unit time period (assumed to be known), $\mathbb{E}$ denotes the expectation (long-term average), and the plus superscript indicates replacing the value of an expression by zero if it is negative.

Table 8.6 Fill rate for Poisson distributed demand.

OUT level (S)	Fill rate
1	0.371
2	0.736
3	0.919
4	0.980

For example, if the lead time is two periods, the review interval is one period and demand is Poisson distributed with a mean demand of 0.4 per period, then the fill rates, for different OUT levels, are shown in Table 8.6 (an example of the detailed calculations is given in Technical Note 8.5).

An OUT level of three units is required to be assured of meeting a fill rate target of 90%. Again, the target will always be exceeded unless it is met exactly, which rarely happens in practice.

8.3.3 Poisson OUT Level when the Mean Demand is Unknown

In realistic situations, the future mean demand level is unknown. It must be forecasted over the protection interval and a variety of forecasting methods may be used for this purpose. Then, depending on the choice of service measure, the methods outlined in Sections 8.3.1 and 8.3.2 can be used, with the forecasted mean standing in for the true (but unknown) mean demand over the protection interval.

In the analysis of normally distributed demand, we found that service levels would be reached exactly if the mean demand were known. With the mean demand unknown, unbiased forecasts do not lead to target service levels being reached, on average. Adjusted safety factors are required to correct for this problem. This issue also arises with Poisson demand but, for this distribution, we also need to take into account the potential overachievement of service level targets, discussed above. Even if the mean demand is known exactly, the service level target is generally exceeded. Returning to the example in Table 8.5, an OUT level of three units is required to reach a 90% CSL target but, in fact, a 96.6% CSL would be attained.

When demands need to be forecasted, the forecasted mean may be lower or higher than the true mean demand over the protection interval. The effect on the OUT level depends on the 'true' OUT level (i.e. the one that is based on the true mean demand).

If the true OUT level is one unit, then under-forecasts will have no effect, assuming that we continue to stock the item. Under-forecasts may have a detrimental effect on the decision on whether to continue stocking an item or to discontinue it, but will have no effect on the OUT level, which will continue to be set at one unit. Over-forecasts on the other hand, may result in the OUT level being amended to two units (or even higher levels), thus leading to over-stocking.

If the true OUT level is two units or higher, then both under- and over-forecasts may have an effect on the estimated OUT level. In our previous example, the true OUT level is three units, giving a 96.6% CSL. An under-forecast may result in an OUT level of two units, giving an 87.9% CSL. An over-forecast may result in an OUT level of four units, giving a 99.2% CSL. This example illustrates a similar asymmetry to the normal distribution: an under-forecast can have a stronger effect on the CSL than an over-forecast. In our example, the CSL is reduced by 8.7% by an under-forecast, leading to an OUT level of two units, but an increase of only 2.6% in CSL by an over-forecast, leading to an OUT level of four units. The overall effect, therefore, of a mix of over- and under-forecasts may be to reduce the overall CSL from that which would have been obtained from the true mean. However, even with such a reduction, the target CSL may still be exceeded.

These remarks have focused on the CSL measure but also apply to the CSL^+ measure and to the fill rate. The asymmetric effect of under- and over-forecasting holds for these measures, just as it does for the CSL measure.

For Poisson distributed demand, the overall effect on service measures of using a forecasted mean instead of the true mean is not straightforward to assess. Consequently, there is no simple adjustment that can be applied, as in the case of normally distributed demand. A simulation analysis can be performed, using real historical intermittent demand data across a whole set of SKUs being modelled by the Poisson distribution. This enables an evaluation of the service levels that would be achieved based on the chosen forecasting method and the assumption of Poisson demand. This type of simulation will be discussed further in the next chapter. It can have three possible outcomes:

1. *The average performance is acceptably close to the target measure*: What constitutes 'acceptably close' is a matter of judgement for supply chain directors and managers. If the difference from the target is deemed to be reasonable, then the organisation should continue to use their forecasted mean demands to stand in for the true means, and no further adjustments are required.

2. *The average performance exceeds the target measure by an unacceptable amount*: In this case, the appropriate remedial action depends on the cause. If overachievement is caused primarily by SKUs with an OUT level of one unit, then this may lead to a recommendation to discontinue some of them and to place no more orders (contractual obligations permitting). If the overachievement is caused by SKUs with an OUT level of more than one unit, then this may lead to a differential approach to setting target service level with, for example, a higher target for some SKUs and a lower target for others. Simulation experimentation may be required to set these targets appropriately.

3. *The average performance is below the target measure by an unacceptable amount*: The first thing to check, in this case, is whether the Poisson distribution is appropriate for the intermittent demand items being assessed. If not, the remedy is to reassess the SKUs and to use an alternative distribution, such as the stuttering Poisson or negative binomial. Again, the performance may be simulated, to ensure that the required service target is met. Any such simulation of a stock control system should be based on real demand data, rather than artificially generated data from a Poisson distribution. This is because service level performance may have been degraded by deviation of real demand patterns from the assumed Poisson distribution.

8.3.4 Summary

The methods for determining the OUT levels for Poisson distributed demand are based on the CSL, CSL$^+$ and fill rate calculations described in Chapter 3. These would generally lead to an overachievement of target service levels, regardless of the measure used, if the mean demand were known. In practice, when the mean demand is not known and has to be forecasted, this overachievement may be offset by the asymmetric effect of forecast errors, if the true OUT level is for two units or higher. If the OUT level is for one unit, then any overachievement cannot be reduced unless an SKU is discontinued and no more stock is ordered. Any adjustments, for example to the target service levels, should be assessed using a simulation of service performance based on real data.

8.4 Compound Poisson Demand

In Chapter 5, we saw that there is good empirical evidence in support of the stuttering Poisson and negative binomial distributions for intermittent demand. These compound Poisson distributions are more flexible than the Poisson, allowing the variance to exceed the mean and giving higher probabilities of larger demand values than would be anticipated by the Poisson.

At the end of Chapter 5, we concluded that both distributions can be specified by their mean and variance. In this section, we start by assuming that these quantities are known. Then we move on to the effect of forecasting these values.

8.4.1 Stuttering Poisson OUT Level when the Parameters are Known

Suppose that demand is independent and identically distributed with parameters of $\lambda = 0.25$ and $\rho = 0.5$. We continue to work with a review interval of one period and a lead time of two periods, giving a protection interval of three periods. Then, demand over this protection interval is stuttering Poisson distributed, with a λ parameter of 0.75 over the protection interval, and a ρ parameter of 0.5.

To evaluate the CSL implications of different OUT levels, we need to calculate the demand probabilities over the protection interval. These probabilities may be found from the following general formulae, which are very similar to Eqs. (5.4) and (5.5), with the only change being that λ is replaced by $(R+L)\lambda$ in Eqs. (8.13) and (8.14).

For zero demand:

$$\mathbb{P}(0) = e^{-(R+L)\lambda} \tag{8.13}$$

and for positive demand ($x \geq 1$):

$$\mathbb{P}(x) = e^{-(R+L)\lambda} \sum_{j=1}^{x} \frac{(x-1)!}{(j-1)!(x-j)!} \frac{((R+L)\lambda\rho)^j}{j!} (1-\rho)^{x-j} \tag{8.14}$$

An illustrative example of the calculations involved in these equations was given in Section 5.3.2 for the special case of $R+L = 1$. The general case for a protection interval of two periods or longer requires a similar approach. Continuing with our example of

Table 8.7 Cycle service levels for stuttering Poisson distributed demand.

OUT level	Probability	CSL	Conditional probability	CSL$^+$
0	0.472	0.472		
1	0.177	0.650	0.267	0.267
2	0.122	0.771	0.217	0.484
3	0.082	0.853	0.163	0.647
4	0.054	0.907	0.117	0.764
5	0.035	0.941	0.081	0.845
6	0.022	0.963	0.055	0.090
7			0.036	0.936
8		.	0.024	0.960

stuttering Poisson demand with $(R + L)\lambda = 0.75$ and $\rho = 0.5$, the probabilities of demand and corresponding CSL values are shown in the second and third columns of Table 8.7 for a range of OUT levels from zero to six units. It is assumed that service level targets of 90% and 95% are of interest and, therefore, CSL calculations are not required for OUT levels of seven or eight units.

In the example shown in Table 8.7, OUT (S) levels of four and six would be required to attain CSL targets of 90% and 95%, respectively. The expected CSL values of 90.7% and 96.3% exceed the targets, as generally anticipated, but only marginally so for the 90% target.

If we wish to set the OUT level to meet a CSL$^+$ target level, then we need to take into account that the demand over the review interval is constrained to be greater than zero. This requires evaluation of a stuttering Poisson distribution over the lead time (two periods in this example) and a truncated stuttering Poisson over the review interval (one period in this example). The conditional probabilities of demand and corresponding CSL$^+$ values are shown in the fourth and fifth columns of Table 8.7. The detailed calculations are given in Technical Note 8.6. The CSL$^+$ measure results in noticeably higher OUT level requirements than the CSL measure in this example. A target of 90% requires an OUT level of four units for the CSL, but six for the CSL$^+$; similarly, a target of 95% requires an OUT level of six units for the CSL, but eight for the CSL$^+$. This is to be expected. The CSL$^+$ measure is stricter than the CSL, as it excludes review intervals with zero demands, thereby necessitating a higher OUT level.

The fill rate calculations for stuttering Poisson demand follow the same approach as that for Poisson distributed demand. Sobel's formula, given in Eq. (8.12), may be used, in the same way as for the (non-stuttering) Poisson distribution. For the calculations to be made, we need to evaluate the stuttering Poisson over the lead time (two periods), as also required for the CSL$^+$ calculations. Additionally, we require evaluation of the stuttering Poisson over the review interval (one period). This is not the same as the CSL$^+$ which requires the truncated distribution over one period. No such truncation adjustment is needed for the fill rate calculation: a period with no demand makes no difference to the numerator or the denominator in the fill rate formula.

8.4.2 Negative Binomial OUT Levels when the Parameters are Known

To evaluate the CSL implications of different OUT levels for the negative binomial, we need to calculate the demand probabilities over the protection interval. These may be found from the general formulae (Eqs. (5.12) and (5.13)), but rewritten (Eqs. (8.15) and (8.16)) with reference to the whole protection interval rather than a single unit of time.

$$\mathbb{P}(0) = \left(\frac{1}{z_{R+L}}\right)^{\mu_{R+L}/(z_{R+L}-1)} \tag{8.15}$$

and for demand values $x \geq 1$:

$$\mathbb{P}(x) = \left(\frac{(\mu_{R+L}/(z_{R+L}-1)) + x - 1}{x}\right)\left(\frac{z_{R+L}-1}{z_{R+L}}\right)\mathbb{P}(x-1) \tag{8.16}$$

where z_{R+L} is the variance to mean ratio over the protection interval. These probabilities allow calculation of OUT levels for CSL and CSL$^+$ systems in the same way as shown for other distributions.

For fill rate systems, similar calculations can be performed for the probabilities of demand over lead time. If the review interval is greater than one period, then additional calculations are needed and Eqs. (8.15) and (8.16) require adaptation, replacing the protection interval by the appropriate period of time. Then, OUT levels may be calculated using the formula of Zhang and Zhang (2007) for a general review interval (of which Sobel's formula is a special case for a unit review interval). Please see Technical Note 3.1 for an explanation of Zhang and Zhang's formula.

The negative binomial will lead to an overachievement of the target service level (CSL or fill rate) in the same way as other discrete distributions such as the Poisson and the stuttering Poisson. Of course, this depends on the data following the assumed distribution and the parameters being known.

8.4.3 Stuttering Poisson and Negative Binomial OUT Levels when the Parameters are Unknown

The mean and variance of the stuttering Poisson and negative binomial distributions are generally unknown and, in real-life situations, may be changing over time. This situation was reviewed in Section 7.3.2, where the forecasting calculations were explained in detail. To recap, the mean demand over the protection interval may be forecasted using any appropriate method for intermittent demand, such as Croston or SBA. As these methods assume no trend or seasonality, a one-step-ahead forecast may be made, and then multiplied by the length of the protection interval.

The variance of forecast errors requires more care. In the previous chapter, we warned against multiplying the variance of one-step-ahead forecast errors by the length of the protection interval. Instead, we suggested directly smoothing the variance of forecast errors over the protection interval (Eq. (7.9)).

If the variance were known, then over- and under-forecasting of mean demand would have a similar asymmetric effect as described for other distributions, with under-forecasting having a stronger effect than over-forecasting. This means that OUT levels (of two units or more) may be affected as previously discussed. The situation is further complicated by the forecast of the variance of forecast error over the protection interval. To gain a full appreciation of the overall effect, a simulation analysis is required.

As before, if the simulated service level is acceptably close to the target, then no further action is required. If the simulated service level is too high, then the same remedies can be applied as for Poisson demand. If the simulated service level is too low, then non-parametric methods may be considered as an alternative (to be discussed in Chapter 13).

8.4.4 Summary

For stuttering Poisson and negative binomial demand, a simulation analysis will reveal the net effect of: (i) over-achievements because of the discrete nature of demand; (ii) under-achievements because of the asymmetric effect of under- and over-forecasting, and (iii) deviations from achievement because of demand not following the assumed distribution. The complexity of the interaction between these effects makes an exact analytical evaluation impractical and a simulation analysis, using real demand data, is recommended for real-world implementations.

8.5 Variable Lead Times

In the previous chapter, we noted the difficulties encountered when addressing variable lead times:

1. Estimation of the variability of forecast errors becomes complicated.
2. The distributional form also becomes more complex, particularly if demand per unit time is stuttering Poisson or negative binomially distributed.

An alternative approach to determining the OUT level, which may be used when there is a variable lead time, is outlined below.

8.5.1 Empirical Lead Time Distributions

Suppose that an empirical distribution of lead time is available, and demand and lead times are independent. The latter assumption is generally reasonable, unless there are exceptionally high demands that lead to supplier delays.

Lewis (1981) noted that the overall CSL can be calculated as a function of the CSLs for each of the potential lead times. To illustrate this approach, consider the case of a highly unreliable supplier, with a target lead time of two weeks, who delivers on time (in two weeks) on 10% of occasions, and late (in four weeks) on 90% of occasions. If inventory is reviewed on a weekly basis, this will mean protection intervals of three and five weeks, respectively. If demand is Poisson distributed, with a known mean demand of 0.4 units per week, then we can find the CSLs over three and five weeks, using the same method as before

Table 8.8 Weighted cumulative probabilities.

Demand	Cumulative probability (3 weeks)	Cumulative probability (5 weeks)	Weighted average (10 : 90)
0	0.301	0.135	0.152
1	0.663	0.406	0.432
2	0.879	0.677	0.697
3	0.966	0.857	0.868
4	0.992	0.947	0.952

(see Table 8.5). The overall CSL is a weighted average, with 10% weight for three weeks and 90% weight for five weeks, as shown in Table 8.8.

Table 8.8 shows the effect of late deliveries on the CSL. If an OUT level of three is adopted, then a CSL of 96.6% would be achieved if all deliveries are on time. This slips to 85.7% if all deliveries are two weeks late, equating to a penalty of 10.9% in CSL. For every additional 10% of deliveries that are on time, there is a gain of 1.1% in CSL, as shown in the final column, where the CSL has improved slightly to 86.8%. Of course, 90% of deliveries being late is an unacceptable level of performance. Its impact will either be a reduced CSL or an increased stock holding (by raising the OUT level). In this case, an OUT level of four would improve the CSL to 95.2% if 90% of deliveries were late by two weeks.

8.5.2 Summary

The approach outlined in this section is much more intuitive than attempting to estimate the variance of forecast error over a variable lead time and to use this as part of a complex probability distribution. The approach does require an empirical lead time distribution. If there is insufficient data for an individual SKU to estimate this reliably, then the distribution may be estimated for a group of SKUs with similar delivery performance, for example from the same supplier.

A similar approach can be adopted for CSL^+ and fill rate systems. As noted in Chapter 7, the information gained from this analysis of the effect of variable lead times can be used to inform discussions with suppliers about the impact of poor delivery performance.

8.6 Chapter Summary

In this chapter, we have seen that the standard methods for finding OUT levels may be readily implemented but are subject to some limitations. Only in the case of the normal distribution is there an approximation formula to allow the necessary adjustments to overcome these limitations.

For the normal distribution, an unbiased estimate of the OUT level does not lead to an unbiased achievement of target service levels, regardless of whether they are CSLs or fill rates. The reason is the asymmetric effect of under- and over-estimating the OUT level for realistic targets; an overestimate has a more modest effect on the achieved service level than an underestimate. This effect can also be observed for the other distributions examined in this chapter. For normally distributed demand, adjusted safety factors may be used. They are a little higher than the standard safety factors, with the greater discrepancies at higher target service levels.

For the three discrete distributions discussed in this chapter, an additional complicating factor is that the lowest OUT level required to attain the target service level, according to the standard methods, will generally exceed the target. This may be offset by the asymmetric effect of under- and over-estimating the OUT level. There are no ready-made adjustment factors that are available for the discrete distributions. Instead, a simulation analysis is needed to assess the effect on service levels. If the overall effect is negligible, then no action needs to be taken. Otherwise, suggestions have been made about setting differential targets for different sub-categories of intermittent SKUs, designed to meet the overall service target.

The case of variable lead time has also been considered. A pragmatic approach has been recommended, based on empirical distributions of lead time. This should be more straightforward to implement than an approach based on the variance calculations for variable lead time discussed in the previous chapter. An alternative approach will be outlined in Chapter 13.

Technical Notes

Note 8.1: OUT Levels for Normally Distributed Demand

The formulae for determining the OUT level, S, for normally distributed demand (mean μ and variance σ^2) to cover a protection interval of a unit time period, are given in Eqs. (8.17) (CSL) and (8.18) (fill rate).

$$S = \mu + \sigma \Phi^{-1}(P_1) \tag{8.17}$$

$$S = \mu + \sigma G^{-1}\left(\frac{1 - P_2}{\sigma/\mu}\right) \tag{8.18}$$

where P_1 and P_2 are the target CSLs and fill rates, respectively; Φ is the standard normal cumulative distribution, and G, sometimes known as the partial expectation function, is defined in Eq. (8.19).

$$G(k) = \int_k^\infty (z - k)\phi(z)\, \mathrm{d}z \tag{8.19}$$

where $\phi(z)$ denotes the standard normal density function, and z is the standardised normal variable, $z = (x - \mu)/\sigma$, described further in the next technical note.

Strijbosch and Moors (2005) noted that Eqs. (8.17) and (8.18) could be written more compactly as $S = \mu + c_\beta \sigma$ (Eq. (8.8)) where $c_1 = \Phi^{-1}(P_1)$ for $\beta = 1$ and $c_2 = G^{-1}((1 - P_2)/(\sigma/\mu))$ for $\beta = 2$. Tables of Φ, the standard normal cumulative distribution function, are widely available. Tables of G, the partial expectation function, have been provided by Aucamp and Barringer (1987).

Note 8.2: Calculations of CSLs for Different OUT Levels

The standardised normal variable, z, measures how many standard deviations the value, x, is from the mean. Referring back to the example given earlier in this chapter, $\mu = 12.16$ and $\sigma = 4$. For an OUT level of $S = 22$, the value of z is given by Eq. (8.20).

$$z = \frac{S - \mu}{\sigma} = \frac{22 - 12.16}{4} = 2.46 \tag{8.20}$$

Referring to normal distribution tables, this equates to a CSL of 99.3%. Similarly, for $S = 18$, we obtain $z = 1.46$. Again, referring to normal distribution tables, this equates to a CSL of 92.8%.

Note 8.3: Adjusted Safety Factors for Fill Rates

Strijbosch and Moors (2005) estimated adjusted safety factors for fill rate systems, as well as for CSL systems, as discussed earlier in this chapter. The adjusted factors apply for normally distributed demand, with the mean demand forecast updated using single exponential smoothing (smoothing constant α) and the mean absolute deviations of forecast errors also updated with single exponential smoothing (SES) (smoothing constant ω). The adjusted safety factors are presented in Table 8.9.

Note 8.4: CSL$^+$ Calculations for Poisson Demand

Suppose that demand is independent and identically Poisson distributed, with a mean demand (per period) of λ. Then, the mean demand over the review interval is $R\lambda$ and

Table 8.9   Adjusted safety factors for fill rates.

			Adjusted factors		
CV	Target FR (%)	Standard factors	$\alpha = 0.15$ $\omega = 0.03$	$\alpha = 0.15$ $\omega = 0.06$	$\alpha = 0.15$ $\omega = 0.09$
0.5	90.0	0.493	0.517	0.519	0.521
	92.5	0.671	0.695	0.698	0.702
	95.0	0.902	0.926	0.932	0.938
	97.5	1.256	1.292	1.305	1.318
1.0	90.0	0.902	0.925	0.931	0.937
	92.5	1.055	1.082	1.090	1.099
	95.0	1.256	1.291	1.304	1.317
	97.5	1.569	1.619	1.641	1.667
1.5	90.0	1.115	1.143	1.153	1.163
	92.5	1.256	1.291	1.303	1.316
	95.0	1.443	1.487	1.504	1.523
	97.5	1.738	1.796	1.826	1.858

Source: Modified from Strijbosch and Moors (2005).

the mean demand over the lead time is $L\lambda$. To calculate CSL^+, it is necessary to find the distribution of demand over the protection interval, $\mathbb{P}(D_{R+L} = y)$, subject to non-zero demand over the review interval because the CSL^+ measure is restricted to those review intervals with some demand. Therefore, we need to calculate the distribution of demand over the review interval, conditional on non-zero demand, $\mathbb{P}(D_R = x | D_R > 0)$, and the (unconditional) distribution of the remaining demand over the lead time, $\mathbb{P}(D_L = y - x)$.

The conditional distribution of demand over the review interval is not Poisson distributed but truncated-Poisson distributed, allowing for the exclusion of zero demand, as shown in Eq. (8.21), for $x = 1, 2, \ldots$

$$\mathbb{P}(D_R = x | D_R > 0) = \frac{1}{1 - e^{-R\lambda}} \frac{e^{-R\lambda}(R\lambda)^x}{x!} \tag{8.21}$$

The distribution of demand over lead time is not constrained to be non-zero, and follows the Poisson distribution, as shown in Eq. (8.22), for $y - x = 0, 1, 2, \ldots$

$$\mathbb{P}(D_L = y - x) = \frac{e^{-L\lambda}(L\lambda)^{y-x}}{(y-x)!} \tag{8.22}$$

Hence, the distribution of the total demand, over the review interval (non-zero demand) plus the lead time, is given by Eq. (8.23), for $y = 1, 2, \ldots$

$$\mathbb{P}(D_{R+L} = y | D_R > 0) = \sum_{x=1}^{y} \left(\frac{1}{1 - e^{-R\lambda}} \frac{e^{-R\lambda}(R\lambda)^x}{x!} \right) \frac{e^{-L\lambda}(L\lambda)^{y-x}}{(y-x)!} \tag{8.23}$$

And the cumulative distribution, which gives the achieved CSL^+, is given by Eq. (8.24).

$$\mathbb{P}(D_{R+L} \leq S | D_R > 0) = \sum_{y=1}^{S} \mathbb{P}(D_{R+L} = y | D_R > 0) \tag{8.24}$$

In the example given in Section 8.3.1, $R = 1$, $L = 2$, and $\lambda = 0.4$. The calculations of the component elements of Eq. (8.23) are shown in Table 8.10. In each cell of this table, the first factor of the product corresponds to the expression in Eq. (8.23) contained in large brackets (with $R\lambda = 0.4$); the second factor corresponds to the remaining expression (with $L\lambda = 0.8$).

Summing across the diagonals of Table 8.10 yields the required sums from Eq. (8.23) and gives the conditional cumulative probabilities of demand over the protection interval, subject to non-zero demand in the review interval. These values are shown in the second column of Table 8.11. Cumulative sums of these probabilities yield the totals from Eq. (8.24) and give the CSL^+ values of the potential OUT levels (S), as shown in the third column of Table 8.11.

Note 8.5: Fill Rate Calculations for Poisson Demand

In this note, we find the fill rate for the demand distribution shown in Table 8.6, for a lead time of two periods, review interval of one period, and an OUT level of two units ($S = 2$). The demand over the review interval follows a Poisson distribution with a mean of 0.4 (and probabilities of 0.268, 0.054, 0.007, and 0.001 of demand for one, two, three, and four units, respectively). The demand over the lead time (of two periods) has a Poisson distribution

Table 8.10 CSL$^+$ component calculations for Poisson distributed demand.

Demand in Week 1 (x)	Demand in weeks 2 and 3 (y − x)			
	0	1	2	3
1	0.813 × 0.449 = 0.365	0.813 × 0.359 = 0.292	0.813 × 0.144 = 0.117	0.813 × 0.038 = 0.031
2	0.163 × 0.449 = 0.073	0.163 × 0.359 = 0.058	0.163 × 0.144 = 0.023	
3	0.022 × 0.449 = 0.010	0.022 × 0.359 = 0.008		
4	0.002 × 0.449 = 0.001			

Table 8.11 CSL$^+$ calculations for Poisson distributed demand.

S	$P(D_{R+L} \leq S \mid D_R > 0)$	CSL$^+$
1	0.365	0.365
2	0.365	0.731
3	0.185	0.916
4	0.063	0.979

with a mean of 0.8, and probabilities of 0.449, 0.359, and 0.191 (= 1 − 0.449 − 0.359) of demand for zero, one, and two or more units, respectively.

If demand during lead time (D_L) is for two units or more, then there is no stock on hand (($S − D_L$)$^+$ = 0) to serve any demand during the review interval (d_{L+1}), and so stockouts will occur if demand is for one unit or more. Similarly, if demand during lead time is for one unit, then stockouts will occur if demand during the review interval is for two or more. Finally, if there is no demand during the lead time, then ($S − D_L$)$^+$ = 2 and there will be stockouts only if the demand is for three or more in period $L + 1$. These considerations are taken into account in Table 8.12, which shows expected shortages for a range of demands (neglecting demand in period $L + 1$ exceeding four units because of the tiny probabilities involved). In each case, the number of units short is multiplied by the appropriate probabilities. For example, consider the cell (top left) representing no stock after the lead time has elapsed (lead time demand for two or more), and demand in period $L + 1$ for one unit. Then, the expected units short is found by taking the shortage of one unit, multiplied by the chance of one unit being demanded during the review interval (0.268), multiplied by the chance of a demand of two units or more during lead time (0.191).

Table 8.12 Fill rate calculations for Poisson demand.

	$(S - D_L)^+$		
d_{L+1}	0	1	2
1	$1 \times 0.268 \times 0.191$ $= 0.0513$	0	0
2	$2 \times 0.054 \times 0.191$ $= 0.0205$	$1 \times 0.054 \times 0.359$ $= 0.0193$	0
3	$3 \times 0.007 \times 0.191$ $= 0.0041$	$2 \times 0.007 \times 0.359$ $= 0.0051$	$1 \times 0.007 \times 0.449$ $= 0.0032$
4	$4 \times 0.001 \times 0.191$ $= 0.0005$	$3 \times 0.001 \times 0.359$ $= 0.0008$	$2 \times 0.001 \times 0.449$ $= 0.0006$
		Total	0.1055
		Fill rate	0.736

In Table 8.12, all the constituent expected shortages are summed, to give 0.1055. Then, Sobel's formula is applied, giving FR $= 1 - (0.1055/0.4) = 0.736$.

Note 8.6: CSL$^+$ Calculations for Stuttering Poisson Demand

To calculate CSL$^+$, as shown in Table 8.7, we must find the probabilities of demand over the review interval and the lead time separately:

1. Probabilities (unconditional) for demand over lead time ($L = 2$), with $L\lambda = 0.5$ and $\rho = 0.5$.
2. Probabilities for demand over the review interval ($R = 1$), with $R\lambda = 0.25$ and $\rho = 0.5$, conditional on demand being greater than zero.

Table 8.13 shows:

1. The unconditional lead time probabilities (in bold text).
2. The conditional review interval probabilities (in bold italic text).
3. The products of these probabilities (in plain text), representing the chances of all combinations of demand over review interval (D_R) and lead time (D_L).

In Table 8.13, the unconditional probabilities of demand over lead time are found from Eqs. (8.13) and (8.14), but using L instead of $R + L$, to recognise that the review interval is being analysed separately.

The conditional probabilities of demand over the review interval are found from Eq. (8.14), using R instead of $R + L$, and dividing by $1 - e^{-R\lambda} = 1 - e^{-0.25} = 0.221$. This is to recognise that the probabilities are conditional on demand over the review interval being greater than zero.

Table 8.13 CSL$^+$ component calculations for stuttering Poisson demand.

D_R	Probability	Lead time demand (D_L)							
		0	1	2	3	4	5	6	7
		0.607	0.152	0.095	0.058	0.036	0.022	0.013	0.008
1	*0.440*	0.267	0.067	*0.042*	0.026	0.016	0.009	0.006	0.003
2	*0.248*	0.150	*0.038*	0.023	0.014	0.009	0.005	0.003	
3	*0.139*	*0.084*	0.021	0.013	0.008	0.005	0.003		
4	*0.077*	0.047	0.012	0.007	0.005	0.003			
5	*0.043*	0.026	0.007	0.004	0.003				
6	*0.024*	0.014	0.004	0.002					
7	*0.013*	0.008	0.002						
8	*0.007*	0.004							

To find the probabilities of demand over the whole protection interval, conditional on non-zero demand during the review interval, we can sum across the diagonals. For example, a total demand of three can be obtained from $D_R = 3$ and $D_L = 0$, or $D_R = 2$ and $D_L = 1$, or $D_R = 1$, and $D_L = 2$. The corresponding probabilities, highlighted in italics in Table 8.13, are 0.084, 0.038, and 0.042, giving an overall probability of 0.163 (after rounding). All other probabilities are found in the same way, giving the results shown in Table 8.7. Further calculations can be made for $D_{R+L} > 8$ but these are omitted from Table 8.13, and from Table 8.7 because the probabilities are small.

9

Accuracy and Its Implications

9.1 Introduction

So far in this book, we have seen that there are a number of choices that can be made regarding inventory policies, demand distributions, and forecasting methods. All of these choices will have an effect on the overall performance of the inventory system.

When choosing forecasting methods, we want to know which is 'best'. To answer this question, we must first pose another, namely, 'What do we mean by best?' One answer seems obvious: the best method is the most accurate method. However, forecasting is not an end in itself; it is a means towards the goal of better organisational performance. So, there is a need to assess not only the accuracy of a forecasting method but also its performance implications.

For inventory management, we need to assess the effects of forecasting on inventory holdings and service, for a given inventory policy and demand distribution. The measures of these effects are examples of accuracy-implication metrics (Boylan and Syntetos 2006).

In short, forecasting methods may be evaluated using:

1. Accuracy measures, focusing on forecasting performance. Accuracy may be measured in terms of the ability to predict mean demand, or to predict the whole demand distribution.
2. Accuracy-implication measures, focusing on organisational performance.

The choice of forecasting method is not the only factor affecting these measures. The accuracy of demand prediction also depends on the choice of distribution. Organisational performance, in terms of inventory levels and service, depends on the forecasting method, choice of distribution, and selection of inventory policy.

Accuracy and accuracy-implication measures are both valuable. Accuracy-implication measures will be the main concern of a forecasting client, such as an operations manager. These measures will highlight to the client when some aspect of organisational performance is improving or declining. However, they will not show *why* the performance has improved or declined. If performance has worsened, is a decline in forecast accuracy one of the causes? If accuracy has declined, why has that happened? These are the main concerns of a forecasting analyst.

Accuracy measures are useful to the analyst in diagnosing why a forecasting method is not sufficiently accurate. For example, inappropriate forecasting methods may be used or

Intermittent Demand Forecasting: Context, Methods and Applications, First Edition.
John E. Boylan and Aris A. Syntetos.
© 2021 John Wiley & Sons Ltd. Published 2021 by John Wiley & Sons Ltd.
Companion Website: www.wiley.com/go/boylansyntetos/intermittentdemandforecasting

their parameters may be set wrongly. These are issues that will need to be addressed by the forecasting analyst.

In summary, although the principal audiences differ, the two types of measure are complementary. Client concerns over accuracy-implication measures can be addressed by analysts looking more closely at accuracy measures.

In this chapter, the main emphasis will be on the prediction of demand and the measurement of the accuracy of forecasts of mean demand. Later in the chapter, the focus shifts to the accuracy of predictions of whole demand distributions, and then on to accuracy-implication measures. Simulation evaluations are discussed, including some of the practicalities involved, before the chapter closes with a summary of conclusions.

9.2 Forecast Evaluation

In forecasting evaluations, it is common practice to measure the forecast accuracy of one-step-ahead forecasts at all points in time, and then to summarise these errors in some way. The most popular summary statistics will be investigated later in this chapter. Before doing so, there are more basic questions to be answered. Firstly, is it appropriate to focus only on one-step-ahead errors? Secondly, should the evaluation be for all points in time or only some?

9.2.1 Only One Step Ahead?

The answer to the first question has already been discussed in previous chapters but it is worth recapping the key points.

For inventory replenishment decisions in periodic systems, it is the forecast accuracy of the cumulative demand over the next $R + L$ periods that is important (and over the next L periods for continuous systems). This equates to the one-step-ahead forecast only if the protection interval is for a single period.

For the stock/non-stock decision, forecasts of mean demand are required over a fixed period of time (e.g. 12 months). This period is determined by the organisation to reflect their own policies on stock ranges. So, again, one-step-ahead accuracy is not sufficient. It is the accuracy of the mean demand forecast over the fixed period of time that is important.

9.2.2 All Points in Time?

In Chapter 2, periodic review systems were discussed. It was found that, if the review interval is of one period, and if forecasts cannot increase after a period of zero demand, then a replenishment will be triggered only if there has been some demand in the most recent period. If there has been no demand, then a forecast may be recalculated but it will not affect replenishment. (This is true for simple moving averages, single exponential smoothing (SES), Croston, and Syntetos-Boylan approximation (SBA). Exceptions include forecasts incorporating promotions, rarely modelled for intermittent demand.) Consequently, for all 'standard' intermittent forecasting methods, we should restrict our evaluations to forecasts made immediately after a demand occurrence.

If the review interval (R) is of two periods or longer then, as discussed in Chapter 2, the relevant forecasts, at the end of a review interval, relate to those intervals in which there has been some demand since the previous review. For example, suppose $R = 2$, and reviews are due at the end of Periods 2, 4, 6, 8, and 10. Suppose, further, that there were demands in only two of the last 10 time periods, in Periods 5 and 8. Then, we are not interested in evaluating forecasts at the end of Periods 2, 4, or 10, but we are interested in forecasts made at the completion of review intervals at the end of Periods 6 and 8. The latter is needed because of the depletion of stock in Period 8; the former is needed because of a depletion in Period 5.

If forecasts are to inform a stock/non-stock decision, then they may be required at any point in time relative to the last demand occurrence, as discussed in Chapter 2. So, in this case, we should evaluate forecast accuracy at all points in time.

9.2.3 Summary

In practice, the same forecasting methods are often used for a range of stock keeping units (SKUs) with varying review intervals and for both replenishment and stock/non-stock decisions. If this is the case, then we may evaluate the accuracy and organisational performance of forecasts at all points in time, and after periods preceded by at least one demand during the last review interval. Similarly, the accuracy over a variety of forecast horizons may be evaluated. This approach ensures that any choice of forecast method is not sensitive to the inventory application, and is robust in the sense of giving good forecasts in a wide range of situations.

9.3 Error Measures in Common Usage

In this section, we examine some of the most frequently adopted error measures for non-intermittent demand. In later sections, we assess their suitability for intermittent demand, using criteria established in Section 9.4.

9.3.1 Popular Forecast Error Measures

The following four measures are commonly used for non-intermittent demand:

1. *Mean error*: Assesses bias, taking into account the direction of errors, and measuring if forecasts have a tendency to be too high or too low on average.
2. *Mean square error*: Assesses the squared magnitude of errors, ignoring their direction, measuring the squared size of differences between forecasts and actual values.
3. *Mean absolute error*: Assesses the magnitudes of errors, ignoring their direction, measuring the average size of differences between forecasts and actual values.
4. *Mean absolute percentage error*: Assesses the magnitudes of errors as percentages of the actual values.

The formulae for these measures will follow later, in Sections 9.3.3–9.3.6. The first measure is based on errors, while the second is based on their squared values. Squared errors

Table 9.1 Mean error, mean square error, mean absolute error, and mean absolute percentage error.

Period	Actual demand	Forecast demand	Forecast error	Squared error	Absolute error	Absolute % error
1	71	71.0	0.0	0.0	0.0	0.0
2	100	76.0	24.0	576.0	24.0	24.0
3	72	95.4	−23.4	547.6	23.4	32.5
4	69	86.4	−17.4	302.8	17.4	25.2
5	85	80.9	4.1	16.8	4.1	4.8
6	73	88.4	−15.4	237.2	15.4	21.1
7	90	84.2	5.8	33.6	5.8	6.4
8	92	92.7	−0.7	0.5	0.7	0.8
9	81	97.3	−16.3	265.7	16.3	20.1
10	67	92.5	−25.5	650.2	25.5	38.1
Mean			−6.5	263.0	13.3	17.3

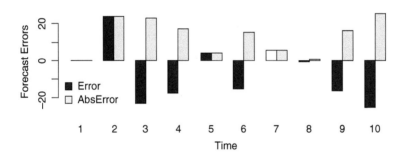

Figure 9.1 Errors and absolute ('Abs') errors.

turn out to be important for the development of classification rules for intermittence, and we return to them in Section 9.8. The third and fourth measures are based on absolute errors, and are often used in practice. To illustrate the application of the error measures given above, consider an example of actual values and one-step-ahead forecasts and their associated errors (Table 9.1).

In this example, in the first time period, the forecast matches the actual observation exactly, and so all error measures are zero. In other periods, if the error is positive it coincides with the absolute error (Periods 2, 5, and 7) but in the remaining periods (3, 4, 6, 8, 9, and 10) the error and absolute error differ (Figure 9.1). Therefore, the mean error (ME) (−6.5) and mean absolute error (MAE) (13.3), calculated over all 10 periods, also differ for this data. The mean absolute percentage error (MAPE) shows that the absolute errors are, on average, 17.3% of the actual observations.

9.3.2 Calculation of Forecast Errors

'Forecast Error' is calculated as: *Actual minus Forecast*. For example, in Period 2, *Error* = 100.0 − 76.0 = 24.0, and in Period 3, *Error* = 72.0 − 95.4 = −23.4. Some forecasters prefer that this should be calculated as: *Forecast minus Actual*. The relative merits of the two methods of calculating forecast error were discussed by Green and Tashman (2008). Those who favour taking forecast error to be *Forecast minus Actual* point out that it is more natural for over-forecasts to be shown as positive errors (e.g. for Period 3, *Error* = +23.4) and under-forecasts to be shown as negative errors (e.g. for Period 2, *Error* = −24.0). Those who favour the calculation of *Actual minus Forecast* contend that it is consistent with a model of the form: *Actual = Forecast + Error*. In Chapter 14, we shall use this form of model in our exploration of model-based methods. Consequently, we adopt the convention that forecast error is calculated as *Actual minus Forecast*.

To be more precise, we can define one-step-ahead forecast error as *Actual minus Forecast (One-Step-Ahead)*. Similar calculations can be made for two-step-ahead forecast errors or, indeed, for errors relating to any forecast horizon. The clarification of the forecast horizon is important. If forecast methods are to be compared, then consistent measures should be used. Otherwise, the results may be misleading because it is often more difficult to attain the same level of accuracy as the forecast horizon lengthens.

In inventory management, we are usually concerned with the error in forecasting cumulative demand over the whole protection interval, rather than the demand in a particular period during the protection interval. This forecast error, over a whole protection interval of length $R + L$ should be distinguished from the $(R + L)$-step-ahead error, which relates only to the final period during the protection interval. In this chapter, most definitions will be for one-step-ahead errors, but these formulae may be readily adapted to h-step-ahead errors ($h = 1, \ldots, R + L$), or to errors over the whole protection interval.

9.3.3 Mean Error

In the previous example, it can be seen from Table 9.1 that over-forecasts (negative errors) are more common than under-forecasts. There are only three under-forecasts and two of them have errors that are quite small. These considerations lead us to expect that the ME will show a tendency to over-forecast. The ME is calculated by totalling all the errors (−64.9 in this example) and dividing by the number of observations (10) to give a ME of −6.49, rounded to −6.5 in Table 9.1. This confirms and quantifies the tendency to over-forecast in a straightforward way. In general, if the calculation is based on N periods, then the ME for one-step-ahead forecasts can be expressed as in Eq. (9.1).

$$\text{ME} = \frac{1}{N} \sum_{t=1}^{N} (d_t - \hat{d}_{t|t-1}) \tag{9.1}$$

In Eq. (9.1), d_t represents the actual demand in Period t and $\hat{d}_{t|t-1}$ represents the one-step-ahead forecast demand for Period t made at the end of Period $t − 1$ (for example, $\hat{d}_{2|1}$ represents the forecast for Period 2, where the forecast was made at the end of Period 1).

9.3.4 Mean Square Error

For one-step-ahead forecast errors, the mean square error (MSE) is defined as in Eq. (9.2), which uses the same notation as the previous equation.

$$\text{MSE} = \frac{1}{N} \sum_{t=1}^{N} (d_t - \hat{d}_{t|t-1})^2 \tag{9.2}$$

Referring back to Table 9.1, we can see immediately that larger errors, for example in Periods 2 and 3, are penalised very heavily using this measure (with squared errors over 500), whereas smaller errors, for example in Period 5, are penalised much less heavily.

An additional measure, often used in practice, is the root mean square error (RMSE). This is calculated by taking the square root of the MSE. In the example in Table 9.1, the RMSE is 16.2 (the square root of 263.0). It has the advantage that it is measured in the same units as the original data, unlike the MSE, which is measured in squared units.

9.3.5 Mean Absolute Error

As already mentioned, the absolute error ignores the sign of the errors and treats all errors as positive. For example, in Period 3, the error of −23.4 is treated as a positive error, +23.4. This absolute error is written as $|-23.4| = 23.4$, where the vertical lines around the number −23.4 denote its 'absolute value'. This error magnitude may be expressed more informally by saying that the forecast for Period 3 is 'out by 23.4'.

The MAE is calculated as the average of all the individual absolute errors, in the same way that the ME is the average of the individual errors. In our example, the MAE is 13.3 (see Table 9.1). The one-step-ahead MAE is expressed in Eq. (9.3), using the same notation as before.

$$\text{MAE} = \frac{1}{N} \sum_{t=1}^{N} |d_t - \hat{d}_{t|t-1}| \tag{9.3}$$

The MAE is a natural measure for non-intermittent demand and one that is easier to explain to non-technical managers than more complex measures.

9.3.6 Mean Absolute Percentage Error (MAPE)

In the final column of Table 9.1, the MAE is shown to be 13.3. Is this a high value? It is difficult to say. One way we can address this question is by expressing the absolute errors as percentages of the actual values to give absolute percentage errors (APEs), as shown in the final column of Table 9.1. For example, the third forecast has an APE of 32.5%, as the absolute error of 23.4 is equal to 32.5% of the actual demand of 72.

The MAPE is calculated as the average of the APEs, as shown in Eq. (9.4), which is valid for strictly positive demands. (See Technical Note 9.1 for discussion of other situations.)

$$\text{MAPE} = \frac{1}{N} \sum_{t=1}^{N} \text{APE}_t = \frac{100}{N} \sum_{t=1}^{N} \frac{|d_t - \hat{d}_{t|t-1}|}{d_t} \tag{9.4}$$

In our example, this formula gives a MAPE of 17.3%, the average of the APEs, as shown in the bottom row of Table 9.1. Hyndman and Athanasopoulos (2020) pointed out that the

MAPE assumes the data to have a 'meaningful zero'. For example, temperatures may be measured in degrees Celsius or Fahrenheit, and the zeroes on these scales are relatively arbitrary. For demand data, the zero is not arbitrary and so percentage calculations are sensible.

The MAPE measure is quite intuitive and is easier to explain to non-technical managers than more sophisticated error measures. It has been adopted by many forecasting software packages, and so will often be encountered in practice.

9.3.7   100% Minus MAPE

In some companies, 100% minus MAPE is taken as a measure of forecast 'Accuracy' (e.g. if MAPE = 17.3%, then Accuracy = 82.7%). This measure is intuitive in some ways; for example, a MAPE of 0% gives Accuracy of 100%. However, an organisation may have erratically demanded SKUs with some forecast errors of magnitude greater than the actual values. This can occur if there are sudden dips in demand and may lead to MAPEs in excess of 100% and negative values of 'Accuracy'. One way of getting round this complication, employed in some organisations, is to replace negative Accuracy results with zeroes. If this is done, then there is no discrimination between MAPEs a little over 100% and those well over 100%.

There are some variants of this measure. Katti (2008) described a measure based on 100% minus APE, which suffers from the problem of APEs in excess of 100%. Gilliland (2010) proposed a different calculation, with the maximum of the forecast and the actual in the denominator, guaranteeing that the Accuracy measure never generates negative results. However, there are problems with replacing the actual by the forecast in the denominator, as will be explained later in this chapter.

Measures based on subtracting an error statistic from 100% do have some advantages. It is arguably more motivating for a demand planner to be aiming to improve an Accuracy measure from 85% to 90% than to reduce MAPE from 15% to 10%. Such measures are often used for management reporting because they are thought to be easy to comprehend. Nevertheless, their interpretation is not necessarily straightforward, especially for erratically demanded products, which are prone to the complications mentioned above. For intermittent demand, there are further difficulties, not least of which is the calculation of APEs, to be discussed in Section 9.5.

9.3.8   Forecast Value Added

Gilliland (2010) introduced a simple, yet powerful, way of presenting forecast accuracy results. He defined FVA (forecast value added) as follows: 'The change in a forecasting performance metric that can be attributed to a particular step or participant in the forecasting process' (Gilliland 2010, p. 82). Suppose that a company's system generates a statistical forecast, which is subject to revision by a forecasting analyst, and may be revised again by a supply chain executive to give the final forecast. Then, the impact of these revisions on the overall MAPE (averaged across all SKUs that have been subject to some revision) can be tabulated, as shown in the example in Table 9.2.

This tabular presentation immediately reveals that the analyst revision step is adding value but the final step of executive revision is actually taking away some of the value added

Table 9.2 Forecast value added (FVA) example.

Process step	MAPE (%)	FVA vs. system (%)	FVA vs. analyst (%)
System forecast	30		
Analyst revised forecast	20	10	
Executive final forecast	25	5	−5

Source: Adapted from Gilliland (2010).

by the analyst. Gilliland (2010) pointed out that if such value-subtracting steps can be identified, then companies can improve their forecasting for free, simply by eliminating that step in the process.

The power of the FVA approach is that it is not restricted to any particular error measure (e.g. MAPE). It can be based on any accuracy measure that is appropriate to the business needs of an organisation. Furthermore, the approach is not limited to judgemental revision. It can also be used to compare the current statistical method with other statistical methods being considered for introduction. These methods may be simpler or more complex, and can be presented in ascending order of complexity to ensure that any additional complications in methods are generating accuracy improvements.

9.3.9 Summary

For non-intermittent demand, the ME, MAE, and MAPE are all useful measures of forecast accuracy. They may be applied to one-step-ahead forecasts, h-step-ahead forecasts (for any forecast horizon, h), or to forecasts of cumulative demand over the whole protection interval. They are quite intuitive, straightforward to calculate, and are often provided as summary error measures by commercial software packages. The MSE measure is less robust to outliers but, as will be seen later, is useful in establishing theoretical properties. Detailed analysis of the value being added or subtracted by various steps in the forecasting process can help to identify those steps that should be removed.

9.4 Criteria for Error Measures

Once an error measure has been accepted, different forecasting methods can be compared. But how should error measures themselves be compared? Davydenko and Fildes (2013) highlighted the following criteria: (1) interpretability, (2) robustness to outliers, and (3) scale independence. These criteria have general applicability, for intermittent and non-intermittent series alike, and are described in Section 9.4.1.

9.4.1 General Criteria

1. *Interpretability*: The measures discussed in Section 9.3 have quite natural interpretations, which make them readily communicable to non-technical managers. This improves the chances that appropriate corrective actions will be taken in the event of a deterioration of forecast accuracy. Not all error measures are so easy to interpret.

2. *Robustness to outliers*: An 'outlier' is an observation that is highly atypical, either because it is very high or very low. Such observations are often associated with large forecast errors and a summary error measure should be robust to these outliers in the sense of not being unduly affected by them. The MSE is not as robust to outlying observations as the MAE, the ME, or the MAPE.

3. *Scale independence*: A measure is scale independent if it is not affected by a change in the scale of the data. Fildes (1992) commented that scale dependence is a serious weakness in a business setting because the units of measurement are often arbitrary. For example, if products are sold in packs of 10, then a scale-dependent accuracy measure will be affected by the decision to record sales in terms of packs or in terms of units within a pack. If an error measure is unaffected by a change of scale, then it is said to be scale independent. The ME and MAE are not scale independent because they are measured on the same scale as the data. The MAPE, on the other hand, is scale independent because the errors are summarised relative to actual demand. This makes it better suited to measuring the average error across many different series, some of which may have demand volumes in the thousands, others in the hundreds, and yet others in tens or units.

9.4.2 Additional Criteria for Intermittence

There are two additional requirements to be added for intermittent series, giving five criteria in all. The fourth applies only to intermittence. The fifth is of general applicability but is particularly important for intermittent demand.

4. *Discrimination at zeroes*: An error measure should be able to discriminate between the accuracy of different forecasting methods when the actual demands are zero. This criterion is not satisfied by some error measures that are in common usage.

5. *Minimisation by appropriate functional*: A final requirement is that an error measure should be minimised by the functional we are seeking to estimate. (A statistical functional is a single number derived from a function or distribution, such as the expected value of the future demand distribution.) For example, the MSE is minimised by the expected (mean) value, making the MSE suitable if it is the mean we are seeking to predict. As we shall see later, some error measures are minimised by the median. This is appropriate if the median demand is being estimated but inappropriate if the mean demand is of interest and it differs from the median.

9.4.3 Summary

We have given five criteria that should be satisfied by error measures for intermittent demand. These criteria are challenging, and we shall see that many of the error measures for intermittence are found wanting when judged against them.

9.5 Mean Absolute Percentage Error and its Variants

The MAPE is a popular error measure but is it relevant for intermittent demand? In this section, we examine the MAPE and its variants, highlighting their limitations for intermittent demand. We return to the ME and MAE measures in later sections.

9.5.1 Problems with the Mean Absolute Percentage Error

The MAPE is an intuitive measure, as discussed earlier. It is robust to outlying high demand values because the actual demand is in the denominator, but less so to outlying low values. It is scale independent: any change of scale affects the numerator and denominator equally, thus cancelling out and leaving the MAPE measure unchanged.

Problems with the MAPE measure arise when there are zero actual demand values. If the absolute error is 2 and the actual value is 10, then the APE is 20%; but what if the absolute error is 2 and the actual value is 0? In this case, it makes no sense to divide 2 by 0, because there is no number, when multiplied by 0, that will give 2 as the answer. So, for intermittent demand, APE cannot be calculated if the actual demand is 0.

By definition, an intermittent demand series must contain at least one zero observation. Referring back to Eq. (9.4), we must have $d_t = 0$ for at least one time period between $t = 1$ and $t = N$. Therefore, for a forecast horizon of one period, we cannot calculate the MAPE because at least one of the observations will have an APE that cannot be calculated. For longer forecast horizons, there will be fewer zero cumulative demands, but no guarantee that all of the cumulative values will be non-zero. Hoover (2006) found that some software packages were reporting MAPEs for intermittent demand by ignoring the time periods when the actual demand is zero. This is a flawed approach as it fails to discriminate between the accuracy of different methods for periods of zero demand. In the study of Willemain et al. (1994), an adapted MAPE was used, whereby the absolute errors are summed and divided by the total demand (T.R. Willemain, personal communication). This is equivalent to the MAE to mean ratio, to be discussed in Section 9.6.1.

9.5.2 Mean Absolute Percentage Error from Forecast

The mean absolute percentage error from forecast (MAPEFF) is an alternative error metric to the MAPE. It alters the MAPE formula by replacing the actual demand by the forecasted demand in the denominator, to give an average 'absolute percentage error from forecast (APEFF)'. The MAPEFF is defined as in Eq. (9.5) for strictly positive one-step-ahead demand forecasts.

$$\text{MAPEFF} = \frac{100}{N} \sum_{t=1}^{N} \frac{|d_t - \hat{d}_{t|t-1}|}{\hat{d}_{t|t-1}} \tag{9.5}$$

Some organisations subtract the MAPEFF from 100% and use this as an accuracy measure. This suffers from the same problems as subtracting MAPE from 100%, discussed earlier.

Kahn (1998) surveyed 40 sales forecasting managers, mainly (75%) from consumer product firms. He found that 14 used the MAPE alone, 10 used the MAPEFF alone, and 2 used both MAPE and MAPEFF. Fildes and Goodwin (2007) noted that two of the companies in their study used a version of the MAPEFF in their software. Green and Tashman (2009) surveyed forecasting discussion-list participants and practitioner journal subscribers. They found that 15% of their 61 respondents thought it is better to use the forecast value in the denominator than the actual value.

Pearson and Wallace (1999) gave the most cogent justification for measures based on 'errors from forecast'. They argued that, while mathematical properties should be taken into account, it is the context of application that should lead the choice of error metric. They pointed out that 'percentage errors from forecast' are intuitive to decision makers and answer the natural question of how well the organisation has done relative to its plan. Of course, when the actual has been realised, it can be helpful to review the 'error from forecast', especially if there are actions that can be taken to influence future actual values (e.g. promotions or discounts). However, if the forecast has been adopted as a plan, then it may be more appropriate to refer to the 'deviation from plan', rather than the 'error from forecast'. Sharpening the terminology may dispel some confusion. Assessing and correcting deviations from plan is an important management activity but is quite distinct from measuring and correcting forecast errors.

In terms of its properties, the MAPEFF measure is scale independent, but less robust than the MAPE to outlying high demand values, unanticipated by the forecast. The MAPEFF lacks a common base in the denominator for comparison of forecasting methods. Suppose the actual demand is 10. Then a method with a higher forecast (e.g. 15) will contribute towards a lower MAPEFF than another method with a lower forecast (e.g. five) even though the absolute errors are the same. As we shall see later, it cannot be recommended for intermittent demand because of its lack of sensitivity to errors when the actuals are zero.

9.5.3 Symmetric Mean Absolute Percentage Error

A further alternative measure to the MAPE is the symmetric mean absolute percentage error (sMAPE). This measure was originally introduced by Armstrong (1985) but was not widely known until it was advocated by Makridakis (1993) and subsequently used in the M3 forecasting competition (Makridakis and Hibon 2000), which did not include intermittent time series.

The sMAPE is defined as follows. The symmetric absolute percentage error (sAPE) is calculated as the ratio of two quantities: (i) absolute error and (ii) average of the actual demand and the forecasted demand. These ratios are calculated for all periods and then averaged to give the sMAPE, as shown in Eq. (9.6) for one-step-ahead demand forecasts.

$$\text{sMAPE} = \frac{100}{N} \sum_{t=1}^{N} \frac{|d_t - \hat{d}_{t|t-1}|}{(d_t + \hat{d}_{t|t-1})/2} \tag{9.6}$$

An alternative formulation, which gets around problems of calculation for negative demands and negative forecasts, is given in Technical Note 9.1. This situation can occur if demands are adjusted by returns. If all demands are non-negative, and all forecasts are strictly positive, then these issues do not arise.

The sMAPE is symmetric in that swapping the values of each of the actual demands and forecasted demands will leave the sMAPE unchanged. For example, if the actual demand is 8, a forecast of 12 gives a sAPE of 4/10 (40.0%), and we would get the same result if the demand is 12 and the forecast is 8, but the APEs would differ (4/8 = 50.0% and 4/12 ≈ 33.3% for the two cases). Therefore, the MAPE is not symmetric in this sense. On the other hand, the sMAPE is not symmetric in its treatment of positive and negative errors (Goodwin and Lawton 1999). For example, if the actual demand is 8, a forecast of 4 gives a sAPE of 4/6 ≈ 66.7%, which differs from the 40.0% value for a forecast of 12. However, this issue does not affect the MAPE. In our example, the APE is 50% in both cases.

The sMAPE is not difficult to explain to non-specialists. It is robust to outlying demand values, providing that these observations are strictly positive, and is scale independent. Like the MAPEFF, the sMAPE lacks a common base in the denominator. Notwithstanding its limitations, the sMAPE has continued to be a popular measure and was used in the M4 Forecasting Competition (Makridakis et al. 2018).

9.5.4 MAPEFF and sMAPE for Intermittent Demand

The MAPEFF and sMAPE measures, as shown in Eqs. (9.5) and (9.6), are defined for series with zero demand periods, provided that none of the corresponding forecasts are zero. These summary measures are shown in the bottom row of Table 9.3.

In Table 9.3, all of the zero actual demands show 100% for the APEFF, and 200% for the sAPE, even though the forecasts are not the same for all zero observations. In fact, when the demand is zero, the APEFF will always be 100% and the sAPE will always be 200% (Syntetos 2001), no matter what (non-zero) value is taken by the forecast.

The insensitivity of the two measures to forecast values, when actual demands are zero, presents some difficulties. Firstly, neither of the measures will detect highly erroneous forecasts. Suppose we made a mistake and entered a forecast of 2.5 as 2500, and the actual value transpired to be zero. Then, the calculations for the two error measures would continue to return 100% and 200%, failing to alert us to the mistake. Secondly, the measures are effective in comparing forecasting accuracy on the non-zero actual values only. If one forecasting method is less accurate than another when the actuals are zero, this will not be identified by the MAPEFF or the sMAPE. Thus, these measures do not offer discrimination between forecast methods when the demand is zero.

A further measure, based on a function of absolute percentage errors, was proposed by Kim and Kim (2016), called the mean arctangent absolute percentage error (MAAPE). It measures forecast errors in terms of angles instead of ratios and, consequently, is less interpretable than the MAPE. It does not discriminate between forecasts when the actual values are zero, always returning the same result in this case. (See Technical Note 9.2 for the MAAPE formula and a more detailed discussion.)

Table 9.3 MAPEFF and sMAPE for intermittent demand.

Period	Actual demand	Forecast demand	Forecast error	Absolute error	APEFF (%)	sAPE (%)
1	0	2.5	−2.5	2.5	100	200
2	10	2.4	7.6	7.6	317	123
3	0	3.3	−3.3	3.3	100	200
4	0	3.1	−3.1	3.1	100	200
5	5	3.2	1.8	1.8	56	44
6	0	3.0	−3.0	3.0	100	200
7	1	2.4	−1.4	1.4	54	82
Mean					119	150

9.5.5 Summary

The MAPE, MAPEFF, and sMAPE error measures are robust to outliers and are scale independent. They also have the advantage of being easy to explain to non-specialists. However, none of the measures can discriminate between the accuracy of forecasting methods when the actual demands are zero. The MAPE cannot even be calculated. The MAPE from forecast and the sMAPE always return the same error values (100% and 200% respectively) for zero demands, regardless of the forecast values.

9.6 Measures Based on the Mean Absolute Error

In Section 9.5, we reviewed scale-independent error measures that fail to discriminate between forecast methods when the actual values are zero. In this section, we examine other approaches to making the MAE measure scale independent but, at the same time, satisfy the criterion of discrimination at zero values.

9.6.1 MAE : Mean Ratio

The MAE can be made scale-independent by dividing it by the mean demand, as recommended by Hoover (2006) and Kolassa and Schütz (2007). This is known as the MAE : Mean ratio, or the MAD : Mean ratio (where MAD stands for mean absolute deviation, another name for the MAE). An example is given in Table 9.4, which summarises the mean demands, MAEs, and MAE : Mean ratios for five SKUs.

Table 9.4 shows that the overall average of the MAEs, 6.4, overstates the typical MAE, which is no greater than three, because of a particularly large MAE for SKU A. This MAE, at 25.0, appears large in comparison to the other SKUs only because the mean demand for the series, 50, is much larger than the others. When expressed as a ratio, in the final column, the value of 0.5 does not seem out of keeping with the other series. The average of the MAE : Mean ratios, 0.453, is a better reflection of the overall performance of the forecasting method on these five series.

Table 9.4 MAE : Mean ratios for multiple series.

SKU	Mean demand	Mean absolute error (MAE)	MAE : Mean ratio
A	50	25.0	0.500
B	5	3.0	0.600
C	6	2.0	0.333
D	2	1.0	0.500
E	3	1.0	0.333
Average		6.4	0.453

The formula for the MAE : Mean ratio, for one-step-ahead forecasts for an individual series, is given in Eq. (9.7).

$$\text{MAE : Mean} = \frac{\frac{1}{N}\sum_{t=1}^{N}|d_t - \hat{d}_{t|t-1}|}{\frac{1}{N}\sum_{t=1}^{N}d_t} \tag{9.7}$$

This measure is defined for any series with at least one non-zero demand. Unlike the MAPEFF and the sMAPE, it does discriminate between methods' accuracy when the actual values are zero. Because the $1/N$ factors cancel in Eq. (9.7), the MAE : Mean ratio is the same as the adapted form of MAPE used by Willemain et al. (1994), mentioned earlier.

Kolassa and Schütz (2007) noted that the MAE : Mean ratio works well for series which are not intermittent but have occasional values close to zero. Suppose that demand is usually between 10 and 20 units per period and suddenly drops to one. An error of five would yield an APE of 500%, whereas the MAE : Mean ratio would be much less sensitive. Kolassa and Schütz (2007) also pointed out that the MAE : Mean ratio can be interpreted as a weighted analogue of the MAPE because it is a weighted average of the APEs, where each APE is weighted by the actual value.

9.6.2 Mean Absolute Scaled Error

Another approach to measuring forecast error is based on a comparison of a method's accuracy with that of the naive method. The naive method is one of the simplest forecasting methods: it takes the next forecast to be the last actual demand. So, if the last demand was 10, then the forecast for the next period's demand is also 10. The naive method is rarely favoured by demand planners, when forecasting at the level of the individual SKU. However, it is often nominated as a benchmark method, on the grounds that a good forecast method should be able to outperform it.

The mean absolute scaled error (MASE) was introduced by Hyndman and Koehler (2006) and recommended by Hyndman (2006) for intermittent demand. To calculate it, we first define in-sample and out-of-sample periods. For example, with 60 periods of data, we may define the first $n = 48$ periods to be in-sample and the last 12 periods to be out-of-sample. The out-of-sample forecast error is calculated for the method and period we wish to evaluate; this is then divided by the in-sample MAE for the naive method.

The formula for the scaled error for period t is given in Eq. (9.8).

$$q_t = \frac{e_t}{\frac{1}{n-1}\sum_{i=2}^{n}|d_i - d_{i-1}|} \tag{9.8}$$

In Eq. (9.8), n represents the length of the in-sample period and t is strictly greater than n to ensure that it is in the out-of-sample period. The average absolute error in the denominator takes into account $n - 1$ absolute errors, from the first naive error at $i = 2$ to the naive error at $i = n$, and is averaged accordingly by dividing by $n - 1$. (A naive forecast cannot be calculated for $i = 1$ if the demand is not known for $i = 0$.) The scaled error is a scale-independent measure. Its absolute value may be averaged over out-of-sample periods, or over a number of series, or both, to give the MASE (Hyndman and Koehler 2006), as shown in Eq. (9.9).

$$MASE = mean(|q_t|) \tag{9.9}$$

The MASE has become a well-established error metric and was used in the calculation of one of the measures employed in the M4 Competition (Makridakis et al. 2018). This competition, like its predecessors, did not include intermittent series.

9.6.3 Measures Based on Absolute Errors

The measures summarised above are based on absolute errors. Wallström and Segerstedt (2010) noticed that minimisation of the MAE resulted in intermittent demand forecasts that tended to be too low, and could even be zero. This was analysed further by Morlidge (2015) who looked at ratio error measures that have the MAE in the numerator. He identified a 'numerator problem', so called to distinguish it from the issues arising from zeroes in the denominator.

The numerator problem is shown most clearly by ignoring the denominator for the moment and examining the MAE by itself. The MAE has the same interpretation for intermittent demand as for non-intermittent demand. It represents the average magnitude of errors between the actual and forecasted values. It is calculated (for one-step-ahead forecasts) using Eq. (9.3). Caution is needed when relying on this measure for intermittent demand forecasting. To illustrate why, we look at the same data as in Table 9.3 but, this time, we compare the previous forecasts with zero forecasts, as shown in Table 9.5. This is done to check if the error measure detects that zero forecasts are of no value for inventory control (Teunter and Duncan 2009).

While the previous forecasts, which ranged from 2.4 to 3.3, may not have been ideal, common sense tells us that it is better than forecasting zero every period. Yet the MAE is reduced from 3.2 to 2.3 by changing to the zero forecast method. Why is this? A closer look at Table 9.5 shows that whenever demand is zero (which happens in four of the seven time

Table 9.5 Mean absolute error for zero forecasts.

Period	Actual demand	Previous forecast	Absolute error	Zero forecast	Absolute error
1	0	2.5	2.5	0	0.0
2	10	2.4	7.6	0	10.0
3	0	3.3	3.3	0	0.0
4	0	3.1	3.1	0	0.0
5	5	3.2	1.8	0	5.0
6	0	3.0	3.0	0	0.0
7	1	2.4	1.4	0	1.0
Mean		2.8	3.2	0	2.3

periods in our example) the zero forecast method has no error, and this pulls down the MAE. So, according to the MAE measure, the zero forecasts are more accurate.

At this point, it is important to highlight the difference between the mean demand and the median demand. The sample median demand is calculated by putting all the demand values in order, from lowest to highest, and finding the middle value. In our example, the middle value of the seven observations (0, 0, 0, 0, 1, 5, 10) is the fourth value, which is zero. The sample mean, on the other hand, is 2.3, which is the same as the MAE (because the absolute error column is identical to the actual demand column in Table 9.5). In this case, the sample median demand of zero is quite different from the sample mean demand of 2.3.

Morlidge (2015) noted that the MAE is not minimised by the best forecast of mean demand. Rather, it is minimised by the best forecast of median demand. (A neat visual explanation of why absolute deviations are minimised by the median was given by Hanley et al. (2001).) For symmetrically distributed demand (for example, following the normal distribution), no issues arise because the mean and the median are identical. For intermittent demand, these quantities may be very different, as in our example. Therefore, it should be no surprise that the MAE is minimised by the zero forecast method. In fact, this will always be true when a majority of the observations are zero.

The organisational implications of adopting a zero forecast would be serious. For example, if demand is represented by the Poisson distribution, then a forecasted mean of zero would also result in a zero order-up-to level. In this case, zero forecasts will translate to zero stock requirements. Then, all demand will be unmet after stocks have been exhausted. Of course, if we have already decided that an item is obsolete, then this would be desirable. But, if not, it makes no sense to stop replenishing stocks. So, in this case, the consequence of the MAE not being minimised by the appropriate functional (the mean demand) is that inventories will not align with organisational goals. To base inventory decisions on forecasts that optimise MAE would be unwise for intermittent demand items.

9.6.4 Summary

For non-intermittent demand, measures based on absolute errors are readily interpretable, and robust to outliers. They can be made scale-independent by scaling relative to mean demand or by the average of the in-sample absolute errors from the naive method.

The MAE : Mean ratio and the MASE both discriminate between forecast methods at zero values. However, neither measure is minimised by the mean demand because the MAE is minimised by the median. This can be problematical for intermittent demand items, for which the mean and median demands may differ quite markedly.

There are two possible remedies to this problem. The first is to complement measures based on absolute errors with bias measures, discussed in Section 9.7. The second approach is to abandon absolute measures and to use measures based on squared errors, to be discussed in Section 9.8.

9.7 Measures Based on the Mean Error

The zero forecast method, discussed in Section 9.6, is a prime example of a biased forecasting method. For intermittent demand, it sometimes under-forecasts (when demand is not zero), and it sometimes forecasts correctly (when demand is zero), but it never over-forecasts. It is unbiased only if all observations are zero. A tendency to under- or over-forecast is not always so easy to detect. In this section, we review some measures that have been designed to identify forecast bias, and discuss their application to intermittent demand.

9.7.1 Desirability of Unbiased Forecasts

Suppose that a forecasting method consistently underestimates the mean demand (the ME is positive) and another method consistently overestimates the mean demand by the same amount (the ME is negative). The implications of the same error in different directions would be very different. In the former case, the underestimation would potentially lead to an out-of-stock situation whereas, in the latter case, the error would result in over-stocking. As already discussed in this book, the backlog cost would typically be (considerably) higher than the inventory holding cost, which means that we would prefer (from a cost perspective) an upwardly biased estimator to a downwardly biased one. This may prompt the question of whether we should prefer a positively biased forecast to an unbiased one. The answer is no. If stockout costs are increasing relative to inventory holding costs, then this should be reflected by an increased service level target (e.g. from 95% to 97.5%) rather than by keeping the target at 95% and deliberately biasing the forecast upwards. Unbiased forecasts are still required, and we need to be able to measure forecast bias to ensure that our methods are unbiased.

9.7.2 Mean Error

The ME was described in Section 9.3.3. For an individual SKU, it is the average of all the forecast errors, with each error retaining its original sign, whether positive or negative. For methods based on size-interval ratios, such as Croston's method, it is important to measure forecast errors in the conventional way, as the differences between actual demands and forecasts. Measures based on comparing the latest forecast with the latest demand size to demand interval ratio are invalid as bias metrics for mean (intermittent) demand forecasts (Boylan and Syntetos 2007).

Like the MAE, the ME is always defined for intermittent demand series. Returning to our example, it is interesting to note the differences in MEs and MAEs between the original forecasts and the zero forecasts (Table 9.5), as summarised in Table 9.6 (to two decimal places).

It is immediately apparent from Table 9.6 that, although zero forecasts have a lower MAE than the original method, they are much worse with respect to the ME. Therefore,

Table 9.6 Mean error (ME) and mean absolute error (MAE).

	ME	MAE
Original forecast	−0.56	3.24
Zero forecast	2.29	2.29

an examination of a bias measure gives a different perspective on the performance of the two forecasting methods.

9.7.3 Mean Percentage Error

For non-intermittent demand series, there is a simple measure to capture the extent of the bias, as a proportion of the actual values, known as the mean percentage error (MPE). It is calculated in the same way as the MAPE except that it is expressed as an average of the percentage errors, rather than the APEs. Each percentage error is the ratio of the forecast error (retaining the original sign) to the actual demand.

For intermittent demand, the percentage error cannot be calculated for any of the zero observations of actual demand. By definition, an intermittent demand series must contain at least one zero observation. So, by the same reasoning as before, we cannot calculate the MPE for a forecast of demand over one period; nor can it be guaranteed that the MPE can be calculated for cumulative demand over longer forecast horizons.

9.7.4 Scaled Bias Measures

The ME can be made scale independent in a similar way to the MAE, by dividing by the mean demand. The calculations are shown in Table 9.7.

In Table 9.7, the absolute value of the ME (|ME|) is divided by the mean demand, for each SKU. This enables the magnitude of the forecast bias to be quantified, regardless of whether it is positive or negative for an individual series. The ratios, as shown in the final column of Table 9.7, are averaged to give the scaled ME, which is 0.193 in our example. If the scaled ME is high, this signals a problem with under- or over-forecasting, and warrants further investigation. Considering the MAE : Mean ratio and scaled ME together enables a more informed comparison of forecasting methods for intermittent demand.

It is also possible to adapt the MASE to be based on forecast errors, rather than absolute errors. For an individual series, the scaled error is calculated as before (see Eq. (9.8)). Then, the mean of the scaled errors is found, instead of the mean of the absolute scaled errors. This can complement the MASE in a similar way that the scaled ME can complement the MAE : Mean ratio.

Table 9.7 Scaled mean error for multiple series.

SKU	Mean demand	Mean error	|ME|	|ME| : Mean ratio
A	50	5.0	5.0	0.100
B	5	−1.0	1.0	0.200
C	6	−2.0	2.0	0.333
D	2	0.0	0.0	0.000
E	3	1.0	1.0	0.333
Average			1.8	0.193

The scaled ME shows the degree of bias, regardless of whether it arises from over-forecasting or under-forecasting. There are other measures that characterise the tendency towards negative or positive bias. Simple measures are the percentages of series with positive and negative bias, although these percentages do not capture the degree of bias. Alternatively, the calculations in Table 9.7 could be performed based on averaging the ratios of ME to mean demand, without taking absolute values of ME. This gives an indication of the overall tendency towards negative or positive forecast bias.

9.7.5 Summary

The ME gives a different view of forecast performance from the MAE. This is valuable for all demand classes but especially so for intermittent demand, for which the MAE may give a misleading impression.

One approach to error evaluation for an individual intermittent series is to examine both the MAE and the ME. If the MAE is low but the ME is high in proportion to it, then the forecasting method may be inappropriate. For multiple series, both the MAE : Mean ratio and the scaled ME may be examined in a similar way to identify weaknesses in forecasting methods.

Using two error measures is useful for diagnosing the reasons for problems with forecasts, but complicates the ranking of forecast methods, which is simpler if a single error measure is used. However, neither MAE nor ME based measures should be used on their own for assessing the accuracy of intermittent demand forecasts. In Section 9.8, further error measures are investigated to assess their suitability when used on their own.

9.8 Measures Based on the Mean Square Error

The MSE has some attractive properties. Firstly, it is minimised by the mean demand (unlike the MAE) and, secondly, it can be decomposed into components relating to forecast bias and forecast variance. The first property is illustrated by re-evaluating the data in Table 9.5. The original method is clearly better at forecasting the mean demand, which is reflected by this method having a lower MSE, of 14.1, than the zero forecast method, with an MSE of 18.0. (MSE calculations are based on Eq. (9.2) and follow the same procedure as in Table 9.1.) The second property, relating to the decomposition of the MSE, will be discussed in detail in the next chapter.

For real-world demand data, the MSE does have some limitations. For an individual series, it can be dominated by one large error arising from an outlier. For example, if forecast errors are usually no greater than 10 in magnitude, then the squared errors will be no greater than 100. If an outlying observation generates a forecast error of 50, then the squared error will be 2500, swamping all other squared errors. Similar difficulties arise, even in the absence of outliers, when a small number of series have squared errors that dominate those of all other series. For example, in an investigation of the results of a major forecasting competition, Chatfield (1988) found that a handful of the 1001 series dominated the calculation of the overall average MSE, leading to potentially misleading findings.

In the following subsections, we take a look at two scale-independent measures based on the MSE, which are designed to be more robust to outlying errors within a series, and less sensitive to a small number of series dominating the overall error measure.

9.8.1 Scaled Mean Square Error

Petropoulos and Kourentzes (2015) proposed a scaled version of the MSE, which is based on the scaled square error, calculated as in Eq. (9.10) for an h-step-ahead-forecast (sSE_h).

$$sSE_h = \left(\frac{d_{t+h} - \hat{d}_{t+h|t}}{\frac{1}{t}\sum_{j=1}^{t} d_j} \right)^2 \tag{9.10}$$

This measure can be used for any forecast horizon (including one-step-ahead, $h = 1$), where it is assumed that the forecasts are made using actual demand data up to, and including, time t.

Petropoulos and Kourentzes (2015) suggested the calculation of a scaled mean square error (sMSE) measure by averaging the scaled square errors across all horizons and series. The sMSE has the advantage that it is not only scale-independent but is also based on the MSE, which has a bias component within it, as will be discussed in Chapter 10.

9.8.2 Relative Root Mean Square Error

Instead of scaling an error measure by the mean demand, another approach is to scale by the same error measure using a different forecasting method. For example, we could calculate, for an individual series, the MAE of method A (the method of interest) to the MAE of method B (a benchmark method). This would not be advisable for intermittent demand because of the problems that arise from using absolute errors, discussed earlier. An alternative would be to calculate the ratio of MSEs or RMSEs. The ratio of RMSEs of method A to method B is defined as in Eq. (9.11) for h-step-ahead forecasts:

$$\frac{RMSE_{A,h}}{RMSE_{B,h}} = \frac{\sqrt{MSE_{A,h}}}{\sqrt{MSE_{B,h}}} \tag{9.11}$$

where the MSE is defined as in Eq. (9.2) but with the one-step-ahead forecast, $\hat{d}_{t|t-1}$ being replaced by the h-step-ahead forecast, $\hat{d}_{t|t-h}$.

This ratio measure is scale independent and is less sensitive to outlying observations in a series than the RMSE itself. The ratios of RMSEs can be averaged across all series to give an overall measure. An alternative approach is to calculate measures based on geometric means. The geometric mean is calculated by multiplying n numbers together, and then taking the nth root. For example, the geometric mean of 2, 2, and 16 is the third (cube) root of 64, which is 4.

Fildes (1992) proposed taking the geometric means of the squared errors for methods A and B, and then using their ratio as a relative error measure; this removes sensitivity to outliers if their effect is multiplicative. This relative measure was used by Syntetos and Boylan (2005) in their evaluation of intermittent demand forecasts. Although the measure worked well in this case, it collapses to zero if only one of the forecast errors is zero. This means that the measure lacks generality (Boylan and Syntetos 2006) and is problematic for assessing accuracy on intermittent demand data (Hyndman 2006).

The ratios of RMSEs can be averaged across all series to give an overall measure. Alternatively, the RMSE ratios can be summarised using a geometric mean across series. In this case, the measure would collapse to zero only if at least one of the series were forecasted perfectly for all observations, giving an RMSE of zero. Whilst this is possible, it becomes more unlikely to occur in practice as the length of errors (per series) increases.

9.8.3 Percentage Best

A simple method of avoiding the difficulties of scale dependence, recommended by Syntetos and Boylan (2005), is to compare the accuracy of a set of forecasting methods and identify which method is most accurate for the highest number of demand series. To use this approach, we firstly need to agree upon the criterion by which one method is said to be more accurate than another. For example, the MSE, or sMSE, can be used for this purpose (although the approach will work for any measure). Then, we need to agree on the methods to evaluate. Suppose we wish to compare three forecasting methods (called A, B, and C) using the MSE as our accuracy measure.

For each demand series, we calculate the MSE of each of the methods and identify which method has the lowest MSE. This is taken to be the 'best' method for that series. Having done this for all series, we can then summarise the percentage of series for which each method is the best. For any measure, not just MSE, a convention needs to be established regarding the inclusion or exclusion of series with ties between methods (Boylan 2005).

A weakness of this approach, however, is that it does not quantify the degree of improvement in accuracy that would be obtained by choosing one method instead of another. For example, it is possible that when method A 'wins', it does so by only a small margin, whereas when method B 'wins', it does so by a large margin. If this is the case, then it is no longer obvious that method A is a better choice than method B, even though it 'wins' for more demand series.

The 'percentage best' approach can be used in conjunction with scale-independent measures such as the sMSE. This will then give an indication of overall performance of a forecasting method as well as the proportion of series best forecasted by that method. If a 'percentage best' analysis reveals some common properties amongst the series for which a particular method 'wins', then this may suggest a classification of SKUs to guide the choice of forecasting method. More formal approaches to SKU classification will be discussed in Chapter 11.

9.8.4 Summary

When assessing the accuracy of intermittent demand forecasting methods across multiple series, scale independent measures are needed to avoid the problem of a small number of series dominating the overall measure. One such metric is the sMSE, which is a promising accuracy measure for intermittent demand forecasting. It does not need a complementary measure, and is straightforward to calculate. This measure, and other scale-independent measures, can be summarised by their averages across multiple series, or in terms of the percentage of series for which a method produces the most accurate forecasts.

9.9 Accuracy of Predictive Distributions

So far in this chapter, we have focussed on the accuracy of point forecasts of expected demand. These are single number forecasts, denoted by $\hat{d}_{t|t-1}$ for the one-step-ahead forecasts of Period t made at the end of Period $t - 1$. These forecasts are essential for stock/non-stock decisions and in estimating the mean of common predictive distributions such as the Poisson or negative binomial. Although good point forecasts of expected values may be necessary for good demand distribution forecasts, they are not sufficient, even if the mean forecast is unbiased. This may be because the variance estimate is poor, or we may have chosen an entirely inappropriate probability distribution.

In this section, we concentrate on the measurement of the accuracy of the whole predictive distribution, as recommended by Willemain (2006) and Snyder et al. (2012). In Chapter 5, we discussed some of the issues in assessing the goodness of fit of demand distributions. Given a history of, say, 24 months, the question was how well the proposed distribution fitted the historical demand data, where that data was used to estimate the parameters of the distribution. In this chapter, we are asking a different question: how well does a proposed distribution fit future demand values? For example, how closely does the distribution, fitted on the previous 24 months of data, fit the demand over the next month?

9.9.1 Measuring Predictive Distribution Accuracy

Suppose that we are predicting that future demand will follow a Poisson distribution with a mean of 0.5 in the next period, and the protection interval is of one period only. Then, following the calculations outlined in Chapter 4, we are predicting zero demand in the next period with probability 60.7%, a demand of one unit with probability 30.3%, a demand of two units with probability 7.6%, and so on. Now suppose that we observe a demand of two units. Whilst the predicted probability of 7.6% is quite low, it is certainly possible to observe a demand of two units if the predicted distribution is correct. The problem is that a demand value of two is also a possibility if the demand is Poisson but with a different mean, or if the demand is following a different probability distribution.

To address this difficulty, we need more than one observation to test. One approach would be to divide the available data history, for an individual SKU, into two parts. The first part is used to update forecasts. For example, with 30 periods of data, we could use the first 24 periods to forecast the mean demand. Then, if we believe that demand follows a Poisson distribution, the mean demand forecast can be used to calculate the predicted demand distribution. We could then check if the remaining six periods of data, in the second part of the data history, conform to the predicted distribution. The trouble is that six observations are still too few to draw any sensible conclusions. In our example, a demand of two units is expected to occur in approximately 1 in 13 periods (7.6%, more precisely). The occurrence or non-occurrence of a demand value of two during six periods tells us very little.

To test a predictive distribution for a single demand series is very difficult, but this becomes more feasible when there are many series to test, as usually occurs in practice. In the following subsections, we review some approaches for doing this.

9.9.2 Probability Integral Transform for Continuous Data

Willemain et al. (2004) proposed using the probability integral transform (PIT) to assess the accuracy of the predictive distribution for a collection of intermittent demand items. To appreciate this method of accuracy assessment, we start with an example of continuous data, rather than the discrete (whole number) data that is more typical of intermittent demand.

Consider the example of fresh fruit sold at a supermarket. If demand is recorded according to weight, then this can be considered as a continuous variable. The weekly demand for a particular type of fruit is unlikely to be intermittent and it is plausible that it can be represented by the normal distribution.

Suppose that our prediction for the weekly demand of bananas at a particular retail store is 1050 kg, with an estimated standard deviation of 150 kg. The next observation (1275 kg) can be converted into a standard normal variable $((1275 - 1050)/150 = 1.5)$. Then, we can find, from normal distribution tables, that this corresponds to a cumulative distribution function (CDF) value of 93.3%. Now, suppose that the retailer has 1000 stores. Then we can find the CDF values of demand for bananas at each of the stores, referring in each case to the predicted means and standard deviations at that store. If our predictive distributions are accurate, then we would expect the 1000 CDF values to be uniformly distributed between 0% and 100% or, more conventionally, between 0 and 1. Now, suppose we allocate each of the CDF values to 1 of 20 equal intervals (0 to 0.05, 0.05 to 0.10, ..., 0.95 to 1.00). Then we would expect there to be an approximately equal allocation to each of the intervals for well-specified predictive distributions. Although the calculations are a little more involved, the same considerations apply to discrete data, to which we now turn.

9.9.3 Probability Integral Transform for Discrete Data

In Section 9.9.2, our attention was restricted to continuous variables. However, in most intermittent demand applications, we are dealing with discrete variables, which can take only whole numbers, including zero of course. Willemain et al. (2004) illustrated how the PIT can be adapted to deal with this situation using the example of Poisson lead time demand with a mean value estimated as 1.3, and with 20 intervals of width 0.05. In this case, the estimated CDF values for 0 and 1 are $\hat{F}(0) = e^{-1.3} = 0.273$ and $\hat{F}(1) = 0.273 + (1.3 \times e^{-1.3}) = 0.627$. If a demand value of 1 is observed, then the count of its occurrence is distributed across the intervals that overlap the range from 0.273 to 0.627. Details of the calculations are given in Technical Note 9.3.

This is repeated for each series and then the distribution of fractional counts can be calculated overall. A disadvantage of using Willemain's allocation of counts for the PIT is that the number of intervals needs to be determined in advance and it is not obvious what the number should be. Kolassa (2016) proposed using an alternative approach, called the randomised probability integral transform (rPIT). Using this approach, the intervals are no

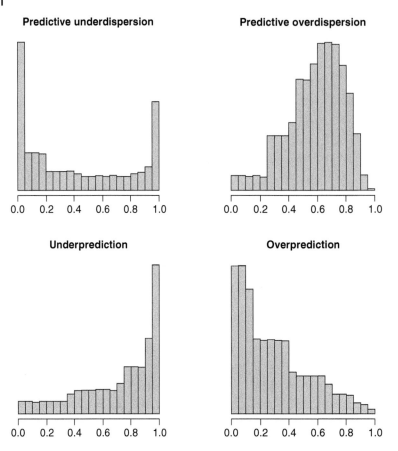

Figure 9.2 Non-uniform distributions of randomised PITs. Source: Diagram by Dr Stephan Kolassa.

longer required to be of equal width, and are determined directly from the estimated CDF. (For further details, see Technical Note 9.4.) Figure 9.2 shows four examples of histograms of rPIT values calculated from discrete data.

The values are not uniformly distributed in any of the four examples in Figure 9.2, indicating that the predictive distribution may be suffering from underdispersion (variance too low), overdispersion (variance too high), underprediction (mean too low), or overprediction (mean too high), according to the shape of the distribution. It is not always so obvious that the distribution is non-uniform, and a chi-square statistical test may be employed in this case.

Boylan and Syntetos (2006) pointed out that, in many applications, our concern is with a particular part of the predictive distribution rather than the whole predictive distribution. This is true in most inventory applications, where the principal concern is with the upper part of the future distribution (for example, from 90% upwards). Testing for uniformity of the PIT or rPIT using a chi-square test may not reject the uniform distribution because the observed distribution is very close to uniform from 0% to 90%, even though it deviates for CDF values over 90%. Kolassa (2016) suggested, instead, using a 'data driven smooth test' (Ledwina 1994; Inglot and Ledwina 2006), available as a package in R, to test for the uniformity of the rPIT more sensitively.

The uniformity of the PIT or rPIT is a necessary but not sufficient condition for the best prediction of a probability distribution. This may be explained with an example. Suppose that we have a Bernoulli demand process, with a time-varying probability of demand occurrence, denoted by f_t. In any period, there is a 50% chance that demand occurrence has a probability of $f_t = 0.9$ and a 50% chance that the probability is $f_t = 0.1$. The weighted probability of demand occurrence is $(0.5 \times 0.9) + (0.5 \times 0.1) = 0.5$. If our prediction of demand occurrence probability is always 0.5, then this will give a uniform rPIT, and is said to be a 'well-calibrated' forecast. But is it the best forecast? If we are able to anticipate the periods of higher probability, our probabilistic forecast would improve. Suppose that we forecast $\hat{f}_t = 0.8$ when the true probability is 0.9 and $\hat{f}_t = 0.2$ when the true probability is 0.1. This seems a better forecast than always using $\hat{f}_t = 0.5$, but this improvement is not detected by tests for a uniform PIT or rPIT.

Gneiting et al. (2007) proposed a strategy of optimising 'proper scoring rules', while satisfying uniformity of PITs. A 'scoring rule' is a penalty function for a probabilistic forecast. It is 'proper' if it is optimised at the best possible distributional forecast. An example of a proper scoring rule is the Brier score (BS), calculated using Eq. (9.12) for variables with only two possible outcomes.

$$\text{BS} = \frac{1}{N}\sum_{t=1}^{N}(\hat{f}_t - o_t)^2 \tag{9.12}$$

where o_t is one if the outcome occurs, and zero otherwise; and $\hat{f}_t$ is the forecasted probability of the outcome's occurrence. For the BS, as formulated in Eq. (9.12), smaller is better. (The score is sometimes formulated with a minus sign, in which case it should be maximised, rather than minimised.) Like other proper scoring rules, such as the log score, the BS rewards 'sharpness'. In this instance, the sharpest possible prediction would be $\hat{f}_t = 1.0$ for periods with demand, and $\hat{f}_t = 0$ for periods without, giving a BS of zero. Of course, such omniscience is unrealistic, but the BS rewards sharper forecasts that are imperfect. In the example above, BS = 0.25 if we always forecast $\hat{f}_t = 0.5$ but this is much reduced, with BS = 0.1, if we were to use probability forecasts of 0.8 and 0.2 for the appropriate periods (see Technical Note 9.5 for calculations). A BS can also be calculated for variables with more than two possible outcomes, as explained in Technical Note 9.5.

Kolassa (2016) advocated the use of a proper scoring rule, in tandem with testing for a uniform rPIT, to assess the accuracy of probabilistic forecasts of intermittent demand. Using this approach, he found that the Poisson underestimated the probabilities of low and high sales on his datasets, and the negative binomial did not perform well for high quantiles.

9.9.4 Summary

The accuracy of the whole predictive distribution should be assessed, across a range of SKUs. There are two aspects to this assessment: calibration and sharpness. Calibration can be assessed by testing for the uniformity of the Probability Integral Transform or randomised Probability Integral Transform. Sharpness can be measured by a proper scoring rule, such as the Brier score.

9.10 Accuracy Implication Measures

If a change is being proposed to forecasting methods, then adoption will depend on an assessment of whether the anticipated benefits are worth the investment of time and money in making the change. The investment costs can be considerable when we take into account acquisition of hardware and software, implementation of the new system, and training of staff.

The most straightforward way of assessing the benefits accruing from a new (or revised) forecasting system is to make the change and then to measure stock holdings and service levels over time. If the change is made as a 'big bang', across all products and locations, then it can take some time for the system to stabilise and can result in great expense if the change was misguided. Another strategy is to pilot a change in the system for a subset of products or locations. In that case, stock holdings and service levels should be monitored not just for the pilot group but also for a control group, to allow an assessment of the effect of the new forecasting system, without being confounded by other factors.

An alternative approach is to simulate inventory performance, based on data that is already available. Simulation facilities are available in some software packages. If not, then a simulation can be conducted off-line, for example using open source software, discussed further in Chapter 15.

9.10.1 Simulation Outline

Before delving into details, it is useful to consider the whole process:

1. Extract the historical demand values for a sample of SKUs.
2. Initialise the stock on hand values for each of the SKUs.
3. Generate forecasts using the current and new methods.
4. Generate inventory settings (e.g. order-up-to levels) based on forecasts using current and new methods.
5. Simulate placement of orders, arrival of orders, depletion of stock, and generation of backorders (or lost sales).
6. Validate simulation using current methods.
7. Calculate summary statistics on stock holdings and service levels.

The details of this process will be discussed in the following subsections. In the meantime, we emphasise the importance of using real demand data. It is possible to generate artificial data using random number generators, based on certain distributional assumptions. For example, we could generate artificial Poisson demand for a range of mean demands. Suppose this is done and then we assess a new forecasting method coupled with a Poisson demand assumption. This will tell us nothing about how well the system works when the demand is not Poisson. If, on the other hand, we use real data, then the performance of the forecasting method coupled with the assumed demand distribution can be assessed.

9.10.2 Forecasting Details

In the simulation of forecasting methods, we should specify not just the names of the method (e.g. Croston) but also how the method is initialised and how the parameters (e.g. smoothing parameters) are selected. Careful documentation of these settings is vital for replication of forecasting methods. Boylan et al. (2015) found that it was not possible to reproduce the results of a well-cited study on seasonal forecasting because of the lack of clarity on such settings. Boylan (2016) highlighted three requirements for reproducible findings:

1. Accessible data.
2. Algorithm or methods specified in sufficient detail.
3. Evaluation metrics fully specified.

These requirements are relevant not only for academic research. They are important in a business context, too. If there is a mismatch between the implemented forecasting methods or metrics and the simulated methods or metrics, then the simulation results may not give a good indication of forecasting performance in practice.

In a similar manner, the distributional assumptions should be clearly specified. If necessary, different combinations of forecasting methods and distributional assumptions can be simulated. Then, the inventory parameters can be generated according to the inventory rule in operation. There is further scope for experimentation in varying the inventory rule itself (e.g. (R, s, S), discussed in Chapter 2, instead of (R, S)).

9.10.3 Simulation Details

In stock-control simulation, there is a need to take into account the treatment of unsatisfied demand, either as backorders or lost sales. If the real system has a mix of backorders and lost sales, then both systems may be simulated. It is also possible to simulate a mix of backorders and lost sales, although complications may arise in deciding how to assign unsatisfied demand to one category or the other.

For evaluation purposes, stocks need to be initialised at the beginning of the out-of-sample period. (They can also be initialised at the beginning of the in-sample period for purposes of validation.) The stock holdings can be initialised with the true stock values, for each of the SKUs included in the simulation study. If this data is not available, then the stock may be initialised at the order-up-to level (S) derived from analysis of the in-sample data.

If the stocks and stockouts (simulated using the current forecast methods, distributional assumptions, and inventory rules) resemble those observed in practice, then this gives confidence that the simulation is a valid representation of the real system. If there are significant discrepancies, then the reasons should be pinpointed. One reason for divergence may be that there have been significant judgemental interventions, either in the forecasts or in the ordering quantities themselves. If there is no significant discrepancy after taking this into account, then we can still have confidence in the simulation as a representation of the inventory system without judgemental intervention.

In the final stage of the simulation process, statistics need to be collected on inventory volumes, inventory values, and service level performance, using an agreed set of measures, both at SKU and aggregate levels (see discussion in Chapter 3). Comparison of inventory-implication measures is not always straightforward and is the subject of Section 9.10.4.

9.10.4 Comparison of Simulation Results

There are two ways in which inventory simulation results may be compared. The first is to convert all the results into financial outcomes, and the second is to use an 'exchange curve' analysis.

The financial approach takes the simulated average inventory valuation and converts this number to an inventory holding cost, to take into account such factors as the cost of capital, cost of space, and risk of obsolescence. There was a fuller discussion of these factors in Chapter 2. Then, the simulated service level is also converted to an inventory penalty cost for backorders or lost sales. As explained in Chapter 3, this is not always a straightforward exercise. However, once this is done, we can compare the different forecasting methods (and distributional assumptions and inventory rules) using a single measure. This measure is the total cost, calculated as the sum of the inventory holding and penalty costs.

An alternative approach is to plot exchange curves of inventory holdings against the preferred inventory service measure. For example, inventory holdings may be plotted against the proportion of unfilled demand, as shown in Figure 9.3.

Figure 9.3 shows that, for a given average on hand inventory, the unfilled rate (1– the fill rate) can differ quite markedly between the three forecasting methods. In the diagram, the lower the unfilled rate the better. One forecasting method is said to dominate another if it is consistently lower than another and, in this example, method 1 (shown in blue) dominates the others. For any target fill rate, we can find the inventory savings that would result by changing from one forecasting method to another. For example, in Figure 9.3, if the target fill rate is 95%, then $1 -$ Fill rate $= 0.05$ and changing from method 2 to method 1 would yield a reduction in 'average on hand inventory' of approximately 300 units. This is another form of forecast value added (FVA), but now expressed in terms of inventory reductions.

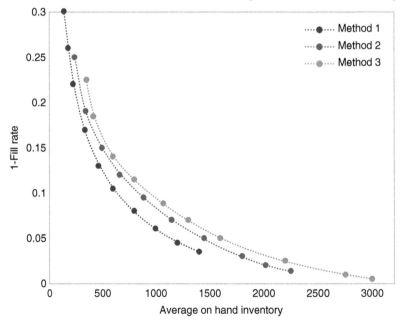

Figure 9.3 Exchange curves.

9.10.5 Summary

Simulation of inventory performance can be a powerful tool for communication with managers. It shows the likely impact of changing forecasting methods, distributional assumptions, or inventory rules. It does so by using real demand data from the organisation, lending greater credibility to the results than purely theoretical calculations.

The results can be presented either in terms of estimated total financial costs or using an 'exchange curve' to show the trade-off between inventory holdings and unfilled demand for a range of forecasting methods.

9.11 Chapter Summary

In this chapter, we have seen that forecast error measures and error-implication measures are complementary. Whilst error implication measures, such as stock holdings and service measures, are the main concern of supply chain managers, forecast error measures are needed to diagnose any reasons for deterioration in these key performance indicators.

Inventory performance is driven by the choice of inventory rules, distributional assumptions, and forecasting methods being employed. If a change in inventory rules is under consideration, then this change can be simulated using real demand data to ascertain if an improvement in performance may be expected.

If the inventory rules are taken as fixed, then problems with stock holdings or service levels may be due to the distribution chosen to represent demand, or the estimates of their parameters derived from demand forecasts. Distributional assumptions may be checked using the in-sample goodness of fit methods discussed in Chapter 5. However, their effect depends on their predictive power, so it is wise to measure the out-of-sample accuracy of the whole predictive distribution. This assessment needs to take into account the discrete nature of most intermittent demand series, and can be applied to non-parametric approaches (to be discussed in Chapter 13) as well as parametric methods.

Measurement of the accuracy of point forecasts of expected demand is beset with traps for the unwary. Measures based on absolute errors are minimised by the median. Minimisation of these measures can result in always recommending zero forecasts, and so absolute error measures cannot be recommended, unless complemented by appropriate bias measures. Three measures which can be used on their own for intermittent demand, across a whole range of demand series, are as follows: sMSE, relative RMSE and percentage best (based on an appropriate measure for individual series).

Technical Notes

Note 9.1 Amended Definitions of MAPE and sMAPE

MAPE: If negative 'demand' values are recorded by an organisation, then the corresponding APEs will also be negative, unless the forecast error is zero. This problem can be overcome by redefining the MAPE according to Eq. (9.13) (Hyndman and Koehler 2006).

$$\text{MAPE} = \frac{100}{N} \sum_{t=1}^{N} \left| \frac{d_t - \widehat{d}_{t|t-1}}{d_t} \right| \tag{9.13}$$

sMAPE: Hyndman (2014) reviewed some misunderstandings about the sMAPE and noted that, according to the definition in Eq. (9.6), the sMAPE can be negative (if $d_t + \widehat{d}_{t|t-1} < 0$) or infinite (if $d_t + \widehat{d}_{t|t-1} = 0$). Replacing the denominator by $(|d_t| + |\widehat{d}_{t|t-1}|)/2$ (Chen and Yang 2004) removes these problems unless $d_t = \widehat{d}_{t|t-1} = 0$. As noted earlier in the chapter, if all demands are non-negative, and all forecasts are strictly positive, then the sMAPE is unaffected by these issues.

Note 9.2 The Mean Arctangent Absolute Percentage Error

Kim and Kim (2016) proposed an error metric for intermittent demand forecasts, similar in spirit to the MAPE, which they called the MAAPE. It is defined as in Eq. (9.14) for one-step-ahead demand forecasts.

$$\text{MAAPE} = \frac{1}{N} \sum_{t=1}^{N} \arctan\left(\left| \frac{d_t - \widehat{d}_{t|t-1}}{d_t} \right| \right) \tag{9.14}$$

where the notation is the same as before. The term to the right of the summation sign is called the 'arctangent absolute percentage error'. It is straightforward to calculate. For example, if the actual demand is 1 and the absolute error is 1, then the APE is 100% (=1). The angle of 45° has a tangent of 1, and so the arctangent APE is 45°. The MAAPE measure is defined for zero demands but is always equal to 90°. Consequently, the MAAPE does not discriminate between the accuracy of different forecasting methods for zero actual values.

Note 9.3 Probability Integral Transform: Fractional Allocation of Counts

If the intervals are defined in advance, then the following example (Willemain et al. 2004) demonstrates the fractional allocation of demand counts, for an observed count of one demand for a single unit, and with estimated values of $\widehat{F}(0) = 0.273$ and $\widehat{F}(1) = 0.627$.

1. Decide on the number of intervals over which demand is to be distributed. Suppose this is 20, giving a first interval from 0 to 0.05 and a last interval from 0.95 to 1.
2. Record demand. Suppose this is for one unit.
3. Identify the range of estimated cumulative probabilities which correspond to this observation. In this example, the range is from 0.273 to 0.627.
4. Identify the intervals overlapping the range. In this example, the first interval is from 0.25 to 0.30 and the last interval is from 0.60 to 0.65.
5. Calculate the estimated probability of the demand. In this example, it is given by: $\widehat{F}(1) - \widehat{F}(0) = 0.627 - 0.273 = 0.354$.
6. Calculate the share of the count value of 1 that should be allocated to each of the intervals overlapping the range.
   - For the interval from 0.25 to 0.30, the allocation is $(0.30 - 0.273)/0.354 = 0.076$.
   - For the six intervals spanning 0.30 to 0.60 the allocation is $0.05/0.354 = 0.141$
   - For the interval from 0.60 to 0.65 the allocation is $(0.627 - 0.60)/0.354 = 0.076$.
7. Record the fractional counts.

Note 9.4 Randomised Probability Integral Transform

Suppose, for one series, the latest observation is y_t. To obtain the rPIT, the first step is to retrieve the latest CDF estimates, $\widehat{F}_t(y_t - 1)$ and $\widehat{F}_t(y_t)$. Then, a rPIT value, $\tilde{p}_t$ is drawn from a uniform distribution between the two CDF estimates, as indicated in Eq. (9.15) (Kolassa 2016).

$$\tilde{p}_t \sim U(\widehat{F}_t(y_t - 1), \widehat{F}_t(y_t)) \tag{9.15}$$

This is repeated over many series to obtain a distribution of rPITs.

Note 9.5 Calculation of the Brier Score

In the example given in Section 9.9, the first probabilistic forecast is: $\widehat{f}_t = 0.5$ for all periods, t. In this case, the components of the BS are calculated as follows:

- If there is demand in period t, then $(\widehat{f}_t - o_t)^2 = (0.5 - 1)^2 = 0.25$.
- If there is no demand in period t, then $(\widehat{f}_t - o_t)^2 = (0.5 - 0)^2 = 0.25$.

The BS is the average of all these values. In this case, the values never vary, regardless of the outcome, and so it follows that BS $= 0.25$.

The second probabilistic forecast is: $\widehat{f}_t = 0.8$ for periods when $f_t = 0.9$ ('high periods'); and $\widehat{f}_t = 0.2$ for periods when $f_t = 0.1$ ('low periods'). In this case, the components of the BS are as follows:

- *High period*: If there is demand, then $(\widehat{f}_t - o_t)^2 = (0.8 - 1)^2 = 0.04$.
- *High period*: If there is no demand, then $(\widehat{f}_t - o_t)^2 = (0.8 - 0)^2 = 0.64$.
- *Low period*: If there is demand, then $(\widehat{f}_t - o_t)^2 = (0.2 - 1)^2 = 0.64$.
- *Low period*: If there is no demand, then $(\widehat{f}_t - o_t)^2 = (0.2 - 0)^2 = 0.04$.

To calculate the overall BS, we need to know how the total number of periods splits into these four categories. In the long-run, the proportions will stabilise at 0.45, 0.05, 0.05, and 0.45, with respect to the same order of categories as above. (These are found by multiplying the probability of high/low periods, 0.5 in both cases, by the probabilities of demand and no demand for each type of period, as given above by f_t for demand and $1 - f_t$ for no demand.) This yields a Brier Score of BS $= (0.45 \times 0.04) + (0.05 \times 0.64) + (0.05 \times 0.64) + (0.45 \times 0.04) = 0.1$.

If there are more than two categories (e.g. occurrence and non-occurrence), say C categories, then the BS is calculated as in Eq. (9.16).

$$BS = \frac{1}{N} \sum_{t=1}^{N} \sum_{j=1}^{C} (\widehat{f}_{jt} - o_{jt})^2 \tag{9.16}$$

where o_{jt} is 1 if category j is observed at time t, and 0 otherwise; $\widehat{f}_{jt}$ is the forecasted probability of category j at time t.

In the context of intermittent demand forecasting, estimated probabilities of demand at time t taking the value j, $\widehat{\mathbb{P}}(d_t = j)$, will start at $j = 0$ and may have no upper bound. In this case, the inner sum extends to infinity and may be written as in Eq. (9.17).

$$BS = \frac{1}{N} \sum_{t=1}^{N} \sum_{j=0}^{\infty} (\widehat{\mathbb{P}}(d_t = j) - \mathbb{1}(d_t = j))^2 \tag{9.17}$$

where $\mathbb{1}(d_t = j)$ takes the value of 1 if $d_t = j$, and 0 otherwise, and $\widehat{\mathbb{P}}$ denotes the estimated probability.

10

Judgement, Bias, and Mean Square Error

10.1 Introduction

In Chapters 6 and 7, we examined statistical approaches to forecasting. This emphasis is appropriate, particularly in the context of intermittent demand, because the sheer volume of stock keeping units requires an automatic solution. In practice, though, software packages almost always allow for user intervention. This means that users of forecasting software packages may override statistical forecasts with forecasts of their own. Whether such overrides are beneficial or harmful to forecast accuracy has been a matter of debate. The evidence will be reviewed in this chapter.

One of the potential disadvantages of overriding statistical forecasts is that the new forecasts may be biased. In fact, the statistical forecasts may be biased themselves if they are not well chosen. Performance measures for bias, including the mean error, were reviewed in Chapter 9. In this chapter, we examine bias in more detail, focusing on its monitoring, and its expectation.

The mean square error (MSE) is a scale dependent measure and is not robust to outliers, as noted in Chapter 9. Nevertheless, it is useful in gaining insights into the components of forecast error, including the expected bias, and is discussed in some depth in this chapter.

The structure of this chapter follows the themes outlined above. We begin with a discussion on judgemental forecasting, reviewing the evidence of its effectiveness for fast-moving products and for products with intermittent demand. Then, we address the issue of forecast bias, looking at its causes and some of its properties. The final section examines the fundamental properties of MSE. This material lays the groundwork for the practical classification rules that are discussed in Chapter 11.

10.2 Judgemental Forecasting

There is some element of judgement in all forecasting. Even if an organisation relies solely on its software to generate forecasts, some judgement would have been necessary in choosing the software package from the alternatives available. When acquired, judgement may have been exercised in deciding how to classify SKUs, and this can affect the forecasting

Intermittent Demand Forecasting: Context, Methods and Applications, First Edition.
John E. Boylan and Aris A. Syntetos.
© 2021 John Wiley & Sons Ltd. Published 2021 by John Wiley & Sons Ltd.
Companion Website: www.wiley.com/go/boylansyntetos/intermittentdemandforecasting

Table 10.1   Reported usage of forecast methods in practice.

Primary forecast method	Sanders and Manrodt (%)	Fildes and Goodwin (%)	Weller and Crone[a] (%)	Fildes and Petropoulos (%)
Judgemental	30	25	26	14
Quantitative or statistical	29	25	29	30
Mix of methods	41	50	44	56

a) Respondents estimated percentages of final forecasts in each category. Averages are reported, with rounding errors resulting in a total of 99%.

method to be used. Similarly, judgement may have been used in deciding on the parameters (such as the smoothing constants) to be applied. Nevertheless, if the forecast itself is then generated using a statistical procedure that has been coded in the software package, then it will be considered as a 'statistical forecast' in this chapter.

Many organisations do not rely solely on computer generated forecasts. In some cases, a forecast may be purely judgemental. For new products, for example, a company may rely on the sales team's forecasts, with no statistical forecasts because of the lack of historical sales data. In other cases, a statistical forecast may be subsequently amended by a demand planner in the light of the planner's judgement about changes in the external environment or changes to the way the product is being marketed.

10.2.1   Evidence on Prevalence of Judgemental Forecasting

A number of surveys have been published in recent decades on the use of quantitative/statistical forecasting methods and judgemental approaches. Sanders and Manrodt (2003) surveyed 240 heads of marketing of US corporations; Fildes and Goodwin (2007) surveyed 144 forecasters attending international forecasting-practitioner conferences; Weller and Crone (2012) conducted an online survey of 200 demand planning professionals from manufacturing companies; and Fildes and Petropoulos (2015) surveyed 47 demand planners and forecasters. The results of the surveys are summarised in Table 10.1.

The findings from the surveys are quite consistent. None of the surveys found quantitative/statistical methods, without any judgemental interventions, to be the dominant approach. No more than 30% of respondents to the first, second, and fourth surveys reported quantitative/statistical methods as primary. In the third survey, it was estimated that only 29% of final forecasts were generated by quantitative/statistical methods alone. It is clear that judgement is used extensively in practice, either on its own or as part of a mix of methods. As it is such an important part of business forecasting practice, it certainly warrants further investigation.

10.2.2   Judgemental Biases

Morlidge (2018) commented that problems with judgemental forecasting are usually revealed in terms of bias, and he categorised the types of human bias as motivational, social, and cognitive.

Motivational biases can be important in many businesses. Managers may deliberately forecast optimistically because it is in their own interests. Suppose sales managers are responsible for judgemental forecasts, and their performance is rewarded if there are high sales but not penalised if there are excessive stock levels. In this situation, an optimistic forecast can contribute to sales managers' rewards. An optimistic forecast will result in high stocks, which will enable high sales if the demand reaches the forecasted level. If demand is much lower, then there will be excessive stocks that may remain unsold, but sales managers will not be penalised for this. This example illustrates the importance of designing appropriate measurement and reward systems.

Social biases can arise in forecast review meetings, when a group of managers meet to consider and agree forecasts and plans. In such situations, there can be pressure to conform to a group view. This may inhibit a manager from expressing a dissenting view on the realism of the forecasts. For example, a manager who is sceptical about the effect of discounting or promotions may not wish to voice these concerns or, if they do, this alternative view may not be taken sufficiently seriously. This is an example of 'groupthink', a term derived from the word 'doublethink', found in George Orwell's novel, *1984*. The Delphi forecasting approach attempts to combat groupthink by anonymising forecasts and their rationale from participants. However, such approaches are often time consuming and rarely used for forecasts of intermittent demand items.

Motivational and social biases can be particularly acute for products that are attracting significant attention from senior managers. Intermittent demand items will rarely be in that category, although they may be part of a product group that is of particular interest.

A further source of bias is known as 'cognitive bias', which arises because of faulty reasoning and insufficient weight being given to evidence that is contrary to a person's expectations. There has been extensive research on the limitations of human reasoning and judgement. The most renowned researcher in this field, Nobel laureate Daniel Kahneman, has challenged the traditional assumption of rationality by his work with the late Amos Tversky on cognitive biases. In his book, *Thinking, Fast and Slow*, Kahneman (2011) considers the following chain of reasoning:

1. All roses are flowers.
2. Some flowers fade quickly.
3. Some roses fade quickly.

College students were asked if the third statement follows logically from the first two. (Note: They were not asked if the third statement is true, merely if it is a logical conclusion of the statements that precede it.) Kahneman reported that a large majority of students endorse this reasoning as valid. Actually, it is not valid because the first two statements include no information about whether roses are among the flowers that fade quickly or not. Therefore, we cannot deduce the third statement from the information in the first two statements, even though the third statement may be true.

This finding is discouraging, as it indicates that when people believe a conclusion to be true, they are also prepared to believe arguments that support it, even when those arguments are invalid. Kahneman summarises this as a 'bias to believe and confirm' (also known as a 'confirmation bias'). This bias is sometimes observed in an organisational setting, when high sales forecasts are justified by managers who have sought confirming evidence and arguments, but have not looked for contradictory evidence, which may temper the forecasts.

This discussion leads us on to optimism bias which, in a forecasting context, is manifested by a tendency to over-forecast positive outcomes (e.g. high sales) and under-forecast negative outcomes (e.g. delays in the duration of projects). In business forecasting, there are factors that may exacerbate optimism bias. There may be a basic confusion between forecasts and targets. Supply chain planning requires accurate forecasts, which are expectations of what will actually happen. Targets, on the other hand, represent a desired state, such as increasing sales by 10% over the previous year. If targets are set ambitiously, and used as forecasts, then optimism bias is very likely to be the outcome.

A further problem is the 'overconfidence effect'. Soll and Klayman (2004, p. 299) defined this phenomenon succinctly: 'When people say they are X% sure about a fact, they are right less than X% of the time'. One form of the overconfidence effect is in terms of people's interval estimates. Consider this example, given by Soll and Klayman: to the question 'When was Charles Dickens born?', a response may be, 'I am 80% sure the answer is between 1750 and 1860'. In this case, the estimated interval from 1750 to 1860 does contain the correct answer (1812). Soll and Klayman (2004) conducted three experiments with just over 100 participants, most of whom were students, posing questions requiring 80% interval estimates. If the participants are accurate at estimating the correctness of their answers, we would expect that 80% of the ranges would contain the correct answers. In fact, the three experiments showed only 39%, 66%, and 55% of the ranges contained the correct answers, demonstrating a strong over-confidence effect.

In the forecasting domain, Bolger and Önkal-Atay (2004) tested students' ability to estimate the accuracy of their forecasts, with each participant being presented with 32 time series and being required to make judgemental interval estimates, for example, 'I am 80% confident that the next observation will be between 100 and 120 units'. The results demonstrated over-confidence but the study also showed that, when presented with the results, the students' estimates of their own accuracy became better in subsequent exercises.

Not all researchers are so pessimistic about the ability of humans to make accurate predictions. Snook et al. (2004) analysed the accuracy of predictions of residential locations of repeat offenders. They compared an actuarial method with the performance of undergraduate students who had been given information on two heuristics (practical problem-solving methods not guaranteed to give the best solution). The first heuristic was 'the majority of offenders commit offences close to home'. The second heuristic was 'the majority of offenders' homes can be located within a circle with its diameter defined by the distance between the offender's two furthermost crimes'. The researchers found no significant differences between the performance of students informed about the heuristics and the more sophisticated actuarial technique.

Wübben and Wangenheim (2008) examined the effectiveness of a simple managerial rule known as the 'hiatus heuristic': if a customer has not purchased within a certain number of months in the past (the 'hiatus'), the customer is defined as inactive, and otherwise active. They analysed prediction of future customer activity, using transaction data from the apparel, airline, and music industries, and found that the heuristic matched or outperformed a complex statistical model.

Both of these examples illustrate the power of heuristics, but do not add to our understanding of judgement that is not aided by heuristic rules. In a forecasting context, heuristics are not always used by planners and Sections 10.2.3 and 10.2.4 contain more direct evidence on the accuracy of judgemental forecasting.

In summary, the findings from experimental research results are somewhat mixed. Some studies show problems with relying on human judgement. Others are more favourable. Most of the evidence has been based on 'laboratory studies'. These are experiments under controlled conditions, with the tasks usually being undertaken by university or college students. Goodwin (1998) summarised the advantages of this type of research and noted that laboratory studies can overcome the limited scope for experimentation and control in the real world. Nevertheless, the findings will not automatically carry across to a practical demand planning setting. It is therefore necessary to assess the accuracy of judgemental forecasts in real-life situations before coming to any firm conclusions on the effectiveness of judgemental forecasting.

10.2.3 Effectiveness of Judgemental Forecasts: Evidence for Non-intermittent Items

There is limited empirical evidence on the accuracy of judgemental adjustments to statistical forecasts. Early studies by Mathews and Diamantopoulos (1986, 1989, 1992) and Diamantopoulos and Mathews (1989) found a tendency for judgement to improve forecast accuracy but noted that it may introduce bias. These studies were all based on the same single company, thereby limiting the generality of the findings.

Blattberg and Hoch (1990) analysed forecasts of coupon redemption rates (three companies) and catalogue fashion sales (two companies). They found that managers' predictive accuracy was comparable to that of the statistical models, and that a simple 50% model plus 50% manager heuristic could improve predictive accuracy of both model and manager alone. However, they did not consider the effect such a rule may have on the future forecasts of the managers if they were aware that their forecasts received only a 50% weighting.

A major study on the effect of judgemental adjustments to statistical forecasts was undertaken by Fildes et al. (2009). The research team analysed the demand forecasts, at SKU level, from four companies in the pharmaceuticals, food, household products, and retailing sectors (labelled as A, B, C, and D, respectively). In total, over 1500 non-intermittent SKUs were examined from the four companies, and almost 70 000 one-step-ahead forecasts were evaluated.

Each of the companies had retained records of their original statistical forecasts as well as their judgementally adjusted forecasts. This good practice in record keeping enabled forecast accuracy to be compared. It is encouraging that many forecasting software systems now have the capability to store judgemental adjustments for further analysis (Fildes et al. 2020).

In order to examine judgemental biases more carefully, separate analyses were conducted by Fildes et al. (2009) for upward adjustments and downward adjustments. The percentage of forecasts that were adjusted was as high as 91% (Company B), with positive adjustments being somewhat more common than negative adjustments overall.

The main finding of the study was that positive adjustments, which increase a statistical forecast, offer a lower improvement in accuracy than negative adjustments, which decrease a statistical forecast. Further analysis showed that negative adjustments tend to reduce the mean bias in statistical forecasts that are too high. Once planners have decided to reduce a statistical forecast, they often produce quite realistic judgemental adjustments. Positive adjustments, on the other hand, tend to be too optimistic, with 66% of judgemental adjustments being too high for Companies A, B, and C. This optimism bias has reduced the benefit of positive adjustments quite markedly for these companies.

The results for Company D showed that positive adjustments were particularly harmful, with severe deterioration of forecast accuracy in many cases. Discussion with the company revealed that, for many SKUs, managers were mixing up demand forecasts with inventory levels required to meet customer service level targets. Inevitably, this confusion led to ill-informed judgemental adjustments. The case of Company D serves to illustrate the importance of adequate training and development of demand planners with responsibility for forecast adjustments.

A further finding was that small adjustments in forecasts have a negligible effect on accuracy. This indicates that small adjustments are not worthwhile and planners' efforts would be better directed elsewhere. This tendency to adjust statistical forecasts unnecessarily was also noted by Franses (2014) in his studies of business and economic forecasting.

In summary, the study by Fildes et al. (2009) offers some encouragement for judgemental adjustment of statistical forecasts. However, the study also demonstrates that 'optimism bias', which is often detected in laboratory studies, is also prevalent in practice. This would suggest that more caution is needed before making positive (upward) adjustments of statistical forecasts than negative (downward) adjustments.

10.2.4 Effectiveness of Judgemental Forecasts: Evidence for Intermittent Items

The study by Fildes et al. (2009) concentrated on faster-moving items. A complementary study was conducted by Syntetos et al. (2009c), which focussed on intermittent demand items from Company A, a pharmaceutical company. The individual demand histories of 138 SKUs from Company A were analysed, all of which exhibited intermittent demand patterns. In all, 4968 forecasts were examined, of which 3659 (74%) were adjusted. This provided the first evidence of the scale of judgemental adjustment of intermittent demand forecasts and showed that, for Company A at least, such adjustments were commonplace. The number of positive adjustments (2039) was greater than the number of negative adjustments (1620), just as it was for faster-moving items (Fildes et al. 2009).

The main conclusions of the accuracy assessments by Syntetos et al. (2009c) were as follows:

1. Overall, judgemental adjustments resulted in an improvement in accuracy.
2. Negative adjustments performed better than positive adjustments.
3. Positive adjustments performed rather poorly, irrespective of their magnitude.
4. Smaller positive adjustments (less than 20 units) improved the accuracy of zero forecasts.

The first two conclusions are entirely consistent with the study on faster-moving demand items by Fildes et al. (2009). The third conclusion is somewhat different: for intermittent demand, there is little evidence of any improvement in forecast accuracy from positive

Table 10.2   Judgemental adjustments: effect on cycle service levels.

CSL target (%)	Statistical forecasts		Adjusted forecasts	
	Stock-holding	CSL (%)	Stock-holding	CSL (%)
95	1684	93.0	1750	95.9
99	2266	95.9	2304	97.6

Source: Based on Syntetos et al. (2009c)

adjustments. An exception to this finding is noted in the fourth conclusion listed above. Zero forecasts must, by definition, be too low if the SKU still has some evidence of demand. For these SKUs, modest uplifts of forecasts are beneficial.

The findings in this study were based on different summaries of absolute errors across demand series. In Chapter 9, we noted some of the limitations, for intermittent demand, of measures based on absolute errors. We also discussed mitigating these limitations by using accuracy–implication metrics, particularly stock holding and service level measures. This strategy was adopted by Syntetos et al. (2009c). In their analysis, two different cycle service level (CSL) targets were used, namely 95% and 99%. An (R, S) stock-control system was simulated, with lead times of one, two, and three periods, and allowing for backorders (to reflect the practice at Company A). The MSE was updated using an exponential smoothing calculation (with smoothing constants of 0.05, 0.10, and 0.15) and was used as an input to a normal distribution of demand over the lead time plus review interval (the latter being fixed at one period). The average results, over all lead times and all smoothing constants are summarised in Table 10.2.

Table 10.2 shows that the improved accuracy of the judgementally adjusted forecasts, noted above, has translated to better CSL performance. For the 95% CSL target, the statistical forecast results in missing the target by 2.0%, attaining only 93.0% CSL, whereas the judgementally adjusted forecasts resulted in a slight over-attainment, at 95.9%. For the 99% CSL target, the statistical forecast results in missing the target by 3.1%, whereas the judgementally adjusted forecasts miss the target by only 1.4%. This may be due to the limitation of assuming a normal distribution of demand over lead time plus review interval. The marked improvement in CSL, by using judgementally adjusted forecasts, comes with an additional 3.9% in stock-holding volume for a 95% target CSL, and an additional 1.7% stock-holding volume for a 99% target CSL.

This study is the only one published, to date, which focuses on the effect of judgemental adjustments to statistical intermittent demand forecasts. It is encouraging that its conclusions on forecast accuracy are broadly consistent with research on faster-moving items, conducted by Fildes et al. (2009). However, the findings from Syntetos et al. (2009c) are based on evidence from just one pharmaceutical company and more studies are needed to give greater confidence in, or to challenge, the study's conclusions.

10.2.5   Summary

Survey-based studies have shown that judgemental adjustments to statistical forecasts are common in practice. The general literature on judgemental predictions comes to somewhat mixed conclusions. Some studies have shown human judges to perform as well as more sophisticated statistical methods. Other studies have pointed to biases that limit the ability of human judges to make accurate predictions.

Regarding judgemental adjustments to statistical forecasts, the most extensive evidence has been presented by Fildes et al. (2009). This study offers some support to both schools of thought regarding judgemental predictions. When human judges decrease a statistical forecast, substantial gains in accuracy have been identified. When judges increase the value of a statistical forecast, any gain in accuracy is diminished, indicating that 'optimism bias' is reducing the benefit of judgemental adjustments.

Specific evidence on judgemental adjustments to intermittent demand forecasts has been provided by Syntetos et al. (2009c). This research came to similar conclusions to the study of non-intermittent demand forecasts by Fildes et al. (2009). It went further, in an inventory context, by quantifying the effect on the CSL, showing an overall improvement in CSL by using judgementally adjusted forecasts, at the cost of some increase in stock holdings.

10.3 Forecast Bias

As we have seen in Section 10.2, poor use of judgement in amending statistical forecasts may lead to biased forecasts. Often these biases are caused by over-optimism, leading to forecasts that are too high on average. If this is so, then we should exercise care in increasing statistical forecasts. Because of the absence of optimism and over-confidence, it may be expected that statistical forecasts will be free from bias. Unfortunately, this is not always true, even though statistical forecasts are often less biased than judgemental forecasts.

Statistical forecasts may be biased because they are mis-specified. This situation arises when a forecasting method is chosen inappropriately. For example, suppose that non-intermittent demand is non-seasonal and following a positive (growth) trend. If an historical average of the data is used as a forecast, then the forecast will be biased. Because the data is exhibiting growth, this average is not a good indication of the current mean demand, but of the mean demand some time ago. As this mean value is lower than the current mean level of demand, the forecasts will generally be too low.

A further reason for bias is that there is an inherent limitation in the method itself. In Chapter 6, we saw two examples of this:

1. Single exponential smoothing has a 'decision point' bias immediately after an 'issue point' (although not when all points in time are considered).
2. Croston's method has an 'inversion bias', which requires correction.

Although there are different causes of forecast bias, the bias is always manifested by a tendency to over-forecast or under-forecast.

10.3.1 Monitoring and Detection of Bias

In Chapter 9, we reviewed some measures of bias, concentrating on the mean error and the mean scaled error. The focus in Chapter 9 was on comparing the bias of different forecasting methods. In this subsection, we assume that the method has been decided upon, but we wish to keep it under review to ensure continued good performance. This is essential because forecasts may operate well for a period of time with little bias but then become strongly biased, especially if the method becomes mis-specified. This is a well-known monitoring problem in statistics, and early solutions were based on cumulative sums (see, for example, Harrison and Davies 1964; Woodward and Goldsmith 1964). The cumulative forecast error at time t (CFE$_t$) is defined as in Eq. (10.1).

$$\text{CFE}_t = (d_t - \hat{d}_t) + \text{CFE}_{t-1} \tag{10.1}$$

Equation (10.1) shows how the measure is the sum of the previous CFE value (at time $t-1$) and the most recent forecast error. Equivalently, the cumulative forecast error (CFE) is the sum of all the previous errors (with positive and negative signs being retained), as shown in Eq. (10.2).

$$\text{CFE}_t = \sum_{i=1}^{t}(d_i - \hat{d}_i) = \sum_{i=1}^{t}d_i - \sum_{i=1}^{t}\hat{d}_i \tag{10.2}$$

The middle expression in Eq. (10.2) shows that the CFE is just the numerator in the mean error. The final expression in Eq. (10.2) shows that a straightforward way of calculating the CFE is to subtract the cumulative forecast from the cumulative demand. An example is shown in Table 10.3, with the cumulative demands and forecasts highlighted in bold.

In Table 10.3, the cumulative forecast is keeping track of the cumulative demand until the sixth period, and this is reflected by low CFEs. The two high demand values in Periods 7 and 9 result in the cumulative forecasts lagging behind the cumulative demand, as shown in Figure 10.1.

Wallström and Segerstedt (2010) introduced a metric called 'periods in stock' (PIS), which is defined in Eq. (10.3).

$$\text{PIS}_t = \text{PIS}_{t-1} - \text{CFE}_t = -\sum_{i=1}^{t}\sum_{j=1}^{i}(d_j - \hat{d}_j) \tag{10.3}$$

Table 10.3 Cumulative forecast error (CFE).

Period	Demand	Cumulative demand	Forecasted demand	Cumulative forecast	Cumulative forecast error
1	1	**1**	0.40	**0.40**	0.60
2	0	**1**	0.52	**0.92**	0.08
3	0	**1**	0.42	**1.34**	−0.34
4	1	**2**	0.33	**1.67**	0.33
5	0	**2**	0.47	**2.14**	−0.14
6	0	**2**	0.37	**2.51**	−0.51
7	10	**12**	0.30	**2.81**	9.19
8	0	**12**	2.24	**5.05**	6.95
9	5	**17**	1.79	**6.84**	10.16
10	0	**17**	2.43	**9.27**	7.73

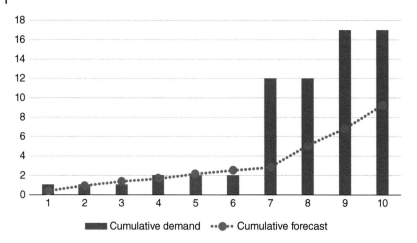

Figure 10.1 Cumulative demands and forecasts.

A positive value of the PIS measure indicates that the forecasting method is overestimating the demand, or inducing periods of excess stock holding. A negative value of PIS is a sign of underestimating the demand, with the risk of periods of stock shortage.

The PIS measure may be interpreted, based on a 'fictitious stock', as the number of periods a unit of the forecasted item has been in stock or out of stock. To illustrate this interpretation, Wallström and Segerstedt (2010) gave the following example. Suppose we forecast ahead for a total of three days (periods) and each day the forecast is for one unit. At the beginning of the first day, one item is delivered to a fictitious stock. If there is no demand during the first day, the result is $PIS_1 = 1$ (whereas a demand of one in the first period results in $PIS_1 = 0$). If the demand is zero in all three periods, then $PIS_3 = 6$. The item from day one has spent three days in stock, the item from the second day has spent two days in stock, and the last item has spent one day in stock. Therefore, the total number of days in stock, for all three items, is six. Wallström and Segerstedt (2010) recognised that this is a simplification of a real stock-control system. However, the metric has the merit that it is related to stock performance even if it does not mirror it exactly.

Kourentzes (2014) introduced a variant of the PIS, called the 'scaled absolute periods in stock' (sAPIS), as a scale-independent measure. It is defined as the absolute value of the PIS divided by the mean demand. This can be calculated for each SKU and averaged across SKUs to give an overall indicator of the consequence of forecast bias.

These cumulative error measures are more responsive to changes in bias than the mean error measure discussed in Chapter 9. Whilst the mean error is an effective measure of performance over a defined period of time, it is slow to react to change, especially if it is based on a long history of errors.

10.3.2 Bias as an Expectation of a Random Variable

Is it possible to quantify the bias of a forecasting method without real-life data? This seems impossible and, in one sense, it is. We cannot know how a method will perform, for any given organisation, until it is tested on real data from that organisation. However, we can analyse how a method will perform on 'synthetic data'. Synthetic data are generated from a hypothetical data generating process, such as $d_t = 10t + \epsilon_t$. This equation shows growth in demand by 10 each period, but this growth in demand is not entirely predictable. The 'residual noise' term, ϵ_t, is chosen from a normal distribution with zero mean and a constant variance (e.g. variance = 4). We can work out the sample mean of a number of selections of residuals from this normal distribution. As the number of selections increases, the sample mean will get closer and closer to the true mean of the distribution, known as its 'expectation', which in this case is zero. So, although individual values may not be close to zero, and sample means will not equal zero exactly, the expectation of each of the residual noise terms is zero.

Suppose that we are at the end of Period 9 and wish to make a forecast for Period 10. Then the data generating process shows that, on average, we would expect the demand to be 100 (but could be higher or lower than that, because of the noise term, ϵ_t). This is the expectation of demand in Period 10 and it may be written as: $\mathbb{E}(d_{10}) = 100$.

Now, suppose that we use the average of the last four periods as our forecast. As mentioned earlier, this forecast is mis-specified for data exhibiting a trend, so we would expect to see that the forecast is biased. To quantify the bias, we need to calculate the expected value of the forecast. The expectations of the observations in Periods 6, 7, 8, and 9 are 60, 70, 80, and 90, respectively; these values follow directly from the data generating process, recalling that $\epsilon_6, \epsilon_7, \epsilon_8$, and ϵ_9 all have zero expected values. The average of 60, 70, 80, and 90 is 75, which is 25 under the expected value of the new observation in Period 10, namely 100. Therefore, the expected bias is 25.

In this example, we have seen how it is possible to quantify bias without using real data. Of course, whether or not this quantity matches real-life experience is another matter. The choice of the best forecasting method remains a question to be resolved using real data. However, the 'synthetic data' approach will help in screening out inappropriate methods for particular data patterns.

10.3.3 Response to Different Causes of Bias

There are three main causes of forecast bias:

1. Judgemental bias.
2. Mis-specified forecast method.
3. Inherent limitation of the method itself.

It is useful to be able to diagnose the reason for forecast bias, as the different causes call for different responses. In the first case, better judgement can be encouraged by better forecasting training, appropriate reward systems (which reward approximately unbiased forecasts and penalise heavily biased forecasts), and better monitoring and feedback systems to enable forecasters to improve their performance.

In the second case, mis-specification may be addressed by improving classification methods, thereby ensuring that appropriate methods are used. This point will be expanded upon in Chapter 11. The final case requires better choice of methods to deal with intermittent demand, avoiding those that show excessive bias.

10.3.4 Summary

The measures that are appropriate for monitoring bias are different to those that are appropriate for measuring overall performance. If monitoring a single SKU, then scale-dependent measures may be satisfactory but, if monitoring across a whole collection of SKUs, then scale-independent measures should be used. If bias is detected, then further probing of the causes of bias can assist in taking remedial action.

It is also possible to examine the bias properties of forecasting methods, based on synthetic data from data generating processes, rather than from real data. This can lead to insights on mis-specification of methods. It can also help us to understand the components of the MSE, as we shall see in Section 10.4.

10.4   The Components of Mean Square Error

In Chapter 9, we looked at some error measures that were suited to fast-moving products, including the mean absolute percentage error (MAPE) and the mean absolute error (MAE). The MAPE is not suited to intermittence. Percentage errors cannot be calculated for zero observations, and the MAPE cannot be calculated for intermittent demand. The MAE is minimised at the median rather than the mean. One error measure that attains its lowest value at the mean, and not the median, is the MSE. We look at how it is calculated, and its properties, in the remainder of this section.

10.4.1   Calculation of Mean Square Error

The calculated MSE, using the same data as in Table 10.3 (with frequent zeroes), is shown in Table 10.4, with squared errors and the MSE highlighted in bold. Absolute errors and the MAE are also shown in Table 10.4.

In Chapter 9, we noted that the MSE is sensitive to large errors. In Table 10.4, a little over 80% of the total squared errors (116.9) comes from just one squared error (94.09), in Period 7. Untypical observations, such as the demand for 10 units in Period 7, tend to be more extreme in intermittent demand than in faster-moving demand. Consequently, MSE is not generally used for performance measurement of intermittent demand forecasts in practice.

However, as noted earlier, MSE does take its lowest value at the mean value (rather than the median) and so will not be optimised by the zero forecast method (always forecast zero). In the example in Table 10.4, the zero forecast would reduce the MAE (from 2.06 to 1.70) but would increase the MSE (from 11.69 to 12.70). The MSE's property of being minimised at the mean makes it a good choice for investigating the properties of forecasting methods using synthetic data, based on hypothetical data generating processes.

10.4.2   Decomposition of Expected Squared Errors

To examine the components of the MSE, we turn our attention from the sample mean of the observed squared errors, as calculated in Table 10.4, to the expectation of the squared errors of the process. The forecast error at time t is $e_t = d_t - \hat{d}_t$, using the same notation as before.

Table 10.4 Mean square error (frequent zeroes).

Period	Actual demand	Forecast demand	Forecast error	Absolute error	Squared error
1	1	0.40	0.60	0.60	**0.36**
2	0	0.52	−0.52	0.52	**0.27**
3	0	0.42	−0.42	0.42	**0.18**
4	1	0.33	0.67	0.67	**0.45**
5	0	0.47	−0.47	0.47	**0.22**
6	0	0.37	−0.37	0.37	**0.14**
7	10	0.30	9.70	9.70	**94.09**
8	0	2.24	−2.24	2.24	**5.02**
9	5	1.79	3.21	3.21	**10.30**
10	0	2.43	−2.43	2.43	**5.90**
Mean	1.70	0.93	0.77	2.06	**11.69**

Suppose that the latest forecast error, e_t, is higher than the expectation of the forecast error, $\mathbb{E}(e_t)$. Then we can visualise the squared error, e_t^2, as shown in Figure 10.2.

The area of the whole square in Figure 10.2 represents the squared error, e_t^2. The area of this whole square is equal to the sum of the areas of the two component squares (A and C) plus the areas of the two component rectangles (B for both). An alternative way

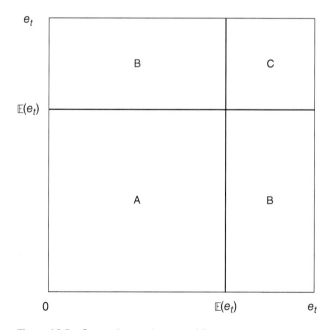

Figure 10.2 Squared error decomposition.

of decomposing the total area is to join the square A to the rectangle B above to form a larger rectangle of area A + B; and then to join the square A to the rectangle B beside it, also giving a larger rectangle of area A + B. Adding these two larger rectangles together results in the square A being counted twice. Therefore, the large square can be decomposed as: C + 2(A + B) − A. This can also be written as in Eq. (10.4).

$$e_t^2 = \left(e_t - \mathbb{E}(e_t)\right)^2 + 2e_t\mathbb{E}(e_t) - \left(\mathbb{E}(e_t)\right)^2 \tag{10.4}$$

The expected squared error $\mathbb{E}(e_t^2)$ can be decomposed (Technical Note 10.1), as shown in Eq. (10.5).

$$\mathbb{E}(e_t^2) = \mathrm{Var}(e_t) + \left(\mathbb{E}(e_t)\right)^2 \tag{10.5}$$

In Eq. (10.5), the first term on the right-hand side is the variance of the forecast errors. It is a measure of the 'erraticness' of forecast errors: the more stable the forecast errors, the lower their variance. The second term on the right-hand side of Eq. (10.5) is the square of the bias. Because of this, Eq. (10.5) is sometimes known as the 'bias–variance decomposition'.

From this result, it may be seen that it is desirable to reduce the error variance and the magnitude of the bias of the forecasts, as both contribute to the expected squared error (which is the long run average found by calculating the MSE). However, it is not always possible to reduce both the variance of the forecast errors and the magnitude of bias, and there is often a trade-off between these two components of the expected squared errors.

In the context of judgemental forecasting, Brighton and Gigerenzer (2015) explain the success of some judgemental strategies using the bias–variance decomposition. They argue that, although judgemental forecasts may be more strongly biased than statistical forecasts, they can sometimes reduce the variance of forecast error to such an extent that the overall squared error is reduced. This is an example of a 'trade-off' where reduction in error variance can be more important than a penalty in forecast bias.

10.4.3 Decomposition of Expected Squared Errors for Independent Demand

In certain circumstances, it is possible to decompose the forecast error variance further so that it includes a term representing the 'residual noise', ϵ_t. This term is random and, therefore, no matter how well we predict, we cannot expect the variance of forecast errors to be less than the variance of the residuals, $\mathrm{Var}(\epsilon_t)$, which is equal to the variance of i.i.d. demand, $\mathrm{Var}(d_t)$. It would be useful if we could include this variance, $\mathrm{Var}(d_t)$, as part of our decomposition, as it will provide a foundation for the classification rules for i.i.d. demand in Chapter 11. So, we assume that the data generating process is such that the expected demand and its variance do not change over time, and demands are independent of previous demand values. In that case, as explained in Technical Note 10.2, the variance of the forecast errors can be decomposed further, as shown in Eq. (10.6).

$$\mathrm{Var}(e_t) = \mathrm{Var}(d_t) + \mathrm{Var}(\widehat{d}_t) \tag{10.6}$$

It should be noted that if demand in the current period is correlated with previous demands (i.e. it is autocorrelated), then this result does not hold. We return to such demand patterns in Chapters 13 and 14. However, if we can be confident that demands are not autocorrelated, then we have the expression for the expected squared error shown in Eq. (10.7).

$$\mathbb{E}(e_t^2) = \text{Var}(d_t) + \text{Var}(\hat{d}_t) + \left(\mathbb{E}(e_t)\right)^2 \tag{10.7}$$

Each of the three components of the right-hand side of Eq. (10.7) deserves close attention.

The first term, representing the *variance of demand*, is not related to the forecasting method. So, no matter what forecasting method is chosen, this component cannot be reduced, unlike the other two components. It may be possible to reduce the variance of demand by other means, for example by following an 'every day low prices' strategy and having fewer discounts and promotional campaigns, as introduced by Walmart in the United States and Tesco in the United Kingdom. It cannot be reduced by choosing a better forecasting method.

The second term, representing the *variance of the forecasts*, is a measure of forecast consistency: the lower the value of this term, the more consistent the forecasts will be. Forecast consistency is reflected by lower MSEs, assuming there is no problem with bias. There is also an indirect benefit for inventory management. More consistent forecasts lead to more consistent orders, and give suppliers no excuse for delays in delivery of shipments, as it is easier to plan production if the orders are consistent in size. However, if there are any structural changes in demand, then a forecasting method that emphasises consistency will often be biased as it will lag behind systematic changes in demand.

The third term represents the square of the *forecast bias*. Although it is desirable to reduce the magnitude of forecast bias, care must be taken that any increase in the variance of the forecasts does not outweigh the benefit from reducing bias.

In summary, Eq. (10.7) can be written in a more interpretable form, as shown in Eq. (10.8).

$$\text{MSE} = \mathbb{E}(\text{Squared error}) = \text{Var}(\text{Demand}) + \text{Var}(\text{Forecast}) + \text{Bias}^2 \tag{10.8}$$

It is desirable to reduce both the variance of forecasts and forecast bias. For example, we found, in Chapter 6, that the SBA method is less biased than Croston's method. The variances of the forecasts, for the two methods, are related by the (exact) formula in Eq. (10.9).

$$\text{Var}(\hat{d}_t^{\text{SBA}}) = \left(1 - \frac{\alpha}{2}\right)^2 \text{Var}(\hat{d}_t^{\text{CR}}) \tag{10.9}$$

where α is the smoothing constant for the demand intervals, and CR denotes Croston's method. As the expression $(1 - \alpha/2)$ is always less than one (for smoothing constants in the range $0 < \alpha \leq 1$), the variance of the forecasts from SBA is always less than the variance from Croston's method. For example, if the smoothing constant is 0.2, then the variance of the forecasts from SBA is 81% of the variance of the forecasts from Croston.

As noted earlier, it is not always possible to reduce both the bias and the variance of forecast error. For example, a more refined version of SBA reduces its bias but at the expense of greater variance (Syntetos 2001).

10.4.4 Summary

In this section, we have seen how to calculate the MSE, based on real data, noting that the measure can be sensitive to just one outlying observation. This makes the MSE problematical for tracking the performance of forecast systems in practice. However, when addressing hypothetical data generating processes, our analysis of the MSE has shown that two of its principal components are forecast error variance and (the square of) forecast bias. If methods can be found to reduce both of these components, then that would be ideal. In some cases, this may not be possible, and we may need to trade off these two quantities, seeking to reduce the overall MSE.

It is also possible to decompose the error variance into its own components, providing that the current demand is independent of previous demands. This decomposition into demand variance and forecast variance shows that, in the long run, we will not be able to reduce the MSE below the demand variance by changing the forecasting method. However, we can look for improvements in forecast variance, keeping an eye on forecast bias, to ensure that the overall MSE is minimised for the hypothetical demand generating process.

10.5 Chapter Summary

We began this chapter by noting that judgemental adjustments of statistical forecasts are very common in practice. The evidence on forecast accuracy shows that such adjustments can improve accuracy, especially when the human judge adjusts the forecasts downwards. However, upward adjustments are usually less beneficial, showing more modest improvements in accuracy, with frequent evidence of 'optimism bias'.

The tendency for biases to creep into forecasts (whether judgemental or statistical) may be countered by monitoring biases over time. Cumulative forecast errors or the 'periods in stock' (PIS) measure may be used for this purpose. Scaled measures are needed if monitoring over a collection of SKUs.

The decomposition of mean square error into error variance and bias components may help to explain the more modest improvements in forecast accuracy when upward adjustments are being employed. The human judges may have reduced the error variance but at the cost of greater bias. For downward adjustments, reductions in bias are more common, yielding greater potential gains in forecast accuracy.

Statistical methods may be improved by reducing error variance and forecast bias. In some cases, it may not be possible to reduce both quantities. However, we may still compare the mean square error of two methods using the bias–variance decomposition. In the case of demand in the current period being independent of demands in previous periods, this analysis can be extended further by decomposing the error variance into its own components. This is a powerful method of analysis for intermittent demand forecasting methods, which will be used in Chapter 11, to help determine appropriate forecasting categorisation rules.

Technical Notes

Note 10.1 Bias–Variance Decomposition

Re-stating Eq. (10.4): $e_t^2 = \left(e_t - \mathbb{E}(e_t)\right)^2 + 2e_t\mathbb{E}(e_t) - \mathbb{E}(e_t)^2$.

The first term on the right-hand side represents the squared deviation of the forecast error from its expected value. High fluctuations in forecast errors will result in high variances.

The magnitude of the second term depends on the size of the individual errors. On average, the errors take the value $\mathbb{E}(e_t)$ itself. Taking expectations of both sides of Eq. (10.4) gives the result shown in Eq. (10.10).

$$\mathbb{E}(e_t^2) = \mathbb{E}((e_t - \mathbb{E}(e_t))^2) + 2\mathbb{E}(e_t)^2 - \mathbb{E}(e_t)^2 \tag{10.10}$$

The first term on the right-hand side of Eq. (10.10) represents the variance of the forecast errors. Therefore, Eq. (10.10) can be re-written in the form of Eq. (10.11):

$$\mathbb{E}(e_t^2) = \text{Var}(e_t) + \mathbb{E}(e_t)^2 \tag{10.11}$$

Note 10.2 Extended Bias–Variance Decomposition

To analyse the error variance further, we start with the following decomposition of forecast errors into three components, as shown in Eq. (10.12).

$$e_t = d_t - \hat{d}_t = (d_t - \mathbb{E}(d_t)) + (\mathbb{E}(d_t) - \mathbb{E}(\hat{d}_t)) + (\mathbb{E}(\hat{d}_t) - \hat{d}_t)) \tag{10.12}$$

In this case, we adopt a more detailed visualisation of the squared error, taking into account each of the three components of Eq. (10.12):

1. Demand minus Expected Demand.
2. Expected Demand minus Expected Forecast.
3. Expected Forecast minus Forecast.

If these three components are added together, then the result is the forecast error. This is shown in Figure 10.3, with the first component on the right-hand side of the horizontal axis (and uppermost on the vertical axis), the second component in the middle of both axes, and the third component on the left-hand side of the horizontal axis (and bottommost on the vertical axis).

If we ignore the four corner squares/rectangles, the remaining area can be expressed as in Eq. (10.13).

$$2(\text{B} + \text{D} + \text{E}) - \text{D} = 2(d_t - \hat{d}_t)(\mathbb{E}(d_t) - \mathbb{E}(\hat{d}_t)) - (\mathbb{E}(d_t) - \mathbb{E}(\hat{d}_t))^2 \tag{10.13}$$

Taking expectations of the right-hand side of Eq. (10.13) results in Eq. (10.14).

$$\mathbb{E}(2(d_t - \hat{d}_t)(\mathbb{E}(d_t) - \mathbb{E}(\hat{d}_t)) - (\mathbb{E}(d_t) - \mathbb{E}(\hat{d}_t))^2) = (\mathbb{E}(d_t) - \mathbb{E}(\hat{d}_t))^2 \tag{10.14}$$

The term on the right hand-side of Eq. (10.14) is the square of $\mathbb{E}(d_t - \hat{d}_t)$ or, expressed another way, the square of the forecast bias. This is the first component of the MSE, and is shown as the third term in Eq. (10.7).

Now, we return to the four corner squares/rectangles. The lower left-hand square, labelled A, has the area shown in Eq. (10.15).

$$\text{A} = (\mathbb{E}(\hat{d}_t) - \hat{d}_t)^2 = (\hat{d}_t - \mathbb{E}(\hat{d}_t))^2 \tag{10.15}$$

Taking expectations of the right-hand side of Eq. (10.15) results in Eq. (10.16).

$$\mathbb{E}((\hat{d}_t - \mathbb{E}(\hat{d}_t))^2) = \text{Var}(\hat{d}_t) \tag{10.16}$$

Thus, the second component, represented as the area of square A in Figure 10.3, is equal to the forecast variance.

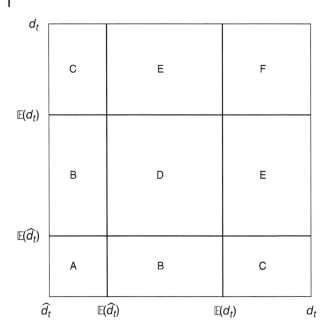

Figure 10.3 (Extended) squared error decomposition.

The upper right-hand square, labelled F, has the area shown in Eq. (10.17).

$$F = (d_t - \mathbb{E}(d_t))^2 \tag{10.17}$$

Taking expectations of the right-hand side of Eq. (10.17) results in Eq. (10.18).

$$\mathbb{E}\left((d_t - \mathbb{E}(d_t))^2\right) = \text{Var}(d_t) \tag{10.18}$$

Thus, the third component, represented as the area of square F in Figure 10.3, is equal to the variance of demand itself, and is shown as the first term in Eq. (10.7). This component is not affected by the choice of forecasting method, and so cannot be reduced by any improvements in forecasting.

The final parts of Figure 10.3 are the two rectangles, of the same area, both designated as C. The total area is given by: $2C = 2(d_t - \mathbb{E}(d_t))(\mathbb{E}(\widehat{d}_t) - \widehat{d}_t)$. Taking expectations, we find that this quantity collapses to zero, assuming independence of demands (which implies that d_t is independent of $\widehat{d}_t$, because $\widehat{d}_t$ is a function of previous demands). Also, please note that the 'area' (2C) can be positive or negative and is, in fact, zero on average.

Summarising, we have found that the expectation of the squared errors has three components of the bias–variance decomposition: (i) forecast bias (squared), (ii) forecast variance, and (iii) demand variance.

This may be written as in Eq. (10.19).

$$\mathbb{E}(e_t^2) = \text{Var}(d_t) + \text{Var}(\widehat{d}_t) + \left(\mathbb{E}(e_t)\right)^2 \tag{10.19}$$

This is the same as Eq. (10.7), shown earlier in the chapter. Subtracting the squared bias from both sides, gives the result shown in Eq. (10.6), presented again here as Eq. (10.20).

$$\text{Var}(e_t) = \text{Var}(d_t) + \text{Var}(\widehat{d}_t) \tag{10.20}$$

11

Classification Methods

11.1 Introduction

Demand forecasting sometimes needs to be performed at a group level for a collection of different items or, indeed, across all the items that are held in stock. This would be the case, for example, when deciding on the mode of transport to distribute products to customers or when investing in a new warehouse, the capacity of which needs to be determined. In such cases, a manager would be interested in the future demand of more than one single item, and the forecasts would typically inform medium- and long-term planning.

As the forecast horizon gets shorter, typically the level of aggregation (the number of items for which an aggregated forecast is required) gets smaller. For inventory management, short-term ordering decisions are at the lowest level of aggregation, namely the individual stock keeping unit (SKU). This necessitates the selection of an appropriate forecasting method for each item. However, a typical organisation holds hundreds or thousands, or in the case of a military entity, like the US Defense Logistics Agency for example, even millions of distinct inventory items.

To streamline the organisation and management of such large collections of items, businesses often utilise classification schemes. Under such a scheme, the items are separated into various classes and common decision processes apply to all items belonging to a particular class or category. (The words 'class' and 'category', as well as 'classification' and 'categorisation', are used interchangeably in this book.)

Of course, classification schemes are needed not only for forecasting. Many other functions, such as warehousing, transportation, and inventory control are addressed through the introduction of classification schemes. In general, classifications are required to support any operational decision that needs to be performed on an item by item basis, such as determining the positioning of an item in a warehouse or determining an appropriate inventory rule to trigger replenishments. In fact, it was not until recently that forecasting-specific schemes were developed. Previously, the forecasting task would be facilitated through schemes that were primarily based on the needs of other organisational functions. Important as they are, we will argue that such schemes bear little relevance to the forecasting task.

Intermittent Demand Forecasting: Context, Methods and Applications, First Edition.
John E. Boylan and Aris A. Syntetos.
© 2021 John Wiley & Sons Ltd. Published 2021 by John Wiley & Sons Ltd.
Companion Website: www.wiley.com/go/boylansyntetos/intermittentdemandforecasting

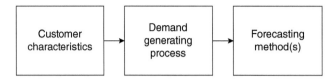

Figure 11.1 Customer demand and forecasting.

For the purpose of forecasting, items should be categorised based on their demand patterns and also, in certain cases, their customer characteristics. This is because the underlying demand pattern of an item, and the characteristics of the customers that generate the demand, should determine the forecasting method(s) to be used to inform stock requirements. This is presented diagramatically in Figure 11.1. (Customer characteristics may also determine cases where reliance upon forecasting may be reduced due to the possibility of obtaining, for example, advance demand information from customers. Such cases will be discussed later in the chapter.)

Items with 'similar' patterns are categorised together and utilise a specific forecasting method (or a set of forecasting methods). To enable this to happen, we must first pose an important question, namely, 'What do we mean by 'similar'?' We know, from previous chapters, that intermittent demand patterns require different forecasting methods from non-intermittent demand patterns. So, a crucial question here would be, 'What constitutes intermittence?' How many zero demands need to be present in a time series for it to be called intermittent? These questions are addressed in detail in this chapter.

In summary, there are two types of classification schemes to facilitate the forecasting task:

1. Classification schemes developed explicitly for forecasting purposes.
2. Classification schemes coincidentally serving the forecasting task.

We start our discussion with the latter category, as this enables the presentation of developments in the area of classification in an appropriate chronological and conceptual order.

11.2 Classification Schemes

Classification schemes are used in almost all inventory systems. Because they are often well established, their appropriateness can sometimes be taken for granted. In this section, we review some of the major purposes of classification and consider how classification criteria can serve those purposes.

11.2.1 The Purpose of Classification

Classification serves a wide range of organisational functions. Depending on the function, some criteria need to be established to allow the classification to take place. For example, warehouse managers are interested in (i) the size of the items, which will determine space usage optimisation; (ii) the price of items, which will determine precautions against theft; and (iii) how often an item is requested, as it makes sense to position fast moving items closer to the pick-up point and slow moving items further inside a warehouse.

Inventory managers are interested in the value of an item, as higher value items have higher inventory holding costs. They will also be interested in the frequency with which an item is 'moving' because the inventory policies needed for items that require frequent replenishments are different from those that are demanded infrequently. Transportation managers would be interested in a classification of items based on size, as they attempt to optimise space usage (e.g. container volume or the volume capacity of a lorry). Along the same lines, sales managers who are interested in maximising revenue would wish to identify the highest revenue generating items, and strategic planners in the after-sales industry would be interested in the current life cycle phase of a product that needs servicing.

11.2.2 Classification Criteria

Once appropriate classification criteria have been established, some method is needed to use them in practice. Assume, for example, that we are interested in the annual sales volume of items, for inventory purposes. This quantity will be used to categorise items, and for the selection of appropriate inventory rules for each of the categories. This means that items with similar annual sales volumes need to be clustered together. This brings us again to the question posed earlier, 'What do we mean by 'similar'?' One approach would be to determine cut-off values in absolute terms. (For example, a low selling category is one associated with an annual sales volume between 0 and 500 units, and a medium selling category relates to annual sales volumes between 501 and 1000 units, leaving all items that sell more than 1000 units per year to be classified as high selling.) You may be wondering where these cut-off values come from. And you would be right to wonder. The values of 500 and 1000 units are ad hoc, and this is the case almost invariably in practical applications. An ad hoc solution, designed for a specific problem, lacks generalisation and so cannot necessarily be applied elsewhere.

Another approach in the example considered above would be to determine the cut-off values in relative (or percentage) terms. Suppose, for example, that we rank all the items in a stock base in descending order of their annual volume: the item with the highest annual sales volume is ranked first, the one with the second highest volume is ranked second, and so on. We may then say that the top 20% of the items, ranked by annual sales, constitute the 'high selling' category, the medium 30% of the items relate to the 'medium selling' category, and the bottom 50% of the items are categorised as 'low selling' ones. This does not overcome the problem of the ad hoc specification of the cut-off points but, as discussed later in the chapter, it does represent a generic pattern of inventories expressed through what is known as the ABC classification. A way of characterising the derivation of these (relative) cut-off values is by referring to them as 'rules of thumb'. Rules of thumb were discussed briefly earlier in this book. Some rules are ill-informed but others, while not being intended to be strictly accurate or reliable for every situation, can be quite robust across different situations. We will see later on that the relative classification discussed above is a widely accepted rule of thumb.

11.2.3 Summary

In summary, different organisational functions require different criteria for classification purposes. Once the criteria have been established, appropriate cut-off values need to be identified to allow the separation of items into various categories. Common decision processes then apply to each of those categories. Two important points arising from Section 11.2 are as follows:

1. The classification criteria need to be linked explicitly to the purpose of the classification exercise.
2. There are various ways of establishing cut-off values for the criteria, ranging from ad hoc to more generally applicable rules, and from absolute to relative specifications.

11.3 ABC Classification

The most commonly applied classification method is known as the ABC classification. In this section, we consider its rationale and its relevance to inventory management and demand forecasting.

11.3.1 Pareto Principle

The ABC or Pareto classification is often used in industry to determine categories of differing importance. It is named after Vilfredo Pareto (1848–1923), an Italian economist and engineer, who observed in 1906 that 80% of the land in Italy was owned by 20% of the population. More generally, it has been empirically observed over the last century that, for many different phenomena, about 80% of the effects come from 20% of the causes, and this has become known as the Pareto principle or the law of the vital few.

In an inventory context, many case studies (e.g. Syntetos et al. 2009b, 2010) have confirmed the validity of the 80 : 20 rule: that about 20% of the items in an inventory base generate about 80% of the sales volume, with 80% of the items generating the remaining 20% of the sales volume. As an extension, more than two categories, typically three but not necessarily so, may be used to control a stock base. Based on a single criterion (most often the annual demand volume, or the annual demand value), all items in a stock base are ranked in descending order. (As discussed in Chapter 1, please note that sales are almost invariably used in industry as a proxy for demand.) The ranked items are then split into three classes, called A, B, and C, with a typical contribution to the annual demand volume (or annual demand value) of about 20%/80%, 30%/15%, and 50%/5%, respectively. More than three categories are sometimes used in practice (Syntetos et al. 2009b).

11.3.2 Service Criticality

The ABC classification by demand value is often used as a proxy for criticality, with the items in class A considered the most critical and thus requiring the highest service levels to avoid expensive backlogs. The demand volume criterion does not take cost into account, which would normally be considered an important aspect of criticality.

As discussed in Chapters 3 and 8, inventory systems are usually driven by a service level target. The ABC classification would then be used to determine what service target we set for each of the three categories, with the highest target set for the A items (say 99%), followed by a lower target for the B items (say 90%), and an even lower one for the C items (say 85%). Higher service targets would then naturally imply higher investments in inventory to support the targeted performance as well as (possibly) the use of different forecasting methods and inventory control rules. In terms of forecasting, methods designed for fast demand items would be used for the A and B items (depending on the inventory base under concern) and intermittent demand forecasting methods would be used for many of the C items.

It has often been argued (e.g. Knod and Schonberger 2001) that the class C items should get the highest service level. This argument (as well as other arguments on the comparatively greater importance of the C items) is based on the collective contribution of these items. When looked at individually, the C items are indeed relatively unimportant. However, when they are considered as a whole, the picture changes dramatically.

A high service level set for the C items would substantially reduce stockouts. The effort and cost of dealing with those stockouts (e.g. by using emergency shipments) may be much larger than the cost of holding more of these items, especially those that are relatively inexpensive. Another important argument is that a major key performance indicator (KPI) in various business contexts (including the third-party logistics industry) is the percentage of order completion, also known as the order fill rate, as discussed in Chapter 3. Of course, orders may be comprised of items from more than one category. Suppose, for example, that we receive 10 orders from 10 industrial customers each consisting of two items. The same best-selling A item is included in all 10 orders and the second item is a different C item in each order. The availability of the 10 different C items is as important as the availability of the particular A item. In fact, if the emergency supply lead times are longer for the C items, the A item may be less important (as it can be replenished faster than the C items, keeping the backorder costs lower).

Moreover, if the SKUs in Class A receive the highest service level (as often happens in practice), and the classification is based on a demand value criterion, then the SKUs with a higher price (and therefore higher holding cost) will have relatively larger stock levels, a situation that is obviously cost inefficient.

The above arguments explain why specialists in commercial ABC applications often find that the demand volume criterion may be more effective than the demand value criterion in reducing inventory costs while maximising service level (R. Pflitsch, personal communication). However, and as discussed above, it makes little sense not to include the value of an item in any inventory related exercise. Surely, the fact that one item costs £1000 while another costs £1 needs to be taken into account. The problem we are faced with is that neither the demand value nor the demand volume criterion has been developed from an inventory perspective and thus may not be particularly effective for inventory management.

11.3.3 ABC Classification and Forecasting

Another major criticism of the ABC classifications relates to the forecasting task. Neither the demand value nor the demand volume criterion is sufficient to characterise the demand pattern of an item or the customer characteristics generating the demand. We do know that, generally speaking, intermittent demand items are amongst the slower moving items, which would correspond to the C category. But suppose, for example, that ABC is being applied in a company operating in the after-sales industry, and all the inventory items are spare parts. As discussed in Chapter 1, spare parts are most often characterised by intermittent demand patterns. In that case, the annual volume or value cannot determine the degree of intermittence, which is sometimes described as 'fast intermittence' (intermittent demand items that move relatively fast) or 'slow intermittence' (intermittent demand items that move very slowly). Of course, it may be that fast intermittent items would be classified as A or B, and slow intermittent items as C. This may be the case, but there are two points to be made here:

1. The average demand size, when demand occurs, may distort our perception of intermittence. Think, for example, of an item that has moved only three times in a year but the average size of the demand, when demand occurs, is 50 units. Now, consider another item that has moved 10 times in a year but the average size of the demand, when demand occurs, is two units. Under the demand volume criterion, the first item may be classified as A (150 units sold in a year) and the second item may be classified as C (20 units sold in a year). However, the first item has demand that is clearly more intermittent.
2. The price of an item may distort the real picture too. In the example discussed above, assume that the price for the first item is £2/unit and the price for the second item is £50/unit. This would result in an annual demand value of £300 (£2/unit × 150 units) and £1000 (£50/unit × 20 units) for the first and the second item, respectively, which would reverse their classification.

11.3.4 Summary

For forecasting purposes, neither the demand value nor the demand volume is a relevant criterion. The former is irrelevant because the choice of the best forecasting method has nothing to do with the price of an item. The latter is also not the most useful because it is not the total volume that would help to determine the right forecasting method but rather how that volume was generated, i.e. the mechanism that determines the frequency of demand arrivals, coupled with the size of the demand, when demand occurs.

Given the above arguments, a classification scheme that captures the constituent elements upon which demand is generated (size and interval) would be useful. Such a scheme, designed specifically to select between forecasting methods, will be discussed in Sections 11.5–11.7.

11.4 Extensions to the ABC Classification

The ABC approach has some drawbacks as a basis for forecasting classification, as discussed above. It also has some limitations for inventory classification, for example when we need to set service level targets for different classes of items. In this section, we concentrate on suggestions to improve inventory classification, without reference to forecasting, before moving to forecasting considerations in subsequent sections of the chapter.

11.4.1 Composite Criterion Approach

A major drawback associated with the demand value and demand volume criteria is that neither of them takes into account the backlog cost (i.e. the cost of expediting stock following a stockout occurrence). By considering such a penalty cost, the criticality of an item may be taken into account. Teunter et al. (2010) proposed a formal criterion for constructing ABC schemes, for order-point order-up-to, (s, S), and order-point order-quantity, (s, Q), inventory systems. The criterion is based on a composite of four factors for SKU i: penalty cost per backordered item (b_i), inventory holding cost per item (h_i), average order quantity (Q_i), and average demand per period (D_i), also known as the 'demand rate'. The use of the term 'formal' indicates that the criterion reflects inventory management considerations, rather than having been developed in an uncritical fashion (along the lines of the demand volume and demand value criteria). The composite criterion, CC_i, for the ith SKU, is defined in Eq. (11.1).

$$CC_i = \frac{b_i D_i}{h_i Q_i} \tag{11.1}$$

The composite criterion can be applied using the following simple steps:

1. Rank all SKUs in descending order of CC_i.
2. Divide the SKUs into classes A, B, and C in increasing sizes of 20%, 30%, and 50%. (More classes can be used as in the single-criterion ABC classifications.)
3. Fix the cycle service level for each class, where A has the highest service level, followed by B, and then C.

A number of points need to be made here. First, both inventory holding and backlog costs are taken into account, which is a very desirable property, as discussed in Chapter 2. Second, the composite criterion ranks an SKU higher if the inventory holding cost is lower. Note that the inventory holding cost is considered in the denominator of the criterion (Eq. (11.1)) and thus the lower its value, the higher the ratio and the higher the positioning of the relevant SKU in the ranked array of items. This addresses the disadvantage of the demand-value criterion discussed in Section 11.3. Third, the demand rate is taken into account; the higher the demand per period, the higher the ranking of an SKU.

The composite criterion has been empirically shown to perform better than the criteria discussed in Section 11.3 (Teunter et al. 2010). It is also more intuitively appealing from an inventory perspective and, in addition, more complex multi-criteria methods, to be discussed below, may be avoided. However, the criterion may not be used in the context of (R, S) policies, which is what we suggest in this book. More research is needed to adapt the rule for such policies. More importantly, the composite criterion was developed with the objective of minimising inventory costs whilst maximising service. Although the demand rate is taken into account, the criterion cannot be used for the purpose of selecting different forecasting methods for each of the resulting categories. The argument is similar to that made in Section 11.3 for the demand value criterion, namely that the selection of a forecasting method to estimate the mean demand has nothing to do with cost parameters.

11.4.2 Multi-criteria Approaches

The use of value, volume, or a composite all fall into the category of a single-criterion classification, which is the most common approach in practice. More complex classification schemes can offer greater flexibility but at a cost of more challenging implementation. Criteria that may be relevant in terms of SKU classifications include, depending on the context: the certainty of supply, the rate of obsolescence, the lead time (and its variability), costs of review and replenishment, design and manufacturing process technology, and substitutability (Syntetos et al. 2011a). Subsequently, multi-criteria classifications may be developed that take some of the above or other relevant factors into account.

Application of multi-criteria approaches is not straightforward, as the importance of the criteria needs to be weighted and combined through structured methodologies like the analytic hierarchy process, with which many managers are unfamiliar. Hu et al. (2018) reviewed the application of multi-criteria approaches for spare parts management and concluded that most of the existing models need to be further developed and validated through empirical studies, before they can be recommended for application in practice.

An alternative to multi-criteria methodologies is multiple-way classifications, for example a two-way classification by purchase cost and demand volume (or by cost and frequency of demands). Such a classification approach, designed specifically for forecasting purposes, will be discussed later in this chapter.

11.4.3 Classification for Spare Parts

Before we close this section, a discussion on the specificities of classification in a maintenance context is required. (Maintenance is further considered in detail in Chapter 12.) In this case, all the SKUs are spare parts and 'criticality' may be determined either informally (along the lines previously discussed in this chapter) or by formal methods such as failure mode, effects, and criticality analysis (FMECA). According to this method, criticality analysis is defined as 'A procedure by which each potential failure mode is ranked according to the combined influence of severity and probability of occurrence' (Department of Defense 1980, p. 3). This approach is often used in the maintenance of industrial equipment or technical systems in general. However, it may also be applicable to service parts for consumers. For example, safety-critical automotive components, such as brakes, would be assigned to a higher criticality category than non-essential automotive accessories.

FMECA is typically complemented by other classification criteria, such as those to be discussed later in the chapter, to allow the specification of appropriate forecasting methods and inventory rules. With regard to the former, important issues (such as the number of hours the equipment has been used) are often expressed as explanatory variables that enable causal forecasting to take place. Causal forecasting is a different approach to extrapolating requirements from those discussed in Chapter 6, which may be termed as time series methods. Causal forecasting will be discussed in more detail in Chapter 12.

In general, statistical forecasting approaches may be broadly divided into two categories:

1. Dependent on explanatory variables (causal methods).
2. Dependent only on the history of the series (extrapolation methods).

A classification of service parts according to the product life cycle can assist in choosing the better approach. The choice of the forecasting approach is mainly determined by the availability of data on explanatory variables, such as the timing of preventive maintenance activities. However, the forecasting approach is also driven by the availability of demand history data which, in turn, is determined by the stage of the service part's life cycle. Causal methods are particularly useful in the initial phase, when the part is introduced, because the lack of an adequate length of demand history precludes the use of extrapolative time-series methods. As more data becomes available, time-series methods like those discussed in Chapter 6 become more relevant.

11.4.4 Summary

Composite measures may offer a useful extension to the classical ABC classifications that rely upon demand value or volume. The measure proposed by Teunter et al. (2010) is meaningful from an inventory perspective but it cannot accommodate the needs of the forecasting function. Multi-criteria classification methods and multiple-way classifications afford other opportunities to capture important inventory aspects, but their implementation is rather challenging. However, a two-way classification scheme (based on criteria that are relevant to forecasting) will be discussed later in this chapter and we will show that it may considerably advance current practices. Finally, an alternative formal way of determining service criticality has been discussed based on the FMECA approach. This is a useful approach for maintenance spare parts. Its implementation requires a thorough analysis of the modes of failures and thus is quite costly. However, it may be justified for industrial maintenance when the cost of downtime is very high.

11.5 Conceptual Clarifications

In practice, a variety of terms are used to describe the demand patterns addressed in this book, including 'slow', 'intermittent', 'sporadic', and 'lumpy'. In one organisation we have worked with, highly variable intermittent demand was called 'lumpy lumpy'. In this section, some key terms are defined more formally, linking them to measurable properties of the demand series.

11.5.1 Definition of Non-normal Demand Patterns

Let us now consider the issue of classification in a forecasting context. In principle, even one zero demand observation in the demand history of an item renders the demand pattern as intermittent. But is just one zero demand sufficient to justify the use of forecasting methods specifically designed for intermittence? Perhaps the answer is 'no', but this depends on how many historical observations are available. If there is only one zero demand out of a total of five observations, then maybe demand is intermittent. But if there is one zero demand out of a total of 25 observations, then maybe demand is not intermittent. This issue constitutes a major problem in industry where ad hoc rules are often used to qualify a pattern as intermittent. Rules like 'An intermittent demand pattern is one that has at least three zero observations out of the last 12' are very often used in practice. A rule like that begs the question 'Why three zero observations and not four or two?'

Further, we discussed in Chapter 5 that the degree of variability present in intermittent demand series relates not only to the degree of intermittence but also the characteristics of the demand sizes, when demand occurs. Highly variable demand sizes are often termed as erratic. But what exactly do we mean by saying 'highly variable'? What is high variability?

Before we attempt to answer two key questions, namely, 'What constitutes intermittence?' and 'What constitutes erraticness?', some conceptual clarifications are required in order to put the more technical discussion in context.

Firstly, we refer to all the demand patterns where demand does not occur in every single period and/or demand is highly variable, to the degree that the normal distribution cannot provide a good fit, as non-normal demand patterns. This terminology allows us to cluster together demand patterns that are difficult to deal with and explore their properties, thereby enabling some further helpful definitions to emerge. An important note here is that, by using this nomenclature, it is not meant that all non-intermittent, non-highly variable demand patterns are necessarily normally distributed. The gamma distribution, for example, is known to offer good results in inventory control. In general, a different distribution may be appropriate, although the normality assumption is reasonable for many real-world cases. This is particularly true when lead times are long, permitting central limit theorem effects (see Chapter 5).

Non-normal demand patterns, then, would cover all the following terms often used in industry: intermittent, sporadic, slow, erratic, clumped, and lumpy. There is a confusion shared amongst practitioners and academics alike as to the exact meaning of these terms. We seek to clarify these terms in Section 11.5.2.

11.5.2 Conceptual Framework

Firstly, sporadicity is an alternative term to intermittence. Both terms refer to the presence of some zero demand observations and the criterion that may qualify a demand pattern as sporadic/intermittent, or not, is the probability of positive demand occurring or, correspondingly, the average inter-demand interval, the average interval between successive positive demand occurrences. Returning to a comment made earlier in this chapter about fast and slow intermittence, the former would relate to an intermittent demand pattern with a 'high' probability of demand occurrence whereas the latter to a pattern with a 'low' probability of demand occurrence. The terms 'high' and 'low' are yet to be quantified; this will take place later in the chapter.

Erraticness refers to the variability of the demand sizes, when demand occurs. Erraticness may be captured in many different ways including the statistical measure of variance (discussed in Chapter 4). Often, it is very useful to express the variance in relation to the mean demand. That would result in the variance to mean ratio or, alternatively, the coefficient of variation (standard deviation to mean ratio). The latter is preferable because it is scale-independent (see Chapter 5) and allows for the specification of cut-off values and this is discussed in more detail in Section 11.7.

When demand is both intermittent/sporadic and erratic, then it is termed as lumpy. If demand is intermittent but not erratic (i.e. the demand sizes are almost constant) then these demand patterns are termed as clumped (Ritchie and Kingsman 1985). Finally, slow

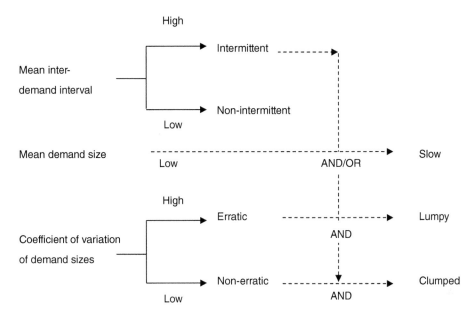

Figure 11.2 Categorisation of non-normal demand patterns. Source: Boylan and Syntetos (2008). © 2019, Springer Nature.

demand will typically be associated with a high degree of intermittence, but not necessarily so. Think, for example, of an item that is requested every period but in very low volumes, say one or two units per period. This would also be a slow demand item, but it would not be intermittent. As previously discussed, this indicates another problem with ABC type classifications when used for forecasting. A demand volume criterion would assign such low-volume non-intermittent items to the C category, but if this category is forecasted using methods developed for intermittent demand items, then the assignment may be misguided.

The discussion conducted above is captured in Figure 11.2 (Boylan and Syntetos 2008) where we present a framework that facilitates conceptual clarifications and qualitative definitions for non-normal demand patterns.

Figure 11.2 allows a conceptual understanding of the various non-normal demand patterns but it cannot be implemented for classification purposes. For that to happen, the relevant cut-off points need to be established first, followed by the specification of different forecasting methods for the various resulting categories.

11.5.3 Summary

Classification for forecasting purposes requires a full comprehension of the characteristics of non-normal demand patterns. In particular, it is essential to understand how the mean (and variance) of inter-demand intervals and demand sizes contribute to such patterns. Clear terminology is also required with regard to the various forms these patterns may take. In this section, we have undertaken this preliminary work so as to enable further discussion on the sources of demand (in Section 11.6) and the proposition of operationalised classification rules (in Section 11.7).

11.6   Classification Based on Demand Sources

Before we attempt to relate forecasting methods to the underlying demand patterns and thus facilitate the development of forecasting-based classification schemes, it is important to discuss how the demand patterns are generated in the first place. What are the factors that lead to demand having specific characteristics? How is demand created? These are the questions that are addressed in this section.

11.6.1   Demand Generation

It is clear that the more potential customers we have (or the bigger the market size), the more frequent demand will be for a particular SKU. It is important to bear in mind that in 'business-to-business' situations, the number of customers may not necessarily be high. In addition, the frequency with which customers request a particular product will also have an effect on how often demand occurs.

Two other important characteristics that shape the demand for a particular product are the heterogeneity of the market in terms of the size of the customers and the variance of the requests that are being placed by each customer. The more variable the market is, in terms of the size of the customers and the requests made by each of those customers, the more variable the demand will be.

Finally, there is one more important characteristic that may influence the demand pattern, which is the correlation between customers' requests. Lumpiness for example may occur in a market with a great number of customers, if their requests are strongly correlated with each other. Correlation may be due, amongst other reasons, to imitation and fashion, which induce similar behaviours in customers so that sudden peaks of demand may occur after periods of no requests.

In summary, the following factors contribute to SKU demand characteristics (for a detailed discussion, please refer to Bartezzaghi et al. 1999):

1. *Number of potential customers*: This indicates the market size.
2. *Frequency of customers' requests*: How often the customers place an order.
3. *Heterogeneity of customers*: Heterogeneous requests occur when the potential market consists of customers with considerably different sizes (e.g. few large customers coexist with a large number of small customers).
4. *Variety of customers' requests*: Variety occurs when a single customer's requests vary in size.
5. *Correlations between customers' requests*: Induced by similar behaviours.

11.6.2   A Qualitative Classification Approach

This above list is by no means exhaustive, but it provides an insightful summary of some key factors behind the mechanism of demand generation. It also offers a framework for analysing forecasting process improvements.

In more detail, the first and second factors determine the intermittence of demand. For those SKUs with very few customers, it may be feasible to liaise directly with them, and to enhance forecasts accordingly.

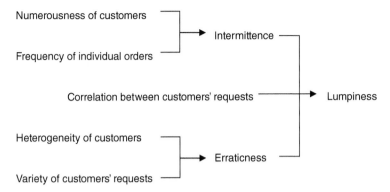

Figure 11.3 Categorisation based on sources of demand characteristics. Source: Boylan and Syntetos (2008). ©2019, Springer Nature.

The third and fourth factors determine the erraticness of demand. For highly irregular orders, it pays to exploit early information at the customer level. Of course, such early indications are not always available, especially when addressing business-to-customer (rather than business-to-business) demand. But early confirmed orders may give a good indication of final orders, and they are especially useful when there is a strong correlation between customers' demands (the fifth factor). The combined effect of all five factors is presented in Figure 11.3 (Boylan and Syntetos 2008).

This classification scheme has two important practical implications:

1. When the number of customers is low, and especially if some of the customers are large, it may be beneficial to enhance forecasting through direct communication with these customers.
2. Early indications of demand in the form of advance demand information is a particularly attractive option for improving the forecasts, particularly for customers with highly variable requests.

These strategies can be very useful in business-to-business environments, where such communication is feasible. For those items without early indicators, forecasting must be undertaken using a purely time-series approach.

11.6.3 Summary

In understanding the sources of demand (how demand is generated), we are able to more readily identify the ways in which the forecasting process can be improved. By logically linking the sources to demand characteristics (intermittence, erraticness, and lumpiness), we can assess whether any useful information may be directly retrieved from customers. This information may then complement time-series forecasts, for example through judgemental adjustment (see Chapter 10).

11.7 Forecasting-based Classifications

A logical definition of intermittence is that a series should have at least one zero observation. Is that the most useful definition from a forecasting perspective? Also, how should we take into account the variability of (non-zero) demand sizes? These are the questions that are addressed in this section.

11.7.1 Forecasting and Generalisation

Forecasting methods are selected on the basis of providing the best possible estimates in accordance with the underlying demand pattern. Before such an exercise takes place, an important question needs to be answered, namely, 'What do we mean by 'the best possible estimates'?' As discussed in Chapter 9, forecasting methods can be compared based on both accuracy and accuracy-implication metrics. The latter relies upon the assumption of a particular inventory rule being in place, and so the accuracy implications of a forecasting method will vary according to the inventory rule. The same is true if the demand forecasts are used for transportation purposes. One routing determination rule will result in different implications than another routing rule. In general, accuracy implications will always be conditioned by the particular rule being used by the organisational function served by the forecasts. That makes it impossible to compare forecasting methods if we are to reach some generalisable conclusions that hold across a number of different rules.

With regard to accuracy measures, we have seen that different measures may lead to different conclusions. A set of measures was suggested in Chapter 9 that are appropriate for intermittent demand forecasting and diagnostic purposes. To determine forecasting classification rules, though, one single measure is needed. That measure should ideally capture as many of the important characteristics discussed in Chapter 9 as possible. It should also be amenable to mathematical analysis to allow the development of generalised conclusions, and this is further discussed below. The accuracy measure that possesses all those attributes is the mean square error (MSE).

The MSE reflects both the issue of bias (previously discussed through the ME) and that of the variance (see Chapter 10). The theoretical importance and unique characteristics of this error measure were explained in Chapter 10 where it was shown that, for independent demand:

$$\text{MSE} = \mathbb{E}(\text{Squared error}) = \text{Var}(\text{Demand}) + \text{Var}(\text{Forecast}) + \text{Bias}^2 \tag{11.2}$$

In Eq. (11.2), $\mathbb{E}$(Squared error) does not denote the sample mean squared error, but the expected value of the squared errors. It is this value that is used in deriving the classification rules discussed below.

MSE was not recommended in Chapter 9 for practical applications for two reasons: its scale dependence and its sensitivity to outlying observations. Scale dependence is most concerning when evaluating multiple series of varying scales. This is not an issue for classification, as each SKU is considered individually. The problem of outliers does not arise, either, because classification rules may be derived based on the underlying demand process in which all observations follow a prescribed process.

The theoretical properties of the MSE (expected value of squared errors) make this measure amenable to mathematical analysis. Under well specified assumptions related to the underlying demand patterns, the variance of demand can be mathematically expressed. The same is true for the bias of specific forecasting methods and the variance of their forecasts. Then, the MSE expression of one estimator can be directly compared to that of another estimator and regions of superior performance can be identified. (Please note that the variance of demand would not influence the comparative performance of different estimators – see also Chapter 10.) Subsequently, forecasting methods can be proposed for the regions where they perform best. If the categorisation rules work well in a wide range of situations, even if the modelling assumptions are not fully met, then the rules identified can be used with greater confidence across a range of companies and industries.

11.7.2 Classification Solutions

The purpose of forecasting-based classifications is to select the appropriate forecasting method(s) to be used for different categories. The major problem associated with classification solutions used in industry is not only that the cut-off values assigned to criteria are ad hoc but also that the selection of the methods is not clearly related to the classification of the demand patterns. If the very objective is to select appropriate forecasting methods, then it would make more sense to compare directly the candidate forecasting methods and then identify regions of superior performance based on the results.

Johnston and Boylan (1996) examined the conditions under which Croston's method (1972) (designed for intermittent demand and discussed in Chapter 6) is more accurate, in terms of MSE, than single exponential smoothing (SES). The authors suggested a rule, on the basis of simulation of a range of realistic lead time conditions and underlying demand patterns, that if the mean inter-demand interval (μ_I) is greater than 1.25 review intervals, then Croston's method should be used, rather than SES. The comparisons were undertaken based on the simulated MSE. This form of classification is based on the premise that it is preferable to identify conditions for superior forecasting performance, and then to categorise demand based on these results. The essence of the rule lies in this approach and the identification of the mean inter-demand interval as a categorisation parameter (rather than the suggestion of a specific cut-off value).

From a forecasting perspective, Syntetos, Boylan, and Croston (2005) re-examined the comparison between methods, such as Croston and SES. This study was based on a comparison of approximate expressions for theoretical (rather than simulated) MSEs for data that follow i.i.d. assumptions; these assumptions were discussed in Chapter 6. This research provided further support for the consideration of the average inter-demand interval as a demand classification variable. In addition, a complementary form of classification was also suggested, by the variability of demand sizes (when demand occurs). In particular, the squared coefficient of variation of demand sizes (CV_S^2) was recommended to define erraticness.

Figure 11.4 shows how a two-way classification scheme (by the average inter-demand interval and the CV_S^2) enables a choice to be made between Croston's method and SES, for the case of issue points only, when there are forecast updates and stock reviews at the end of every period ($R = 1$). (Recall, from Chapter 6, that SES has different properties when issue point forecasts or forecasts at all points in time are considered.) Similar schemes, based on four quadrants, can be constructed to compare SES with the Syntetos-Boylan approximation (SBA), and Croston with SBA. This four-quadrant approach was introduced by Syntetos, Boylan, and Croston (2005), and is abbreviated to the SBC classification method.

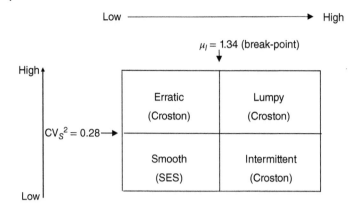

Figure 11.4 Categorisation by mean square error: SES (issue points, $R = 1$) vs. Croston.

Please note that the definition of demand patterns follows from the identification of regions where methods perform comparatively better. The demand patterns with low intermittence and erraticness, which correspond to a superior performance of SES, are termed as 'smooth'.

The scheme discussed in Figure 11.4 also has important implications for the selection of an appropriate distribution to represent demand. Theoretical distributions, such as those discussed in Chapters 4 and 5 will be appropriate for the 'erratic', 'smooth', and 'intermittent' demand categories. However, the high variability present in the 'lumpy' demand category may require non-parametric approaches such as bootstrapping (to be discussed in Chapter 13).

The four-quadrant classification approach is quite intuitive and easy to implement, but care is needed in specifying the cut-off values. Although the approach can be used for any two methods for which MSE expressions may be obtained (exact or approximate), the cut-off values depend on which methods are being compared. For example, the cut-off values for SES vs. Croston (Figure 11.4) are not the same as the values for SES vs. SBA (Figure 11.5 in Technical Note 11.1). Also, if SES is one of the methods being compared, then clarity is needed on whether the comparison is for issue-points only (as in Figure 11.4) or for all points in time. Finally, there have been some modifications to the four-quadrant approach, to refine the comparison between Croston and SBA, and between SES and SBA (see Technical Note 11.2).

11.7.3 Summary

In this section, we have argued that if the objective of SKU classification is to select appropriate forecasting methods, then it makes sense to compare directly some possible estimators to identify regions of superior accuracy performance. Then, the SKUs can be classified, according to their demand patterns, based on the results of the forecast comparison. To do so, an appropriate error measure needs to be specified that captures as many important forecast accuracy characteristics as possible and is amenable to mathematical analysis. The latter aspect ensures (i) the derivation of the classification rules in a mechanistic fashion (i.e. without any human involvement) and (ii) the generalisation of such rules across a wide range of situations. The MSE was shown in Chapter 10 to meet the following requirements:

1. It reflects both bias and variance related concerns.
2. It is a mathematically tractable error measure.

The solutions discussed in this section enable the selection of forecasting methods to precede and drive the categorisation of demand patterns and have been shown empirically to add considerable value to organisations dealing with intermittent demand items (e.g. Ghobbar and Friend 2002; Regattieri et al. 2005; Rego and Mesquita 2015). They are also being utilised by such supply chain software developers and consultants as Blue Yonder, Implement Consulting, LLamasoft, and Syncron.

11.8 Chapter Summary

Classification is an essential precursor to forecasting. It should enable the separation of large numbers of items into categories within which common forecasting methods can be employed. However, the majority of classification schemes used in industry have not been developed specifically for forecasting purposes.

ABC-type schemes, which attempt to prioritise the service criticality of a large collection of items, suffer from some major drawbacks not only with regard to forecasting but with regard to inventory management in general, as they have not been developed from an inventory perspective. Extensions, such as a composite measure developed by Teunter et al. (2010), should account for inventory improvements although they are not relevant to the forecasting function. The same is true for classification schemes used in a maintenance context that attempt to identify the potential modes of failures of spare parts. For the purpose of forecasting, items should be categorised based on their demand patterns and/or their customer characteristics. Both approaches have been shown in this chapter to be valuable for different reasons.

- The former approach enables the derivation of generalisable, operationalised definitions of criteria (such as intermittence and erraticness) that may be used in an automated fashion to classify SKUs. (Operationalisation is the translation of abstract concepts into indicators or measures, enabling observations to be made, as defined by Popper (1959).)
- The latter approach (classification based on customer characteristics), enables higher level considerations such as the reduction of reliance upon forecasting and the exploitation of advance demand information where possible.

These approaches are complementary and should allow considerable improvements in the forecasting task of modern organisations.

Technical Notes

Note 11.1 Classification Rule for SES and SBA

We outline how the two-way classification is derived for the choice between SBA and SES (for issue points only, $R = 1$), assuming independent and identically distributed demand. In this case, the approximate bias of SES estimates (see Chapter 6) is given by Eq. (11.3).

$$\text{Bias}_{\text{SES}} \approx \frac{\mu_S}{\mu_I}(\alpha(\mu_I - 1)) \tag{11.3}$$

The variance of the SES estimates (for issue points only, $R = 1$) was given by Rao (1973), who corrected the original formula by Croston (1972). The variance expression, which includes terms up to second order, is shown in Eq. (11.4).

$$\text{Var}_{\text{SES}} \approx \alpha^2 \sigma^2 + \frac{\alpha(1-\alpha)^2}{2-\alpha}\left(\frac{\mu_I - 1}{\mu_I^2}\mu_S^2 + \frac{\sigma_S^2}{\mu_I}\right) \tag{11.4}$$

This approximate bias of the SBA estimates (see Chapter 6) is given in Eq. (11.5).

$$\text{Bias}_{\text{SBA}} \approx -\frac{\alpha}{2}\left(\frac{\mu_S}{\mu_I^2}\right) \tag{11.5}$$

The approximate variance of the SBA estimates is shown in Eq. (11.6), up to terms of third order (Syntetos 2001). (A more refined approximation, using terms of higher orders, was derived by Syntetos and Boylan (2010).)

$$\text{Var}_{\text{SBA}} \approx \frac{\alpha(2-\alpha)}{4}\left(\frac{\mu_I - 1}{\mu_I^3}\left(\mu_S^2 + \frac{\alpha}{2-\alpha}\sigma_S^2\right) + \frac{\sigma_S^2}{\mu_I^2}\right) \tag{11.6}$$

Then, approximate MSE expressions related to these two methods can be calculated and compared directly in order to identify regions of superior performance, i.e. regions where the MSE of one method is found to be lower than that of the other. Syntetos (2001) established the condition in (11.7) for the MSE of SBA to be less than the MSE of SES (issue points only) for $\mu_I > 1$.

$$\frac{\sigma_S^2}{\mu_S^2} > \frac{(\mu_I - 1)((1-\alpha)^2/(2-\alpha) + \alpha(\mu_I - 1) - \alpha/4(\mu_I - 1)\mu_I^2 - (2-\alpha)/4\mu_I)}{\alpha(\mu_I - 1)/4\mu_I + (2-\alpha)/4 - \alpha\mu_I^2 - \alpha(1-\alpha)^2\mu_I/(2-\alpha)} \tag{11.7}$$

A similar analysis has been undertaken, to compare SBA and SES (all points in time). Syntetos, Boylan, and Croston (2005) showed that this results in the inequality in (11.8) for SBA to have a lower MSE than SES, for $\mu_I > 1$.

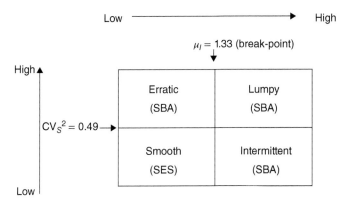

Figure 11.5 Categorisation by mean square error: SES vs. SBA.

$$\frac{\sigma_S^2}{\mu_S^2} > \frac{\mu_I(\mu_I - 1)(4\mu_I - (2 - \alpha)^2) - \alpha(2 - \alpha)}{(2 - \alpha)(2\mu_I^2 - \alpha\mu_I) - 4\mu_I^3} \tag{11.8}$$

Both of the inequalities, (11.7) and (11.8), contain three key parameters: the mean demand interval (μ_I), the squared coefficient of variation of the demand sizes ($CV_S^2 = \sigma_S^2 / \mu_S^2$) and the smoothing constant (α). Cut-off values can now be determined, for μ_I and CV_S^2, for which both inequalities (11.7) and (11.8) hold over the range of smoothing constants $0.05 \le \alpha \le 0.20$, which are most commonly applied in practice. This results in the classification scheme shown in Figure 11.5.

A similar approach has been taken for comparing the MSEs of SES with Croston, and Croston with SBA. The conditions under which the MSE of one estimator (called X) is less than another (called Y) carry across from one period to the whole protection interval $(R + L)$ for i.i.d. demand. If $MSE_{X,1} < MSE_{Y,1}$ (where the subscript '1' denotes a single period), then the inequality in (11.9) follows immediately.

$$Var_{X,1} + Bias_{X,1}^2 < Var_{Y,1} + Bias_{Y,1}^2 \tag{11.9}$$

Multiplying both sides of this inequality by $(R + L)^2$ gives (11.10).

$$(R + L)^2 Var_{X,1} + ((R + L)Bias_{X,1})^2 < (R + L)^2 Var_{Y,1} + ((R + L)Bias_{Y,1})^2 \tag{11.10}$$

Inequality (11.10) states that, for i.i.d. demand, $MSE_{X,R+L} < MSE_{Y,R+L}$, thus showing that the classification rule for a single period carries across to the whole protection interval.

Note 11.2 Refined Classification Rules

A more refined approximate classification for comparing Croston and SBA was proposed by Kostenko and Hyndman (2006). They showed that an approximate condition for SBA to have lower MSE than Croston is given by the following inequality: $CV_S^2 > 2 - (3/2)\mu_I$. Some empirical support for this condition, in comparison to the Croston-SBA cut-off points proposed by Syntetos, Boylan, and Croston (2005), was offered by Heinecke et al. (2013).

Petropoulos and Kourentzes (2015) noted that in a comparison of SES with SBA, the four-quadrant rule should be over-ridden in the case of non-intermittent demand. SES should be preferred to SBA in this case, as SBA is biased for non-intermittent demand, whereas SES is unbiased. This also applies to a comparison of Croston and SBA because Croston produces the same forecasts as SES when demand is non-intermittent.

12

Maintenance and Obsolescence

12.1   Introduction

As previously discussed in this book, intermittent demand forecasting is particularly relevant in a maintenance context. In this chapter, we move beyond forecasting methods that are applicable to intermittent demand items in general, to emphasise some issues specifically related to spare parts. Their need arises whenever a component fails and has to be replaced (corrective maintenance) or when a replacement is made to forestall future problems (preventive maintenance).

So, in summary, the former type of demand is relevant to our discussion and is addressed Spare parts demand arising from corrective maintenance, after a failure has occurred, is stochastic and requires forecasting. Demand arising from preventive maintenance for equipment is scheduled (since we know when such maintenance activities are due) and thus deterministic, at least in principle. However, a qualification is needed here. Although the timing of preventive maintenance activities is known well in advance, the important thing is that the relevant spare parts requirements for the equipment is also communicated in advance to the stockist. When specialist departments within a company perform maintenance activities this will typically be the case. Usually, this would also be true when an external vendor undertakes maintenance tasks on an organisation's behalf, as it is beneficial for both parties for such information to be shared. Although there are exceptions to the rule, it is fair to assume that demand in these situations is deterministic.

So, in summary, the former type of demand is relevant to our discussion and is addressed in this chapter. The latter is not subject to estimation but rather to appropriate scheduling methodologies and is not pursued further. The difference between these two types of demand is conceptually similar to that discussed in Chapter 2, when referring to independent and dependent demand. The former arises out of customers' needs (which in a spare parts context are due to failures) whereas the latter is deterministically generated from the requirements at a higher level in the bill of materials. So the same item is needed for completely different purposes: in the former case to satisfy independently generated demand (that requires forecasting) and in the latter to support production (that requires scheduling). (For further discussion, please refer to Technical Note 12.1.)

Intermittent Demand Forecasting: Context, Methods and Applications, First Edition.
John E. Boylan and Aris A. Syntetos.
© 2021 John Wiley & Sons Ltd. Published 2021 by John Wiley & Sons Ltd.
Companion Website: www.wiley.com/go/boylansyntetos/intermittentdemandforecasting

In Section 12.2 we examine, in more detail, different maintenance contexts, before we outline the organisation of the remainder of this chapter.

12.2 Maintenance Contexts

Fortuin and Martin (1999) categorised the contexts for service logistics as follows:

1. Technical systems under client control (e.g. machines in production departments, transport vehicles in a warehouse).
2. Technical systems sold to customers (e.g. telephone exchange systems, medical systems in hospitals).
3. End products used by customers (e.g. TV sets, personal computers, motor cars).

In the first context, there is usually a specialist department within the client organisation performing maintenance activities and managing spare parts inventories. In the second, a specialist department within the vendor organisation will generally undertake these tasks. In both cases, large amounts of information are available to the vendor, or can be shared with the vendor. This information may include scheduled (preventive) maintenance activities, times between failures, usage rates, and condition of equipment, all of which may help to explain the demand generated by equipment failures. When a wealth of data is available, it is possible to identify explanatory variables, which may be used to predict the demand for spare parts. This will be discussed further in Section 12.3 of this chapter.

In the third context, parts are used by consumers and much less information is available. Fortuin and Martin (1999, p. 957) commented, 'Clients are anonymous, their usage of consumer products and their 'maintenance concept' are not known'. Most demand arises from purely corrective maintenance (e.g. on TV sets, personal computers), which is required in the case of a defect. Even when preventive maintenance occurs (e.g. on motor cars), prediction is complicated by the 'maintenance concept' of consumers being unknown. For example, customers may not bring in their cars at the correct time for a service, or may not bring them in at all. In many practical situations where end products are used by consumers, the vendor must gauge demand for service parts from the demand history alone. In this case, demand for an stock keeping unit (SKU) may be decomposed into regular components (e.g. from direct customers) and irregular or lumpy components (e.g. from warehouses and wholesalers) (Kalchschmidt et al. 2006).

Demand arising from maintenance requirements is often intermittent and therefore shares the characteristics discussed in this book so far. However, there are two additional issues that need to be taken into account in a spare parts context:

- The first issue is that of obsolescence. To consider this in more detail, the concept of the life cycle of a product or component needs to be understood and how it affects forecasting and inventory requirements.
- The second issue relates to the specific characteristics of the spare parts demand generation process that differ from those of other intermittently demanded SKUs.

These issues are considered in Section 12.4 where relevant time series approaches to forecasting are also presented.

12.2.1 Summary

Intermittent demand for spare parts poses a considerable challenge to those responsible for managing inventories. Demand for such items may be generated because of equipment failure and a distinction needs to be drawn between maintaining such equipment (whatever that may be) in a preventive way, and fixing failures, as they occur, in a corrective way. Preventive maintenance activities are known well in advance and, as long as they are appropriately communicated to the stockist of spare parts, they result in demand that does not need to be forecasted. Corrective maintenance, on the other hand, needs to be anticipated. In Section 12.3 we address causal forecasting for spare parts requirements, followed in Section 12.4 by an examination of some time series methods specifically designed to deal with obsolescence and spare parts characteristics. These methods attempt to bridge the gap between forecasting and inventory, a gap that was first considered in Chapter 2. We close with a discussion on the integration between forecasting and stock control in a spare parts context and beyond.

12.3 Causal Forecasting

Causal forecasting has not been addressed thus far in this book. So, before we discuss how this may be utilised for spare parts, a general introduction is given to the main characteristics underlying its implementation. Unlike extrapolative time series methods that rely solely on past demand history to forecast future demand, causal methods rely on some information other than the demand itself that has some explanatory power, which can help explain the volume of demand now and in the future. Consider, for example, the relationship between the weather (temperature in particular) and the consumption of cold drinks in a retail store. It does make sense to assume that the warmer the weather is going to be the more cold drinks we are going to sell. So if we manage to establish a relationship between the temperature (degrees Celsius) (independent variable, explanatory) and the sales of cold drinks (dependent variable, to be forecasted), an accurate weather forecast for tomorrow would help us predict how much we are going to sell on that day.

As it happens, the relationship discussed above is useful and, indeed, some efficient inventory management arrangements in the retailing sector are heavily dependent upon good weather forecasts. Of course, more than one explanatory variable may be present; for example, the expenditure related to our weekly advertising campaigns (that is known in advance) may also be found to be a good predictor of sales of cold drinks next week. So, more than one variable may be useful in predicting demand, but this does not change the nature of the forecasting process, which remains causal.

Explanatory variables may be identified in a deductive or an inductive way. In the former case, a conceptually appealing association between demand and one or more independent variables is identified and then tested on real data to check its validity and predictive power. Of course, not all conceptually appealing relationships will always work in practice. So, although it makes sense to assume that the number of people arriving daily by tram to the city centre of Budapest may help explain demand at a particular retail store, this may not always be safely used for forecasting purposes.

Alternatively, and given the wealth of data currently available in most organisations, relationships may be tested (without any good a priori case) and explanatory variables that have a good predictive power identified. In this case, an inductive approach may reveal previously unnoticed associations and the power of such an approach becomes increasingly evident in the current era of 'big data'.

'Big data' has been credited with offering organisations immense opportunities for improving their forecasting capabilities (see, e.g. Boone et al. 2019). The considerable volume, variety, and velocity with which unstructured information can be collected nowadays have the potential to increase predictive power. However, it has also been argued that such an abundance of information may lead to devastating effects if data is forced to reveal patterns that are simply not there, and people have been wrongly developing the notion that 'everything is connected to everything' (Syntetos et al. 2016a). Consequently, information may be vulnerable to dubious interpretations and some tendency to sacrifice logical thinking to support some spurious relationship between the consumption of apples in Turkey and the time it takes to grow oranges in the UK.

Despite the above, it is clear that well thought-out inductive approaches offer the opportunity to uncover important explanatory variables, and thus may lead to significant improvements in forecasting. Deductive approaches, on the other hand, typically offer the most natural interpretation of a causal framework. We are yet to see how the two approaches can be best combined for intermittent demand.

12.3.1 Causal Forecasting for Maintenance Management

What would the important variables be in a maintenance context to help us predict the occurrence of failures that precipitate the demand for spare parts? And, are those variables likely to have a reasonable amount of data to facilitate such a prediction? These are the main questions addressed in this subsection.

Demands for spare parts are triggered by equipment breakdown, which is influenced by how equipment is used and how it is maintained (Kennedy et al. 2002). This implies that the occurrence of demand for spare parts at any time may be linked to equipment maintenance operations and may depend on some explanatory variables (Hua et al. 2007). However, historically there have been very few causal forecasting applications in the area of maintenance management. This may be explained, partly at least, by the fact that the data required for such an exercise may be very substantial in volume and thus very demanding in terms of storage capacity. Consider, for example, sensor data that relate to consecutive measurements (every two minutes) of the condition of all the main assemblies used in a windmill (condition monitoring). Such information would obviously be very helpful in terms of demand prediction, but storing the relevant data would not have been possible some years back, although it is now and, of course, will become even easier in the future. This is one reason why research on evaluating the relationship of independent (explanatory) variables with spare parts demand has been very limited.

With the wide application of management information systems in equipment maintenance and spare parts inventory management, more information and data about explanatory variables are now available to improve forecasting accuracy. For example, information on the maintenance policy, preventive maintenance records, and emergent part replacement records of each piece of equipment can be very helpful in the forecasting task. Thus, we expect more research to be conducted in this area in the near future. We provide an overview, below, of the main studies that have appeared so far in the literature.

Ghobbar and Friend (2002) investigated the sources of intermittent demand behaviour, as measured by the average demand interval (ADI or μ_I) and the squared coefficient of variation of the demand sizes (CV_S^2). (Recall from the previous chapter that these are the recommended parameters to use for demand and forecasting classification purposes; see Section 11.7.) Their analysis was based on data relating to 35 repairable parts for aircraft from Aerei da Trasporto Regionale, British Aerospace, and Fokker. The researchers assessed the dependence of ADI and CV_S^2 on three maintenance-related characteristics, namely: (i) the aircraft utilisation rate, (ii) the component overhaul life, and (iii) the type of primary maintenance process (hard-time or condition-monitoring, discussed below). Historical data were available for these characteristics and they are all plausible factors behind demand behaviour.

Firstly, the higher the aircraft utilisation rate, the lower the interval between successive demands will be, and the higher the demand sizes (and their variability). Similarly, the component overhaul life may help explain the observed demand patterns. For a big item, for example, with a long life, maintenance is determined by flying hours/landings and this helps the movement of aircraft parts into periodic maintenance tasks to be smooth and systematic.

With regard to the maintenance processes, hard-time is defined as the preventive maintenance process in which known deterioration of an item is limited to an acceptable level by the maintenance actions carried out at periods related to time in service. This time may be calendar based, or based on a variable such as the number of landings (in the particular case considered by Ghobbar and Friend 2002). On the contrary, condition-monitoring is not a preventive maintenance process, but rather one in which information on items, gained from operational experience or actual measurements, is collected, analysed, and interpreted on a continuing basis as a means of implementing corrective procedures. It is reasonable to suppose that such maintenance processes may influence demand for spare parts.

The analysis by Ghobbar and Friend (2002) found the utilisation rate, the component overhaul life, and the maintenance process had a (statistically significant) relationship with CV_S^2. Hard-time was found, as expected, to lead to a reduction of the CV_S^2 in contrast with condition-monitoring, which leads to high levels of erraticness. The aircraft utilisation rate had a (statistically significant) relationship with ADI although the other factors were not found to be statistically significant. However, further analysis of these factors, and their interaction, may be fruitful, given the evidence presented by Ghobbar and Friend (2002).

Understanding the explanatory effect of relevant maintenance factors, such as those discussed above, on the demand patterns (as determined by the CV_S^2 and the ADI, μ_I) is important for two reasons. First, management may try to act on the demand sources to reduce the levels of lumpiness (e.g. by reducing or increasing the mean time between overhaul, or focusing on components with high failure rates such as condition-monitored ones). Second, understanding the sources of lumpiness is necessary in order to choose the proper forecasting method, as discussed in Chapter 11. In fact, the arguments made here are very similar to those made in Chapter 11 when discussing customer-generated rather

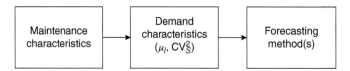

Figure 12.1 Maintenance generated demand and forecasting.

than maintenance-generated demand (see Figure 11.1). In Figure 12.1, we summarise the relationships discussed above.

In a further study, Ghobbar and Friend (2003) showed how forecast accuracy depends on various characteristics of the demand process, including the forecast horizon, as well as the primary maintenance process (Technical Note 12.2). Hard-time components were found to have more effect on forecast accuracy than condition monitoring.

Hua et al. (2007) used two zero-one explanatory variables, plant overhaul and equipment overhaul, to help predict demand of spare parts in the petrochemical industry. They compared the performance of their method to two time-series approaches (single exponential smoothing [SES] and Croston, described in Chapter 6) and the bootstrapping method developed by Willemain et al. (2004) (to be considered in detail in Chapter 13) on the demand data of 40 types of spare parts and found their method to perform best. This is not surprising; if we manage to relate the demand to the physical process generating it, through the use of appropriate explanatory variables, then it should be possible to increase forecast accuracy.

12.3.2 Summary

Causal forecasting can be very helpful in a corrective maintenance context where a plethora of explanatory variables are typically available to help predict demand for spare parts. However, and despite the intuitive appeal of causal forecasting for maintenance spare parts, not much has been done in terms of scientific research or empirical evaluations. (For a comprehensive review on this topic, please refer to Van der Auweraer et al. (2019).) This can be attributed to the information technology (IT) storage requirements associated with relevant explanatory variables that until recently were not affordable. Recent IT advancements mean that more and more relevant information can be easily stored and utilised and we anticipate a considerable increase of academic work in this area.

12.4 Time Series Methods

Having discussed the relevance of causal forecasting in a spare parts context, we now consider two key time-series related advancements in this area. The first addresses an important concern in spare parts management, namely that of obsolescence. The second attempts to capture granular maintenance related information and incorporate it in the forecasting process.

12.4.1 Forecasting in the Presence of Obsolescence

Obsolescence is a natural issue to consider in a spare parts context and should be distinguished from deterioration and perishability (Technical Note 12.3). Every product will typically follow a life cycle, whether short or long, and so do the spare parts that serve the functioning of the product. The main phases of the life cycle of a product or spare part are depicted in Figure 12.2.

After its 'launch' to the market, a product will typically experience increasing sales ('growth'), which will then stabilise during the 'maturity' phase, before falling off in the final phase ('decline') of its life cycle. Products are often in high demand after their introduction to the market due to their new features and, typically, strong advertising campaigns that complement their launch. Subsequently, they reach a maturity stage when companies enjoy a high degree of sales, until new products enter the market and thus sales start naturally declining. This final phase is extremely important from an inventory perspective, given that enough needs to be stocked to satisfy future customer demand but not too much because, at some (unknown) future point in time, sales will be discontinued and any leftover quantities can only be discarded. In addition to its economic implications, this issue also raises important concerns about the environmentally friendly disposal of the leftover inventories (please refer also to our discussion in Chapter 1).

It is natural, then, that any indication as to when that point in time is to arrive can only be beneficial for forecasting purposes. This is more important for spare parts than for original equipment. The latter have clearer (market) indications as to when sales are starting to decline (and eventually stop) and companies themselves can regulate the final phase of the life cycles by means of introducing technologically advanced versions of their own products ('revival'). For spare parts though, and unless there are specific warranty periods, there is a great degree of uncertainty as to how long they will be required for servicing the original products.

Despite the importance of this issue, obsolescence has not been appropriately addressed when developing forecasting methods for spare parts demand. An exception is a method proposed by Teunter, Syntetos, and Babai (2011), hereafter TSB (Teunter–Syntetos–Babai).

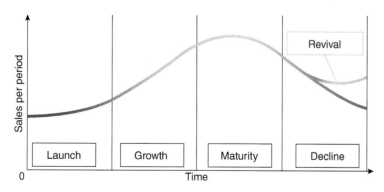

Figure 12.2 Life cycle stages.

In the description of this method, we use a 'demand occurrence' variable, denoted by o_t, which takes the value of 1 if demand occurs at time t and 0 if demand does not occur at time t. The other notation is given below:

- d_t is demand at time t;
- $\widehat{d}_{t+1}$ is the estimate of mean demand for period $t+1$, made at the end of period t;
- s_t is the actual size of demand in period t;
- $\widehat{s}_{t+1}$ is the exponentially smoothed estimate of mean demand size for period $t+1$, updated only when demand occurs, using a smoothing constant α (between 0 and 1). NB: this is a change from the notation in Chapter 6, where $\widehat{\mu}_{S,t+1}$ was used to denote this estimate.
- $\widehat{p}_{t+1}$ is the exponentially smoothed estimate of the probability of demand occurrence, updated at the end of every period (regardless of whether demand has or has not occurred in that period). The estimate is for period $t+1$, made at the end of period t using a smoothing constant β (between 0 and 1).

The TSB method operates as shown in Eqs. (12.1) and (12.2).
If $o_t = 1$ then:

$$
\begin{aligned}
\widehat{s}_{t+1} &= \widehat{s}_t + \alpha(s_t - \widehat{s}_t) \\
\widehat{p}_{t+1} &= \widehat{p}_t + \beta(1 - \widehat{p}_t) \\
\widehat{d}_{t+1} &= \widehat{p}_{t+1}\widehat{s}_{t+1}
\end{aligned}
\tag{12.1}
$$

else if $o_t = 0$ then:

$$
\begin{aligned}
\widehat{s}_{t+1} &= \widehat{s}_t \\
\widehat{p}_{t+1} &= \widehat{p}_t + \beta(0 - \widehat{p}_t) \\
\widehat{d}_{t+1} &= \widehat{p}_{t+1}\widehat{s}_{t+1}
\end{aligned}
\tag{12.2}
$$

producing unbiased forecasts, if we consider all points in time.

Please note that two different smoothing constants are explicitly suggested as part of the method's implementation; this is because the demand probability is updated more often than the demand size. The former is updated in every time period, whereas the latter is updated only after a demand occurs. The probability is adjusted upward in periods with positive demand and downward in periods with zero demand. After many periods with zero demand and therefore many downwards adjustments, the TSB estimate for the probability of having positive demand approaches zero, and therefore, the estimate of the mean demand per period approaches zero as well. As discussed below, this is a desirable feature in the final phase of an item when we are primarily concerned with whether we should continue stocking the item or not. However, if we are concerned with how much and when to order, for an item that has not yet reached the end of its life cycle, then the TSB forecasts are less relevant. In Figure 12.3 we show the mean demand forecasts produced by the TSB and Croston's method for a highly intermittent demand series.

Because the forecast of the mean demand is updated in every period, the TSB method is able to react more quickly than Croston to situations with sudden obsolescence or with an increasing risk of obsolescence. If an item suddenly becomes obsolete (e.g. for a spare part because equipment is taken out of operation) and demands no longer occur as a result, then the TSB method will adjust its estimates towards zero as described above. On the contrary, neither Croston nor the Syntetos-Boylan Approximation (SBA) method will be able to

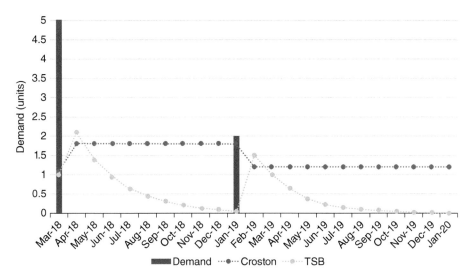

Figure 12.3 TSB and Croston forecasts.

react and will stick to the pre-obsolescence estimates. In less extreme situations where the demand rate decreases (e.g. because a competitor enters the market), the Croston and SBA methods do react. However, the adjustment does not happen until positive demands occur and hence will be rather slow, especially if demand intervals are long. The TSB method responds more quickly by adjusting forecasts in every period, thereby allowing close monitoring of when a particular item becomes obsolete and thus when we should stop stocking the item. The method's strength lies in the natural linkage between all point forecasts and stock/non-stock decisions, which are highly relevant in the final phase of an item's life cycle.

However, it is important to note that if we consider issue points only, then the TSB method is biased, for the same reason that SES is biased. That bias can lead to inflated replenishment orders, with the strongest bias effect if inventory is reviewed every period (see Chapter 6). Further, suppose that an item in the maturity stage faces highly intermittent demand and the TSB method is used to decide when and how much to replenish. Since the mean demand forecast becomes close to zero after many periods with no demand, we may eventually end up raising no orders for that item, which is surely mistaken.

Babai et al. (2014) examined the empirical forecasting and inventory replenishment performance of TSB on data from the automotive industry and the Royal Air Force. They showed that if demand data are stationary and the emphasis is on all points in time rather than issue points only, the TSB method is associated with a lower (empirical) bias than both Croston and SBA. However, its inventory implications were found to compare less favourably to those of the other methods, highlighting the previously discussed problems associated with TSB when used for replenishment purposes.

Babai et al. (2019) proposed a 'modified SBA method', the logic of which switches between SBA and TSB depending on the time since the last demand. In periods with positive demand, the method updates the demand size, demand interval, and mean demand estimates using SBA. In periods with zero demand, a check is made on whether the elapsed time interval since the last demand has become strictly greater than the most recently estimated mean demand interval. This is likely to happen when the risk of obsolescence increases. If the elapsed time does not exceed the interval estimate, then the smoothed demand sizes and intervals remain unchanged. On the other hand, if the elapsed time does exceed the most recent interval estimate, then the interval is updated in every period (in accordance with the logic of TSB). The performance of the 'modified SBA method' was tested empirically and the results showed that it may be a good alternative to SBA or TSB when there is a risk of obsolescence.

An alternative to the TSB method, introduced by Prestwich et al. (2014b), is known as hyperbolic exponential smoothing (HES). This method is based on smoothed demand sizes and demand intervals, but differs from Croston and SBA by being updated after a zero demand, taking into account the number of periods since the last non-zero observation. If the most recent smoothed demand size is $\hat{s}_{t+1}$ (smoothing constant α), the most recent smoothed demand interval is $\hat{\tau}_{t+1}$ (smoothing constant β), and the number of periods since the last positive demand is τ_t, then the HES forecast is defined as in Eq. (12.3) (Prestwich et al. 2014b).

$$\hat{d}_{t+1} = \frac{\hat{s}_{t+1}}{\hat{\tau}_{t+1} + \beta(\tau_t - 1)/2} \tag{12.3}$$

These forecasts decay hyperbolically when there is no demand. The HES method is approximately unbiased for stochastic intermittent demand (over all points in time) and is unbiased for non-intermittent demand.

Prestwich et al. (2014b) compared the accuracy of the HES and TSB methods on theoretically generated data. They obtained mixed results, suggesting greater robustness of HES but better performance by TSB in their obsolescence experiments. Further empirical work is needed to understand the relative merits of the TSB and HES methods in practice.

12.4.2 Forecasting with Granular Maintenance Information

Romeijnders et al. (2012) proposed a two-step time series methodology for forecasting the demand for spare parts using information on component repairs. This two-step forecasting method separately updates the average number of parts needed per repair and the number of repairs for each type of component. Instead of forecasting parts demand directly based on the part demand history, the method starts at the component level. For each component type, it updates the number of repairs in every period using SES. The average demand per repair is updated separately only at the end of those periods when some repair has taken place (also using SES); at other periods, the average demand remains the same. The product of the estimated number of repairs per component and the number of parts needed per repair gives the estimated number of parts related to a specific component. Adding these requirements over all relevant components gives the total predicted demand for the spare part under concern (see Technical Note 12.4 for the mathematical formulation of the method).

The performance of the method was evaluated in an extensive empirical study based on 10 years of repair operations at Fokker Services. Despite the method being able to capture information at a more granular level, it performed very similarly to TSB, SES, and the simple moving average. This may be attributed to several causes, the most plausible of which is that most parts are contained in many different components, and hence there is an inherent risk of compounding forecast errors when using this method. Nevertheless, Romeijnders et al. (2012) also showed that additional information on when components are repaired (from planned maintenance/overhaul operations) may reduce the inaccuracy of the method by up to 20%, while other methods are not able to incorporate this information.

This study is interesting because it sheds light on the sources of the demand behaviour we observe for spare parts. The methods discussed in Chapter 6, and also the TSB method discussed above, base their forecasts directly on the demand history at the part level. By doing so, they ignore the underlying process of repair operations that explains (at least partly) the typical intermittent and lumpy nature of spare parts demand. There is no demand for a part of a certain type unless a component containing such parts is repaired (intermittence) and, for a particular part, more than one may be needed to complete a repair (lumpiness).

12.4.3 Summary

When discussing intermittent demand forecasting in Chapters 2 and 6, we established the difference between all and issue points forecasts only, emphasising the comparative importance of the latter for stock replenishment purposes. We focussed on the situation when the inventory review interval is of one period ($R = 1$). In this case, forecasts produced at the end of demand occurring periods are those utilised for replenishment purposes. If these forecasts are biased, as is the case with SES and Croston for example, then excessive stock will be held to meet a prescribed service level. However, in the final phase of a spare part or any product's life cycle, all points in time become more relevant. This is because a decision is required on whether an SKU should no longer be replenished. A decision is needed, at a particular point in time, as to whether we should stop stocking an item, which is the stock/non-stock decision discussed in Chapter 2. A forecast of the mean demand, updated in every period, should allow us to monitor closely the declining phase of demand and eventually lead to the decision of not replenishing the stocks of that item any longer.

The development of the TSB and HES methods reflects an important inventory-related concern, namely that of obsolescence. Similarly, the development of the method proposed by Romeijnders et al. (2012) reflects the maintenance operations of many organisations, and it attempts to capture the underlying process that generates spare parts demand. More empirical evidence is needed before we are able to comment conclusively on these methods' utility in practice. Nevertheless, the methods share an important characteristic: their development is motivated by the context in which the methods are to be utilised. Although this seems obvious, we argue in Section 12.5 that such contextual motivation of methods' development is often ignored in the area of statistical forecasting.

12.5 Forecasting in Context

The maintenance context provides an interesting opportunity for considering an important requirement when developing forecasting methods: that of taking into account the context in which the method is to be used. We argue that this context can be established by answering two key questions (see also the first and third boxes of Figure 12.4).

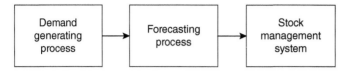

Figure 12.4 Forecasting in context.

1. How does the demand arise? What is the demand generating process and what are the factors (if any) that may help explain the demand behaviour?
2. How is the forecast used? Forecasting is never an end in itself and the forecasts are always to be translated into some sort of decision. In this book we are concerned with forecasting for inventory management decision-making.

Understanding the demand generating process is a first step towards establishing the context in which forecasting takes place, and both causal and extrapolative methods may help advance the current state of the art in spare parts demand forecasting. Causal methods should see greater popularity in the near future due to IT advancements that permit the easy storage and retrieval of large amounts of relevant explanatory information. Similarly, time series methods are increasingly accommodating very fine levels of granularity. We are yet to see much evidence on the empirical performance of such methods. The data is there, but an important question is, 'Does it help to achieve greater forecast accuracy and better inventory performance?' As the degree of information exploited increases, a method should be more accurate in terms of its bias (or lack thereof). However, it may also become over-sensitive to demand fluctuations, thus having a greater forecast variance. We can speculate that this may be the problem with the method discussed in Section 12.4.2.

How much information is useful for forecasting purposes? There seems to be a point beyond which information is harmful rather than beneficial. More information to include in the forecasting process implies more parameters to estimate for forecasting purposes, often requiring more complex forecasting models and methods. So, TSB may perform better than a simpler alternative (SES) because it uses more relevant information, but it may also perform better than a more complex alternative (Romeijnders et al. 2012) because it does not use too much relevant information!

The received wisdom in the statistical theory of prediction (e.g. Hastie et al. 2009) is that simple methods tend to have large bias and small variance and complex methods tend to have small bias and large variance. Both bias and forecast variance contribute (either explicitly through the MSE, or implicitly) to the forecast error, as discussed in Chapter 10. Future research in the area of intermittent demand forecasting should reveal what constitutes 'simple' and 'complex' and how the best trade-offs are achieved.

A further important issue, as discussed in the beginning of this section, is establishing the decision-making process that the forecasting function serves. In the area of inventory management, forecasts translate into decisions of whether or not to replenish stock, and if so by how much. Although it seems obvious that the decision-making process should have some influence on choice of forecasting method, or at least on forecast method evaluation, this is the exception rather than the rule in the academic literature. Forecasting is almost always treated as if it is an end in itself, which is never the case in practice. Arguably, reflecting the decision-making dynamics into the process of building a forecasting method is not a

Consider subsequent (stock control) computations

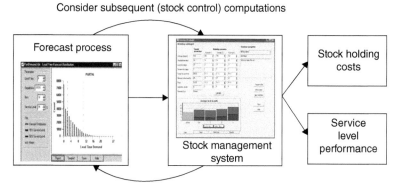

Consider preceding (forecasting) computations

Figure 12.5 Inventory-forecasting interactions. Source: Adapted from Boylan and Syntetos (2006).

straightforward thing to do. However, relevant features may be implicitly considered as with the issue of obsolescence when developing the TSB method. Alternatively, simply appreciating that accuracy metrics should be accompanied by accuracy-implication metrics may be a step in the right direction.

The fact that a forecasting method may be more accurate than another method does not necessarily mean that this performance superiority will be sustained in terms of inventory performance, usually measured by the stock holding cost and achieved service levels. Although method X may be more accurate than method Y (however forecast accuracy is measured), it may be that method Y results in more cost-efficient inventory solutions than method X, when both are used in conjunction with the same demand distribution and inventory rule, say an OUT policy. This is not only because the forecasting methods have been presumably built on the basis of minimising some given forecast error function but also because the OUT policy (or any inventory policy for that matter) has been developed by assuming that the demand distribution, and all its parameters, are known.

In summary, inventory theory generally assumes that there are no preceding stages of computation, whereas forecasting theory usually assumes that there are no subsequent stages of computation – please refer also to Figure 12.5. At the time of writing, the interactions between forecasting and inventory control are not well understood. It is clear that inventory theory needs to be revisited to take into account (demand) estimation error, and forecasting theory needs to be (re-)evaluated to take into account accuracy-implication metrics.

12.6 Chapter Summary

In this chapter, we moved beyond intermittent demand forecasting in general, to address some issues that are of importance in a spare parts context in particular. Spare parts that serve maintenance processes and are often at great risk of obsolescence.

In a maintenance context, a plethora of explanatory variables may be available to help predict spare parts demand and causal forecasting is particularly relevant in these cases.

Big data appears to have considerable value for maintenance and reliability analysis, and it is reasonable to expect that information gathered in an almost continuous fashion, say through sensors, will help better prediction of failures and more efficient organisation of maintenance operations. However, this remains a speculation at the time of writing. Empirical evidence is lacking and more research is required to turn such speculation into a trustworthy conclusion.

Further, three time series methods that build upon the developments considered in Chapter 6 were also discussed in this chapter. The TSB (Teunter, Syntetos, and Babai 2011) and HES (Prestwich et al. 2014b) methods update forecasts at the end of every period, to address the issue of obsolescence. The method developed by Romeijnders et al. (2012) exploits granular maintenance related information.

In this chapter, we have also discussed the importance of specifying the context in which forecasting takes place. This is both in terms of the process that generates the demand that is input into the forecasting calculations, and in terms of the decision-making process that forecasting serves. In doing so, the value of increasing volumes of potentially useful (demand) information was debated, and the need for furthering our understanding on the interactions between forecasting and stock control was highlighted.

Technical Notes

Note 12.1 Preventive and Corrective Maintenance

It is important to note that preventive and corrective maintenance requirements are sometimes bundled together, resulting in lumpy demand patterns faced by the stockist. The heterogeneity of these requests (very low volume requests generated by genuine failures coupled with larger batch requests for the same item for servicing a number of machines in a preventive way) results in patterns that are difficult to forecast, assuming that information about preventive maintenance has not been communicated to the supplying source (internally or externally). Although this is a problem in its own right, and goes some way to explain why intermittent demand may sometimes be lumpy, it is not considered further here. It is clear that splitting up these two streams of demand (and communicating the known part to the stockists, as previously discussed) may be very beneficial for planning purposes.

Note 12.2 On-condition Monitoring

One additional primary maintenance process was considered: on-condition. This requires that an appliance or part is periodically inspected or checked against some appropriate physical standard to determine whether it can continue in service. The purpose of the standard is to remove the unit from service before failure during normal operation.

Note 12.3 Deterioration, Perishability, and Obsolescence

The terms 'deterioration', 'perishability', and 'obsolescence' are sometimes used interchangeably in the literature but do, in fact, have distinct meanings. Deterioration refers to the process of decay, damage, or spoilage of a product, so that the product loses its value and can no longer be sold or used for its original purpose. In contrast, an item with a fixed lifetime perishes once it exceeds its maximum shelf lifetime and then must be discarded. Obsolescence refers to 'writing off' or 'writing down' the value of the on-hand inventory because its demand has declined so much that the inventory is perceived as having no value, or having a reduced value.

Note 12.4 Forecasting of Spare Parts Based on Component Repairs

The method proposed by Romeijnders et al. (2012) operates as follows. For each component type, $c = 1, \ldots, C$, the estimates of the number of repairs at time $t + 1$, denoted by $\hat{r}^c_{t+1}$ and the average demand for the spare part per repair, also at time $t + 1$, denoted by $\hat{d}_{t+1}$, are updated separately at the end of period t using Eqs. (12.4) and (12.5).

$$\hat{r}^c_{t+1} = \hat{r}^c_t + \alpha(r^c_t - \hat{r}^c_t) \tag{12.4}$$

$$\hat{d}^c_{t+1} = \begin{cases} \hat{d}^c_t & \text{if } r^c_t = 0 \\ \hat{d}^c_t + \beta \left(\frac{D^c_t}{r^c_t} - \hat{d}^c_t \right) & \text{if } r^c_t > 0 \end{cases} \tag{12.5}$$

where α and β are smoothing constants ($0 \le \alpha, \beta \le 1$) and D^c_t is the total parts demand (across all repairs) for components of type c at time t. Note that the forecast of the average demand per repair is not updated at the end of time periods without repairs. The forecast of parts demand used only for component of type c is given by Eq. (12.6).

$$\hat{Y}^c_{t+1} = \hat{r}^c_{t+1} \hat{d}^c_{t+1} \tag{12.6}$$

By adding these forecasts over all (relevant) components, we obtain the final parts demand forecast, as shown in Eq. (12.7).

$$\hat{Y}_{t+1} = \sum_{c=1}^{C} \hat{Y}^c_{t+1} \tag{12.7}$$

13

Non-parametric Methods

13.1 Introduction

In previous chapters, we have adopted a parametric approach to the characterisation of uncertain demand. This presupposes that future demand can be well represented by a distribution with parameters that are unknown but may be forecasted using past data. This approach is reasonable if a distribution can be found that satisfies the criteria introduced in Chapter 4:

1. Empirical evidence in support of its goodness of fit.
2. Intuitive appeal in terms of a priori grounds for its choice.
3. Flexibility to represent different types of demand patterns.
4. Computational ease.

The most basic requirement is the first. Unfortunately, this requirement is often not met for a significant proportion of stock keeping units (SKUs). This problem was illustrated in Chapter 5, where we reviewed some empirical evidence on goodness of fit. Demand over a single period was well fitted by the stuttering Poisson distribution for over 90% of SKUs (Table 5.3). However, this figure dropped to 72% for the Royal Air Force (RAF) dataset when considering demand over lead time (Table 5.4), leaving 28% of SKUs not well fitted by this distribution.

In a situation like this, we can look to other distributions to fill the gap, but need to take care not to overcomplicate the allocation of SKUs to probability distributions. (Indeed, the flexibility criterion was introduced to avoid this type of complication.) Another possible solution would be to use a three-parameter distribution, such as the geometric-Poisson-gamma or the logarithmic-Poisson-gamma, introduced in Chapter 7 for demand over variable lead times. Typically, though, these distributions lack an a priori justification for fixed lead times.

An alternative approach is to abandon the search for a parametric distribution. By following this approach, the data are not assumed to follow any standard probability distribution. Instead, direct methods are used to assess the distributions required for inventory management. These methods are the focus of the current chapter. We begin with the empirical distribution function (EDF), to forecast the distribution of demand over a single period. Then, we move on to forecasting the distribution of demand over the whole protection

Intermittent Demand Forecasting: Context, Methods and Applications, First Edition.
John E. Boylan and Aris A. Syntetos.
© 2021 John Wiley & Sons Ltd. Published 2021 by John Wiley & Sons Ltd.
Companion Website: www.wiley.com/go/boylansyntetos/intermittentdemandforecasting

interval using the methods of non-overlapping blocks (NOB) and overlapping blocks (OB). Alternative non-parametric methods, based on resampling of previous observations, are introduced and some limitations are discussed, leading on to extensions that have been implemented in commercial software. The chapter concludes with a review and summary of the strengths and weaknesses of non-parametric methods.

13.2 Empirical Distribution Functions

In this section, we consider the problem of estimating the demand or sales values for which the cumulative distributions attain predetermined targets (e.g. 90%, 95%, or 99%) when the protection interval is a single period. We move on to multiple periods in later sections of this chapter.

The EDF is based on calculation of cumulative frequency percentages. Let us consider the unit sales for a product over the last 36 months (Product C in Chapter 1 of Makridakis et al. 1998), shown in Figure 13.1.

The intermittent sales history, depicted in Figure 13.1, is summarised in Table 13.1, including the frequencies, cumulative frequencies, and cumulative frequency percentages of sales values over the last 36 months. The third column is a 'running total' of the frequencies from the second column. For example, the cumulative frequency for a sales value of three is the running total, $25 + 4 + 2 + 2 = 33$, and tells us that there were 33 months when the sales value was less than or equal to 3. The final column converts the cumulative frequencies to percentages. For example, the cumulative frequency percentage for a sales value of 3 is $(33/36) \times 100 = 91.7\%$; similarly, for a sales value of 2, it is 86.1%. Therefore, 3 is the 90th percentile of the sales distribution, meaning that it is the lowest value for which a cumulative frequency percentage of 90.0% is attained or exceeded.

The linkage between the first column of observations and the final column of cumulative frequency percentages in Table 13.1 is sometimes known as the empirical distribution function (EDF). It is usually denoted by $\hat{F}$ where the hat-symbol is used to distinguish it from F,

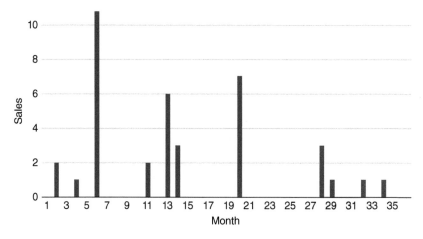

Figure 13.1 Intermittent series.

Table 13.1 Cumulative frequency percentages.

Sales	Frequency (months)	Cumulative frequency	Cumulative frequency (%)
0	25	25	69.4
1	4	29	80.6
2	2	31	86.1
3	2	33	91.7
4	0	33	91.7
5	0	33	91.7
6	1	34	94.4
7	1	35	97.2
8	0	35	97.2
9	0	35	97.2
10	0	35	97.2
11	1	36	100.0

the true (but unknown) cumulative distribution function (CDF). Table 13.1 indicates that $\hat{F}_1(3) = 91.7\%$, where the subscript 1 denotes that the EDF refers to demand over a single period.

13.2.1 Assumptions

We would now like to use the (known) EDF $(\hat{F})$, over the last 36 months, as a predictor of the (unknown) CDF (F) over the next month. To take this leap, we must make two assumptions:

1. The CDF has been unchanged over the data history and will remain unchanged over the next month.
2. The observation in the next month is independent of the observations in previous months.

The first assumption will be retained in this chapter, with further discussion in the chapter summary. The second assumption will be relaxed later in this chapter in the discussion on extensions to resampling methods. In the meantime, the assumption will be retained. In this case, our previous example would have a forecasted 90th percentile of three units. For a cycle service level (CSL) driven system, this may then be translated to an order-up-to level, S, of three units, for a protection interval of one period.

13.2.2 Length of History

A practical problem that must be addressed is to decide on the length of data history to use. As discussed in Chapter 5, there are two opposing factors:

- The shorter the history, the more difficult it is to estimate high percentiles with any degree of reliability. This is true for any time series but the problem is exacerbated for erratic or lumpy demand. In this type of demand, the presence or absence of just one or two very high values in a short data history can strongly affect the estimates of high percentiles.
- The longer the history, the less likely it is that the CDF has remained unchanged over that period. If demand has been slowly declining, then the EDF, based on the whole history, is likely to overestimate the probabilities of higher demand values in the near future.

The trade-off between these two factors is not usually clear cut. However, the performance of estimates may be compared using simulation methods, based on real historical data and various lengths of data history, using the approaches discussed in Chapter 9.

13.2.3 Summary

Empirical distribution functions (EDFs) have some qualities that make them attractive for practical implementation. Although the four criteria highlighted in Section 13.1 were proposed for parametric distributions, it is instructive to review EDFs against them. They are certainly intuitively appealing, and probably more so than parametric distributions. They are more flexible than parametric methods because they can represent any shape of distribution function. Moreover, they are simple to compute. Hence, they satisfy the second, third, and fourth criteria very well.

With regard to the first criterion, goodness of fit, it may seem that EDFs will always outperform parametric distributions. By definition, they are a perfect fit to the historical data. However, this is to miss the point of the criterion. What is important is goodness of fit to the demand over the forecast horizon. Historical goodness of fit is only a proxy for this. If the data history is short, then an EDF will not always give good estimates of higher percentiles. Also, if a parameter such as the mean is changing over time, then a good parametric forecasting method will tend to keep up with these changes, whereas a non-parametric approach may lag behind. Consequently, there is no guarantee that EDFs will be more accurate than parametric distributions. The empirical approach becomes more beneficial for longer demand histories, more stable demand distributions, and situations in which none of the parametric distributions is a good fit to the data.

13.3 Non-overlapping and Overlapping Blocks

In Section 13.2, we restricted attention to situations where the protection interval was of one period. This meant that percentiles of demand during one period could be obtained directly from the EDF. As we move to longer protection intervals, alternative methods are required, the simplest of which are non-overlapping and overlapping blocks.

13.3.1 Differences Between the Two Methods

The overlapping blocks (OB) and non-overlapping blocks (NOB) methods are based on straightforward calculations. An example of monthly demand is given in the second column of Table 13.2. The three-month OB and NOB methods give the results shown in the last two columns of the table.

Table 13.2 Three-month overlapping blocks (OB) and non-overlapping blocks (NOB).

Month	Demand	OB	NOB
1	0		
2	**0**	1	1
3	**1**	1	
4	**0**	6	
5	5	5	5
6	0	6	
7	1	3	
8	2	3	3
9	0	2	
10	0	2	
11	2	22	22
12	20	22	
13	0	21	
14	1	6	6
15	5	6	
16	0	15	
17	10	12	12
18	2	12	
19	0	4	
20	2	2	2
21	0	3	
22	1	1	
23	0	2	2
24	1		

The NOB method is so called because each total is based on distinct blocks, with no over-lapping periods. The three-month totals shown in the fourth column of Table 13.2 convert a monthly time series into a quarterly time series.

The OB method is based on non-distinct blocks. Periods 1, 2, and 3 are used for the first calculation. The second calculation is based on Periods 2, 3, and 4, as highlighted by the numbers in bold type in the second and third columns of the table. Each block (of length two periods or more) overlaps the next and, depending on the block-length, may overlap some later blocks too. The cumulative frequency percentages for both OB and NOB are shown in Figure 13.2, based on the demand data in Table 13.2 and the same calculation method as before.

Figure 13.2 shows the cumulative frequency percentages from the OB method to be a little smoother than those from NOB. This is often the case, unless the data is highly sparse, because the OB method is based on more blocks.

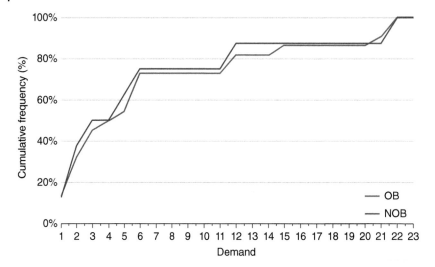

Figure 13.2 Cumulative frequency percentages: three-month overlapping blocks (OB) and non-overlapping blocks (NOB).

13.3.2 Methods and Assumptions

Forecasts from the OB and NOB methods are based on similar assumptions to those discussed earlier for the EDF: (i) the CDF has been unchanged over the data history and will remain so over the whole of the forecast horizon (not just the next period) and (ii) the total demand over the forecast horizon is independent of previous observations. In the following discussion, the forecast horizon is always taken to be the protection interval. The blocks are set to be the same length as the protection interval, so that the results are immediately applicable to inventory calculations.

13.3.3 Practical Considerations

In practice, the number of observations available may not be an exact multiple of the length of the protection interval. For example, suppose that the protection interval is of three periods, and 23 periods of demand history are available.

For the NOB method, the usual practice would be to use the 21 most recent observations to form seven blocks. As noted above, an assumption is made that the empirical distribution over an historical period is a good representation of the distribution over the forecast horizon. This assumption is most realistic if the most recent information is used.

For OB, no data is lost if the length of demand history is not a multiple of the length of each block. In this sense, OB makes better use of the data. One side effect of the method is that not all periods in the demand history are used equally frequently. In our example in Table 13.2, Periods 3–22 (inclusive) are used three times, Periods 2 and 23 are used twice, and Periods 1 and 24 are used only once (in the first and final block, respectively).

13.3.4 Performance of Non-overlapping Blocks Method

From a statistical perspective, the accuracy of the non-parametric methods discussed in this chapter can be assessed in terms of their bias and variance as estimates of the true, but unknown, CDF, assuming that demand per period is independent and identically distributed (i.i.d.).

The NOB method is unbiased as an estimator of the true CDF for i.i.d. demand. This means that the expected value, denoted by $\mathbb{E}$, of NOB estimates will match the true CDF value for any block-length (m) and any demand value (y) as shown in Eq. (13.1).

$$\mathbb{E}(\widehat{F}_m^{\text{NOB}}(y)) = F_m(y) \tag{13.1}$$

The graph of NOB cumulative frequency percentages shown in Figure 13.2 exhibits step-changes and is far from smooth. Of course, this is due to the small number of blocks, only eight in this case, which are being used to estimate the percentages. If we had looked at an earlier sequence of eight blocks, then we may have seen a quite different graph even if the true (unknown) CDF had not changed at all over the whole history.

In general, we would anticipate that the variance of the estimate of the CDF of demand would reduce as the number of blocks increases. This is reflected in Eq. (13.2), showing the variance of CDF estimates, using non-overlapping blocks of length m to predict the CDF, over the next m periods, if the total demand in each block is independent of total demand in other blocks. This condition holds, for any block-length, if demand per period is i.i.d.

$$\text{Var}(\widehat{F}_m^{\text{NOB}}(y)) = \frac{F_m(y)(1 - F_m(y))}{k} \tag{13.2}$$

In Eq. (13.2), k represents the number of non-overlapping blocks. If the number of observations (n) is divisible by the block-length (m), then $k = n/m$; if not, then k is the whole number (integer) part of n/m (sometimes written as $k = \text{INT}(n/m)$). Equation (13.2) shows us that, for given values of y and m, the variance is inversely proportional to the number of blocks.

It may be objected that, for Eq. (13.2) to be useful, we would need to know the value of the CDF of demand over m periods, but that is exactly what we are trying to estimate! This objection is correct. Nevertheless, the equation will be useful in gaining some insights into the comparison of NOB and OB methods, as will be shown in Section 13.4.

13.3.5 Performance of Overlapping Blocks Method

Like NOB, the OB method is unbiased as an estimator of the true CDF, for all block-lengths (m) and demand values (y), for i.i.d. demand, as shown in Eq. (13.3).

$$\mathbb{E}(\widehat{F}_m^{\text{OB}}(y)) = F_m(y) \tag{13.3}$$

In this regard, then, there is no difference in performance between OB and NOB. For a block-length of two periods ($m = 2$), the variance of the CDF estimate using OB is given by Eq. (13.4) for i.i.d. demand (Boylan and Babai 2016).

$$\text{Var}(\widehat{F}_2^{\text{OB}}(y)) = \frac{F_2(y)}{k} + \left(\frac{(k-2)(k-1)}{k^2} - 1 \right) F_2(y)^2 + \frac{2(k-1)}{k^2} \Theta_1(y) \tag{13.4}$$

In Eq. (13.4), k represents the number of overlapping blocks ($k = n - m + 1$). The theta function, $\Theta_1(y)$, represents the chance that two blocks of two periods, with a partial overlap of one period, both have total demands not exceeding y. The theta function is affected by the homogeneity of the data. If a particular value (e.g. demand of one unit) becomes more common, then the theta function will increase. As a series becomes more intermittent, it also becomes more homogeneous because of the commonness of zeroes and, therefore, the theta function will increase. The calculation of the theta function is illustrated in Technical Note 13.1.

A general expression for the variance of the OB estimate, for any block-length, is given in Technical Note 13.2. The variance depends on the same factors as for NOB, namely the number of blocks (k) and the true CDF (F), but it also depends on the block-length (m) and a set of theta functions. For block-lengths longer than 2, we need to take into account differing degrees of partial overlap. For example, if the block-length is 4, we must consider partial overlaps of one, two, and three periods, each with its own theta function. In each case, the theta function represents the chance that two partially overlapping blocks both contain totals that do not exceed a certain value. In general, for a block-length of m, there are $m - 1$ partial overlaps that must be taken into account.

The formulae given in Technical Note 13.2, which apply for any block-length, show that the OB estimates become less variable as the theta functions decline and the demand becomes more varied. It will not usually be necessary to calculate the theta functions in practice. Their main application is in theoretical analyses of the conditions under which the OB method will yield CDF estimates of lower variance than the NOB method.

13.3.6 Summary

The OB method is as easy to use as the NOB method. Also, just like that method, it is unbiased for i.i.d. demand. In this section, we have seen that it is possible to obtain formulae for the variance of the non-overlapping blocks and overlapping blocks CDF estimates, for i.i.d. demand. The variance expressions are not necessarily useful for direct application but rather for deriving insights into the comparative performance of OB and NOB, as discussed in Section 13.4.

13.4 Comparison of Approaches

An obvious practical question is whether to use the OB or NOB approach. One way of making this choice, given that both methods produce unbiased CDF estimates, is to find the conditions under which one method produces less variable CDF estimates than the other, for i.i.d. demand. These conditions will be given in this section and the associated technical notes. We shall see that in most situations, but not all, OB produces less variable estimates than NOB.

13.4.1 Time Series Characteristics Favouring Overlapping Blocks

Boylan and Babai (2016) compared the variance of the CDF estimate from NOB (Eq. (13.2)) with the variance of the CDF estimate from OB (Eqs. (13.7) and (13.8), both given in

Figure 13.3 Proportional reduction in variance of CDF estimates by using OB instead of NOB ($m = 2$, $y = 2$) for Poisson demand, as a function of mean demand (λ) and length of history (n). Source: Boylan and Babai (2016). © 2016, Elsevier.

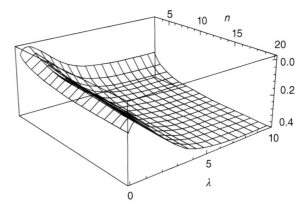

Technical Note 13.2). For i.i.d. demand, and a block-length of two periods, the OB estimate has lower variance than the NOB estimate if the inequality in 13.5 holds.

$$\Theta_1(y) < \left(\frac{n-1}{2n}\right) F_2(y) + \left(\frac{n+1}{2n}\right) F_2(y)^2 \tag{13.5}$$

where n (assumed to be even) is the length of the demand history. A general inequality, for any block-length, is given in Technical Note 13.3.

Boylan and Babai (2016) found that, under most circumstances, OB was less variable than NOB for a block-length of two periods. However, for very short demand histories (e.g. of only four periods) and highly intermittent data, NOB may be less variable. This is shown in the top-left corner of Figure 13.3, where there is a small advantage to NOB.

Closer scrutiny of the inequality in (13.5) gives some hints as to the effects of the length of history and demand intermittence on the relative performance of the OB and NOB methods. The right-hand side of the inequality will be higher for longer demand histories, indicating that such histories may be more favourable to OB. The left-hand side will tend to be higher for more intermittent demand, indicating that greater intermittence may favour NOB.

Figure 13.3 shows the proportional reduction in variance of CDF estimates by using OB instead of NOB for the special case of Poisson distributed demand. In the figure, the demand has mean λ, the demand history is of length n, the block-length is of two periods ($m = 2$), and the CDF is estimated for a demand value of two units ($y = 2$). Figure 13.3 confirms that, for a block-length of two periods, OB is most beneficial for longer demand histories (n) and higher mean demand values (λ), corresponding to less intermittence. It also shows that considerable reduction in the variability in estimates can be achieved by using OB instead of NOB for i.i.d. demand, for a block length of two periods. Even greater reductions can be achieved for a block-length of three periods (Boylan and Babai 2016).

The analytical results in this section assume i.i.d. demand. These assumptions do not always hold in practice, but the OB method may still be beneficial. Evidence on real data, not necessarily conforming to i.i.d. assumptions, is reviewed in Section 13.4.2.

13.4.2 Empirical Evidence on Overlapping Blocks

Porras and Dekker (2008) conducted a detailed empirical analysis of spare parts from a Dutch petrochemical complex. Each spare part had 55 months of demand history. The spare parts were classified into four categories, with most of the intermittent items being in Class 1 (parts with only 0 or 1 as demand values, comprising 2226 SKUs) or Class 2 (total demand, over 55 months, greater than 0 and less than 60 – but with some demand values other than 0 or 1, comprising 5185 SKUs). They equated the block-length to the (actual) lead times in months, rounded up if necessary. An (s, NQ) inventory system was used in conjunction with OB. This is similar to the (s, Q) system described in Chapter 2, where a quantity, Q, is ordered when the inventory position falls below s, but differs if the quantity, Q, is not sufficient to bring the inventory position up to s, in which case the order quantity is doubled ($N = 2$), and if this is not sufficient, it is tripled ($N = 3$), and if this is not sufficient, it is quadrupled, and so on. The order-point, s, was determined using the estimated lead time demand (LTD) distribution, and the order quantity, Q, was based on economic order quantity (EOQ) calculations (see, for example, Silver et al. 2017, for discussion of the EOQ).

Porras and Dekker (2008) analysed the effect of estimation methods on the CSL, fill rate and inventory costs of the organisation, where the costs take into consideration ordering and inventory holding. They found that, for Class 1, the OB approach was able to attain high CSLs and fill rates. It also achieved lower costs than a method based on an assumption of Poisson demand, coupled with an $(S - 1, S)$ inventory policy. For Class 2, the OB method was able to achieve an improvement in the fill rate as well as an inventory cost saving compared to the system in operation at the petrochemical complex.

Boylan and Babai (2016) compared the performance of the OB and NOB methods using a dataset from the US jewellery industry. They analysed 4076 intermittent demand SKUs over a year (52 weeks of demand). The lead time was fixed as one week. An order-up-to (R, S) inventory policy was used, with reviews every week ($R = 1$). The system was driven by a target CSL, with unmet demand being backordered. Target CSL values of 80%, 90%, and 95% were employed, with experimentation of three demand history lengths (6, 12, and 24 weeks) and two block lengths (two and three weeks). The researchers compared the performance of the OB and NOB methods using trade-off curves of inventory holding volumes and backorder volumes. They found little difference between the performance of OB and NOB for shorter demand histories (6 and 12 periods). For a length of 24 periods, OB showed marginally lower backorders for a target CSL of 95% and aggregation of two periods. For aggregation of three periods, OB showed more noticeable reductions in backorders for target CSLs of 90% and 95%.

Zhu et al. (2017) sought to improve the OB method, noting that the method has difficulty in attaining high service level targets. They used an empirical extreme value theory (empirical-EVT) approach to model the tail of the LTD distribution. Their study was based on the same automotive dataset of 3000 spare parts used by Syntetos and Boylan (2005) and 2549 spare parts from the aircraft component dataset analysed by Romeijnders et al. (2012), with a lead time of three periods for the former, and five periods for the latter. The researchers assessed the ability of Croston, Syntetos–Boylan approximation, and the empirical-EVT method to achieve CSL targets, without consideration of total inventory costs. For the automotive dataset, empirical-EVT gets closer to the target than the original empirical (OB) method. However, it does not perform quite as well as Croston or SBA. For the aircraft component dataset, the empirical-EVT performs better than the original empirical method; it also gets closer to the target CSL than SBA and performs similarly to Croston's method.

13.4.3 Summary

The performance of OB and NOB has been analysed. Theoretical results have been established, comparing the variance of the CDF estimates of the two methods, assuming i.i.d. demand. These results give some insights into the conditions favouring NOB, namely very short histories and highly intermittent demand. Analysis of Poisson distributed demand shows that, under most circumstances, the method of OB has CDF estimates with lower variance than NOB. The theoretical evidence, then, is in favour of the OB approach.

Empirical evidence remains scarce. Two studies have examined the inventory performance of the OB approach, and shown some promising results. A third study, on the empirical-EVT method, shows that there is potential in combining non-parametric methods with extreme value theory.

13.5 Resampling Methods

The OB and NOB approaches both retain the original sequence of demand observations within their blocks. They can be used even if the i.i.d. assumption does not hold, although some analytical results no longer apply.

We can move away from methods based on blocks of consecutive periods, if it is reasonable to assume that demand per period is i.i.d., and form blocks of non-consecutive observations from the demand history. For example, to form a block of three periods, we may select the 2nd, 11th, and 19th observations from a history of 24 periods. The issue now is how to make these choices. An approach based on random selection is outlined in Section 13.5.1.

13.5.1 Simple Bootstrapping

Returning to the monthly demand data given in Table 13.2, we need to estimate the probabilities of demand over the protection interval. Suppose that this is for three months. The bootstrapping method works by resampling from the historical demands, as illustrated in Table 13.3, which shows ten replications (or 'reps') of the resamplings.

Having observed 24 recent monthly observations, we are now simulating possible future demands in Months 25, 26, and 27. Using the bootstrapping technique, three previous periods are selected randomly. In the first resample, representing the first possible future scenario, Months 1, 3, and 9 are selected (see Table 13.3). Such random selection may be achieved in any programming language by multiplying a random number by 24, and rounding it up to the next whole number, where the random number should be uniformly distributed between 0 and 1. The selection of Months 1, 3, and 9 means that one future scenario is for the demands in these periods to reoccur (demands of 0, 1, and 0, respectively, see Table 13.2) as demands in Months 25, 26, and 27.

In the eighth replication, the 23rd observation has been selected twice, to represent demand in both Months 25 and 26. This is permissible in bootstrapping, as the resampling is 'with replacement'. We can imagine a container with 24 numbered balls. When one is chosen (23 in this case), it is then replaced, with a one in 24 chance of it being chosen again

Table 13.3 Resampling from previous observations.

	Observation resampled			Demand resampled			
Rep	Month 25	Month 26	Month 27	Month 25	Month 26	Month 27	Total
1	1	3	9	0	1	0	1
2	8	16	2	2	0	0	2
3	12	11	20	20	2	2	24
4	16	22	13	0	1	0	1
5	6	4	1	0	0	0	0
6	4	14	3	0	1	1	2
7	20	3	9	2	1	0	3
8	23	23	22	0	0	1	1
9	15	11	9	5	2	0	7
10	5	14	1	5	1	0	6

on the next occasion. A brief examination of Table 13.3 shows that some of the previous months appear to be over-represented (e.g. Month 1 is chosen three times) whereas others are not selected at all (e.g. Month 7). This is a sampling effect due to the small number of replications, only 10 in this example. If this number were to be increased, then the effect would be diminished.

Suppose that, instead of only 10 replications, we undertake 10 000 replications. The total demand results from each of these 10 000 replications are then sorted, from the lowest to the highest. If the first 1618 replications in the sorted list have a total demand of zero, then this gives an estimate of the chance of the total demand being zero of 16.18%. Also, if the next 2203 replications have a total demand of one, this gives an estimate of 22.03% of the chance of total demand being one. As the first 3821 observations are either 0 or 1, the estimate of the cumulative probability for a value of 1 is 38.21%, representing the chance of the total demand being either 0 or 1. A full set of results is shown in Figure 13.4.

Figure 13.4 shows that bootstrapping can produce smoother cumulative frequency percentages than NOB or OB. If we were to undertake another set of 10 000 resamplings, then we would obtain slightly different results from the bootstrapping method. However, the differences would indeed be slight. We can generally be satisfied that 10 000 replications is sufficient for the level of intermittence of demand observed in most practical inventory management applications, although some experimentation is advisable to check that each full set of replications produces very similar results.

The random selection of observations used in bootstrapping ignores the original sequence. This is legitimate if the observations are i.i.d. If this is not the case, then OB may be better because this method retains the sequence of observations from the original data.

13.5.2 Bootstrapping Demand Sizes and Intervals

Viswanathan and Zhou (2008) proposed an alternative bootstrapping method, sometimes referred to as the VZ method. The objective is the same as simple bootstrapping, namely to

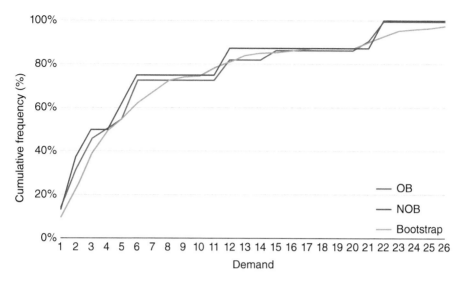

Figure 13.4 Cumulative frequency percentages (OB, NOB, and bootstrap).

predict the distribution of demand over the next protection interval. Instead of resampling demand from individual periods, the method works by resampling demand intervals and demand sizes separately. The VZ method is as follows:

1. Initialise the *time horizon* and *demand size total* to be zero.
2. Resample a demand interval. Update the *time horizon* by adding the sampled demand interval.
3. If the *time horizon* is less than or equal to the protection interval, then resample a demand size, add to the previous *demand size total*, and go to Step 2; else if the protection interval has been exceeded, then go to Step 4.
4. Repeat, 1000 times, steps 1, 2, and 3.
5. Sort the 1000 results and generate the distribution of demand over the protection interval.

The 1000 replications suggested by Viswanathan and Zhou (2008) is less than the 10 000 replications recommended earlier for simple bootstrapping, but the two numbers are not directly comparable because the VZ method resamples demand intervals and sizes rather than demands from individual periods. As before, it is advisable to check that different full replications produce similar results.

This procedure will be illustrated with the data from Table 13.2. In that table, the 13 observed demand sizes were as follows: 1, 5, 1, 2, 2, 20, 1, 5, 10, 2, 2, 1, 1. The 12 observed demand intervals were: 2, 2, 1, 3, 1, 2, 1, 2, 1, 2, 2, 2. The VZ method is executed, with ten replications ('reps') of the loop containing Steps 1, 2, and 3, for a protection interval of three periods ($R + L = 3$), as shown in Table 13.4.

In the first resampling, a demand interval of one period is resampled and, with it, a demand size of 5. The time horizon advances to the end of the first period. Then, in the same replication, a further demand interval of one period is resampled and, with it, a demand size of 1. The time horizon advances to the end of the second period. At this point, it is

Table 13.4   VZ resampling method ($R + L = 3$).

Rep	Interval resampled			Size resampled			Total demand
	First interval	Second interval	Third interval	First size	Second size	Third size	
1	1	1	2	5	1		6
2	2	2		2			2
3	1	1	1	1	10	5	16
4	3			2			2
5	2	2		1			1
6	2	3		2			2
7	1	2		5	2		7
8	2	4		1			1
9	2	1		20	1		21
10	3			5			5

possible that there may be another demand within the protection interval of three periods. However, the next resampled demand interval is for two periods, taking the time horizon beyond the end of the third period. Therefore, no demand size is resampled and the total of the resampled demands is 6. The remaining replications in Table 13.4 illustrate some of the combinations of demand intervals and demand sizes that may be resampled using the demand sizes and intervals listed above.

The VZ method assumes that the lengths of successive demand intervals are independent, successive demand sizes are independent, and sizes and intervals are mutually independent (for example, a large demand size is no more likely after a long demand interval than after a short demand interval). These conditions will be satisfied if demand per period is i.i.d.

13.5.3   VZ Bootstrap and the Syntetos–Boylan Approximation

Zhou and Viswanathan (2011) compared the non-parametric VZ method with the parametric SBA method, using industrial data from an aerospace company. They analysed 50 SKUs, each of which had 72 months of demand history, with the first 48 months being used to generate estimates and the remaining 24 months to compare performance. The SBA method was used to forecast the mean demand, with the variance being estimated using the smoothed mean square error formula of Syntetos and Boylan (2006) (see Chapter 7). Two applications of SBA were employed, based on negative binomial and normal distributions of lead time demand.

In their empirical analysis, Zhou and Viswanathan (2011) used an (R, S) periodic order-up-to system, with reviews every period. The system was driven by a CSL measure, with a target CSL of 95%. Lead times of one, three, and six months were analysed. The researchers found that the VZ method was able to attain results that were closest to the target CSL, but at a considerable penalty in terms of the average inventory cost. They found the negative binomial application of SBA to give higher CSLs for the longer lead times (three and six months) but with greater inventory cost than the normal distribution application of SBA. They concluded: 'The bootstrapping method is inferior to the parametric approach for the industrial data' (Zhou and Viswanthan 2011, p. 484). The main reason was that the 48 months of historical data used to generate VZ estimates was not sufficient to allow accurate estimation of the distributions of demand sizes and intervals.

Hasni et al. (2019) examined the VZ method by simulating inventory costs based on an (R, S) inventory system, with $R = 1$, as used by Zhou and Viswanathan (2011). They found, using theoretically generated demand data, that VZ had a lower inventory cost than SBA when the coefficients of variation of both demand intervals and demand sizes were less than or equal to 0.5. They found that shorter lead times tended to favour SBA, whereas longer lead times tended to favour VZ. They also conducted an empirical analysis of 5000 SKUs from the RAF, each with 84 months of demand history, and using actual lead times. The system was driven by fill rate requirements, with backordering to holding cost ratios of 5, 10, 50, 100, and 200 being tested. Demand was assumed to be negative binomially distributed. The analysis showed SBA to have a lower total inventory cost than VZ for a backordering to holding cost ratio of five, with a saving of approximately 9% if the same initial inventory is used for all SKUs and a saving of approximately 23% when different initial inventories are used. The dominance of SBA was sustained for higher backordering to inventory cost ratios. These findings were consistent with the results on theoretically generated data because of the preponderance of series in the RAF dataset with coefficients of variation greater than 0.5.

13.5.4 Extension of Methods to Variable Lead Times

In Chapter 7, we considered the problem of variable lead times. The main focus was on parametric distributions that take the variable lead time into account. Discussion on bootstrapping methods was postponed to this chapter.

Both of the bootstrapping methods outlined in this section can be extended to variable lead times. The first step is to construct an empirical distribution of item-specific lead times (Willemain et al. 2004). Then, resampling from this distribution, and adding the appropriate (fixed) review interval, will give the sampled protection interval for the particular resampling.

For the simple bootstrapping method, it is straightforward to resample demands from previous observations, with the number of observations resampled being dictated by the length of the sampled protection interval. The VZ method also proceeds as before, except that the time horizon is checked against the sampled protection interval, rather than the fixed protection interval.

13.5.5 Resampling Immediately After Demand Occurrence

Teunter and Duncan (2009) proposed an adaptation to the bootstrapping approach, which addresses the service level requirements of the CSL^+ measure. This is the cycle service level measure based on replenishment cycles with some demand, introduced in Chapter 3.

Teunter and Duncan (2009) assessed the fraction of orders that arrive on time, thereby restricting attention to those cycles with some demand. They noted that an order in a period is triggered by a demand, and a bootstrapping method will need to be adjusted to allow for this. In their paper, a periodic review system was employed with a fixed review at the end of every period ($R = 1$). Also, these authors based their analysis on a protection interval of length L (rather than length $L + 1$) because they assumed that an order placed in period t will arrive in time to satisfy the demands of period $t + L$. (They remarked that if a period is a working day, then this could be achieved using overnight deliveries.)

Teunter and Duncan's adaptation of simple bootstrapping, under the conditions described above, is to insist that the first resample be drawn from those periods with positive demand, with the remaining $L - 1$ resamples drawn in the usual way from the entire demand history.

These adaptations are needed for systems driven by the CSL^+ measure. They are not required if the CSL measure is used because the CSL measure is not restricted to cycles with some demand. In this case, unmodified bootstrapping methods may be used.

13.5.6 Summary

Resampling methods require quite intensive computation for just one series, but this is becoming less of an issue as computing processing capability continues to grow. The methods outlined in this section have a number of practical advantages: (i) ease of coding, (ii) intuitive to explain, and (iii) results are consistent with previous observations, and do not depend on theoretical distributions that may be difficult to justify (e.g. Poisson, normal).

Analysis of the bootstrapping method of Viswanathan and Zhou (2008) shows that it is most promising for demand series that are weakly variable both in terms of demand intervals and demand sizes. The empirical evidence on industrial data sets is less encouraging, showing that the SBA method can yield lower total inventory costs. Some further evidence on a modification of the VZ method will be reviewed later in this chapter. No empirical evidence has been found on the simple bootstrapping method. This approach has been extended, to overcome some of the limitations of the method. Empirical evidence on the extended method will be considered in Section 13.7. In Section 13.6, we discuss the limitations that motivated the extensions and modifications of simple bootstrapping.

13.6 Limitations of Simple Bootstrapping

As we noted earlier, the simple bootstrapping method rests upon assumptions of demand being i.i.d. In this section, we discuss the need to allow for demand being autocorrelated and the future possibility of demand taking values not previously observed.

13.6.1 Autocorrelated Demand

In the example of simple bootstrapping in Section 13.5, each observation was resampled without any reference to previous resamplings. Returning to the analogy of the container of numbered balls, each drawing was independent of previous drawings. In the context of intermittent demand for products, this assumption may not always be correct. For example, short demand intervals may be followed by further short demand intervals (positive interval autocorrelation), high demand sizes may be followed by low demand sizes (negative size autocorrelation), or long demand intervals may be followed by low demand sizes (negative cross-correlation between demand intervals and sizes). This is all hypothetical. Is there any empirical evidence for such autocorrelations and cross-correlations?

Willemain et al. (1994) examined the demand patterns of 54 products, all intermittent, drawn from the electrical equipment, jet engine tools, veterinary health, and consumer food sectors. They found: (i) all interval autocorrelations for the consumer food items were positive; (ii) all size autocorrelations for the veterinary health products were negative; and (iii) all cross-correlations for electrical equipment were negative. However, they also noted that it can be difficult to estimate autocorrelations and cross-correlations, owing to the sparseness of intermittent demand data. Only two correlations in their datasets reached statistical significance at the 5% level.

Eaves (2002) conducted more extensive research on consumable parts for the RAF. He analysed over 12 000 RAF line items and decomposed the series into sizes and intervals. He concluded that up to a quarter of items are significantly autocorrelated and/or cross-correlated (at the 5% level). Nikolopoulos et al. (2011) examined autocorrelation of 5000 intermittent demand items from the RAF. The researchers did not decompose the series into sizes and intervals; instead, they analysed the demand series themselves. They found little correlation between the series and the same series lagged by one period (demand autocorrelation of lag one).

Altay et al. (2012) analysed the demand patterns of more than 4500 aircraft service parts from the US Defense Logistics Agency. They found that about 22% of items had significantly autocorrelated demand intervals, 27% had significantly autocorrelated demand sizes, and 35% had statistically significant cross-correlations (at the 5% level). This is the strongest evidence, to date, of autocorrelations and cross-correlations in intermittent demand data.

Overall, the evidence for violation of the independent demand assumption is mixed. One consistent finding is that the majority of intermittent series show little autocorrelation or cross-correlation and, for such items, the independence assumption may be maintained. However, there is growing evidence that this assumption may not be correct for a sizeable minority of intermittent series. This means that we may need to consider alternative approaches to the simple bootstrap for such series. These will be discussed in Section 13.7.

13.6.2 Previously Unobserved Demand Values

Even if the underlying distribution remains unchanged, there may be values that are not incompatible with the current distribution of demand but have not yet been observed. Using a simple bootstrapping procedure will mean that these values will not be generated, as they are not part of the historical data being resampled. Suppose we had just the last ten observations from the example in Table 13.2 (Periods 15–24), as shown in Table 13.5.

If only this data were available, then resampling for Periods 25, 26, and 27 would never generate demands of 20 for any of these individual periods. However, we know that a demand of 20 is feasible as it has been observed previously (in Period 12, see Table 13.2). Furthermore, although a period with a demand value of 6 has never been observed throughout the whole history (Periods 1–24), it would not be unreasonable to suppose that

Table 13.5 Most recent 10 observations from Table 13.2.

Period	15	16	17	18	19	20	21	22	23	24
Demand	5	0	10	2	0	2	0	1	0	1

this value could be observed in the future, especially since values of 1 and 5 have been observed. This is an inherent weakness of simple bootstrapping, although adaptations are available to address it. These will be reviewed in Section 13.7.

13.6.3 Summary

For many SKUs, the assumption of i.i.d. demand is reasonable. However, there is growing empirical evidence that, for a significant minority of SKUs, this assumption is not correct. It would be helpful to have adaptations of simple bootstrapping that address some of the limitations of assuming i.i.d. demand. Similarly, extensions may be needed to allow the generation of values not previously observed to enrich the bootstrapped samples.

13.7 Extensions to Simple Bootstrapping

In this section, we discuss two extensions to simple bootstrapping, suggested by Willemain et al. (2004). The first, Markov chains, addresses potential dependence between demand occurrences. The second, 'jittering', addresses the possibility of observing demand values in the future that have not been observed in the past.

13.7.1 Discrete-time Markov Chains

A discrete-time Markov chain is a system that undergoes transitions from one state to another over discrete (whole number) periods of time. For example, suppose that each day is labelled as 'Dry' or 'Rainy', abbreviated as D and R, and we have observed the following sequence of days: D, D, R, D, R, R, R, D, D, R, D, D, D, D, R, R, R, R, R, D, R, D, D, R. Inspection of this time series reveals that there appear to have been more 'streaks' of dry days (and also of rainy days) than would be expected if these states were not correlated over time. In other words, there appears to have been a tendency for a dry day to be followed by another dry day and, similarly, for a rainy day to be followed by another rainy day.

Now suppose that we wish to record a day with a demand occurrence as '1' and a day without a demand occurrence as '0', and we have the following sequences of actual demands over 28 days: 1, 5, 1, 2, 0, 0, 0, 1, 2, 0, 1, 5, 1, 1, 0, 1, 0, 0, 0, 3, 2, 0, 0, 1, 6, 0, 0, 0. This can be transformed to a sequence of demand occurrences by replacing any non-zero demand value by 1, to indicate that demand has occurred in that period: 1, 1, 1, 1, 0, 0, 0, 1, 1, 0, 1, 1, 1, 1, 0, 1, 0, 0, 0, 1, 1, 0, 0, 1, 1, 0, 0, 0.

We can calculate four conditional probabilities, which show the chance of demand (or no demand) today, given that there was demand (or no demand) yesterday. The four conditional probabilities that are relevant in this case are shown in Table 13.6.

Table 13.6 Conditional probabilities of demand occurrence.

	Demand today	No demand today
Demand yesterday	9/15 = 0.600	6/15 = 0.400
No demand yesterday	5/12 = 0.417	7/12 = 0.583

In each case, the calculations are based on counts. Of the 15 days with demands, there were 9 occasions when the next day also saw a demand, and 6 when not. Of the 13 days with no demands, we must discount the last observation, as we do not know what happened on the next day. Of the remaining 12 days, 5 were followed by a day with a demand, and 7 were not.

13.7.2 Extension to Simple Bootstrapping Using Markov Chains

Recognising that demand occurrence may show dependence on the previous demand occurrence, Willemain et al. (2004) proposed that this pattern could be incorporated into the bootstrapping method, with resampling taking place in two stages:

- *Stage 1*: Resample the occurrence (or non-occurrence) of demand, taking into account the occurrence (or non-occurrence) of demand in the previous period.
- *Stage 2*: Resample the size of demand if Stage 1 yields demand occurrence.

The bootstrapping approach with a Markov chain model of demand occurrence proceeds as follows for Stage 1:

1. Generate a random number from a uniform distribution between 0 and 1.
2. Check the most recent period of the demand history to see if there was a demand or not.
3. If there was a demand, then compare the random number to the probability of demand today given that there was demand yesterday. If the random number is lower, record a value of 1 for demand occurrence; else, if it is higher, record a value of 0.
4. If there was not a demand, then compare the random number to the probability of demand today given that there was no demand yesterday. If the random number is lower, record a value of 1 for demand occurrence; else, if it is higher, record a value of 0.

In this process, we no longer randomly sample one of the previous periods. Instead, we take account of the conditional probabilities when simulating the occurrence (or non-occurrence) of demand.

Stage 2 is more straightforward. Resampling occurs only if a demand occurrence has been generated by Stage 1. All that is required is to make a random selection from those previous periods in which demand occurred. Both stages are completed for each period in the forecast horizon. This is then replicated many times.

The whole procedure is illustrated in Table 13.7, for a horizon of two periods, and showing just four replications ('reps'), with conditional probabilities as calculated in Table 13.6, and recalling that there was no demand in the final period (Period 28).

For the first resampling, the conditional probability of demand occurrence in Period 29 is 0.417, because there was no demand in Period 28. As the random number (Rand = 0.410)

Table 13.7 Simple bootstrapping with Markov chain extension..

| | Demand occurrence | | | | Demand size | | | | |
| | Period 29 | | Period 30 | | Period 29 | | Period 30 | | |
Rep	Rand	Occurs	Rand	Occurs	Sample	Size	Sample	Size	Total
1	0.410	1	0.556	1	2	5	14	1	6
2	0.342	1	0.798	0	21	2			2
3	0.936	0	0.369	1			20	3	3
4	0.587	0	0.921	0					0

is in the range from 0 to 0.417, this corresponds to a demand occurrence, indicated by a '1' in the 'Occurs' column. For Period 30, the conditional probability of demand occurrence is 0.600 because we have just simulated a demand occurrence in Period 29. As the next random number (Rand = 0.556) is in the range from 0 to 0.600, this again corresponds to a demand occurrence. The simulation of demand occurrences in the second, third, and fourth replications is conducted in exactly the same way.

The generation of demand sizes occurs only when there has been a simulated demand occurrence. The sizes are generated as in simple bootstrapping, except that the random selections are restricted to previous periods with non-zero demands (there were 15 such periods in this example). The resampled periods are shown in the 'Sample' columns and the resampled demand sizes are shown in bold type in the 'Size' columns, with the total of the demand sizes over Periods 29 and 30 shown in bold in the 'Total' column.

This whole process is repeated many times (say 10 000). We would then have 10 000 total demand values, which may be put into order to allow estimation of the CDF and relevant percentiles, as in simple bootstrapping.

Hua et al. (2007) developed an approach to extend the modelling of intermittent demand occurrence to include the effect of explanatory variables such as equipment overhaul or plant overhaul. For series with strongly autocorrelated demand occurrences, they used a similar approach to Willemain et al. (2004), modelling demand occurrence as a Markov chain, without reference to explanatory variables. For other demand series, they used algorithms taking explanatory variables into account to generate bootstrapped demand occurrences. They analysed 40 kinds of spare parts from a petrochemical enterprise in China, measuring accuracy in terms of the absolute percentage error of lead time demand (LTD) forecasts (not defined when LTD = 0). They also measured the accuracy of demand occurrence predictions over lead time using an 'Error Ratio of occurrences of Non-zero demand Judgements' (ERNJ), defined as follows:

$$\text{ERNJ} = \frac{1}{L}\sum_{h=1}^{L}|\tilde{y}_{t+h} - y_{t+h}| \tag{13.6}$$

where L is the lead time, y_{t+h} is one if there is a demand occurrence, and zero if not; similarly, $\tilde{y}_{t+h}$ is one if there is a bootstrapped demand occurrence, and zero if not. The ERNJ metric is calculated for each bootstrap replication and averaged to give an overall measure.

Hua et al. (2007) found promising improvements in forecasting accuracy by using their approach instead of the Markov bootstrapping method (Willemain et al. 2004). They noted, however, that their method depends on the number of non-zero demands in the historical data set not being too small.

13.7.3 Jittering

As previously noted, one of the limitations of the simple bootstrapping method is that plausible values, which have not yet been observed, cannot be resampled and will not appear in the bootstrapped sample.

Willemain et al. (2004) proposed a modification to the simple bootstrap (or to the Markov chain extension) called 'jittering'. The modification works as follows:

1. Resample a (positive) demand value, X, using the simple bootstrap method (or Markov chain extension).
2. Generate a standard normally distributed random variable, Z, with mean 0 and variance equal to 1. (Z can be generated using a standard function in most programming languages.)
3. Calculate a jittered value, J, using the formula: $J = 1 + \text{INT}(X + Z\sqrt{X})$, where the INT function rounds a decimal number down to a whole number (e.g. INT(5.7) = 5).
4. If this value is negative, leave the original value, X, unaltered; otherwise, replace X by the jittered value, J.

The second and third steps of this approach are designed to shift the original resampled value, X, by a randomly generated quantity, $Z\sqrt{X}$. Completion of these steps may generate a value that has not previously been observed, thus addressing the issue highlighted earlier in this chapter. The quantity Z may be negative and so it is possible that $Z\sqrt{X}$ may reduce the original value, X, to such an extent that it becomes negative. Now, it does not make sense to have a negative demand (assuming we are not taking into account returned goods). Hence, the final step is included to prevent such a negative value being returned. Willemain et al. (2004) noted that there are some circumstances in which jittering should not be used. They gave the example of a beer that is sold only in packages of 6, 12, or 24 cans, in which case every total demand value should be divisible by 6. In this case, the jittering operation may be omitted.

The simple bootstrapping approach, with Markov chain and jittering extensions, form the method proposed by the three authors, Willemain, Smart, and Schwarz (Willemain et al. 2004), and is sometimes called the WSS method. This is part of the algorithm implemented by Smart Software, as described in the US Patent (Willemain and Smart 2001).

The Viswanathan and Zhou (VZ) method can also be adapted to include a jittering procedure. Rego and Mesquita (2015) suggested that the VZ method could be modified in two respects. Firstly, they adopted the modification of Teunter and Duncan (2009), insisting that the first resample be drawn from those periods with positive demand (see also Hasni et al. 2019). Secondly, whenever a positive demand is drawn, it is subject to a jittering procedure.

13.7.4 Limitations of Jittering

The process of jittering introduces a bias into the forecast of demand sizes. It does so for two distinct reasons, as explained below.

The formula $J = 1 + \text{INT}(X + Z\sqrt{X})$ has an expected (mean) value of $\mathbb{E}(J) = \mathbb{E}(X) + 0.5$. This arises because the process of taking only the integer part of $X + Z\sqrt{X}$ reduces it by an amount between 0 and 1. Assuming that this reduction is uniformly distributed between 0 and 1 gives an average reduction of 0.5. After adding the value of 1 to $\text{INT}(X + Z\sqrt{X})$, as required by the jittering formula for J, we end up with an average increase of 0.5. Therefore, the formula introduces an upward bias of 0.5. To overcome this problem, Rego and Mesquita (2015) proposed taking the integer part of $0.5 + X + Z\sqrt{X}$. This simple adaptation removes the bias in the original formula.

The final jittering step includes retention of the original (un-jittered) values if jittering would generate a negative demand value. We are now effectively sampling from a truncated normal distribution of Z, with highly negative values of Z (which would generate negative values of J) being replaced by zero. This introduces a second bias because the mean of the Z values is no longer zero, but a value that is greater than zero. This bias is reduced, but not eliminated, if the original demand value is not retained, but replaced by 1, as suggested by Rego and Mesquita (2015).

13.7.5 Further Developments

Further enhancements of the bootstrapping approach have since been implemented, based on grouping items into clusters (Willemain and Hartunian 2013). This introduces the possibility of revising downwards the probability of a non-zero demand observation if an SKU is associated with a cluster showing a decline in its total demand. It addresses the basic concern, discussed earlier in the chapter, of assuming that the demand distribution is stationary and unchanging over time. The cluster-based processing method has some attractive features but it is difficult to judge its effectiveness until empirical evaluations have been published in peer-reviewed outlets.

13.7.6 Empirical Evidence on Bootstrapping Methods

Smith and Babai (2011) provided some historical background to the development of the WSS method and its implementation in Smart Software. They noted that a presentation on the performance of the method was delivered by Charles Smart, the CEO of Smart-Corp, at the 2002 conference of the American Production and Inventory Control Society (Smart 2002). This reported financial benefits for an aircraft maintenance organisation, which identified potential inventory-holding cost savings of $3 million per year. It also reported that the aftermarket business unit of NSK Corporation increased on-time delivery service levels to 98% and saved $1 million, with a further $3 million of savings projected. (Further information on the NSK case had been provided by Smart and Willemain 2000.)

A comparison of the WSS and Croston methods was conducted by Willemain et al. (2004) using demand data from nine different companies in a variety of sectors: aviation, marine, computing, microwave communications, electronics, hardware, industrial refrigeration, and heavy equipment. In all, over 28 000 SKUs were used in the investigation, with demand histories that ranged from 24 to 60 months. The evaluation was made using fixed lead times for all SKUs, set at one, three, and six months. For Croston's method, the classic formula was used to forecast the mean demand per period, with a common smoothing parameter for demand sizes and demand intervals, and forecasts initialised using the time to the first demand and the size of the first demand. The variance of demand per period was estimated using the standard sample variance formula, with no exponential smoothing. The mean and variance estimates were used as inputs to a predicted normal distribution of demand over lead time.

Willemain et al. (2004) compared the LTD distributions predicted by the Croston and WSS methods with the LTDs that transpired, using the probability integral transformation technique (see Chapter 9). They found that the WSS method produced LTD distributions that were better predictors than Croston's method coupled with the normal distribution. Although the accuracy of the WSS method decreased with lead time, it remained more accurate than Croston. Gardner and Koehler (2005) challenged the findings of Willemain et al. (2004) because of the way Croston was implemented, especially: (i) the assumption of normally distributed demand, (ii) lack of recognition of the bias of Croston's method, and (iii) use of the sample variance formula when more appropriate alternatives are available. It should also be noted that the comparison was not extended to inventory holding or service level implications.

Porras and Dekker (2008) analysed the effectiveness of the WSS method from an inventory perspective. They examined the total inventory cost savings using the WSS method for two demand classes, using the same classes and experimental setup described earlier in the chapter. Two analyses were conducted. The ex-post analysis used all of the available data for fitting, whereas the ex-ante analysis withheld some data from fitting. The ex-ante analysis is more appropriate, both scientifically and practically because, as the authors acknowledged, in reality the future demands are unknown. In both ex-ante and ex-post analyses, the OB method achieved greater inventory cost savings than the WSS method, with both methods realising fill rates of 90% or higher.

Rego and Mesquita (2015) analysed 10 032 SKUs from a Brazilian automotive manufacturer, with six years of demand history. They compared the simple moving average and the Syntetos–Boylan approximation (linked to normal, gamma, and negative binomial distributions) with the adapted VZ bootstrapping method, including the modification of Teunter and Duncan (2009) and a jittering procedure. When jittering, they took the integer part of $0.5 + X + Z\sqrt{X}$ (where X is the original demand and Z is a standard normal variable), and replaced any negatively generated values by 1. These forecasting methods were applied using an (s, NQ) inventory policy, with inventory control parameters revised either monthly or semi-annually, and target fill rates of 80%, 90%, 95%, and 99%. Lead times were not taken as fixed but treated as probabilistic, based on a triangular distribution (see Chapter 4) governed by minimum, most probable, and maximum lead times. The forecasting methods were evaluated using a trade-off between total inventory costs and realised fill rates. This evaluation was undertaken using the four-quadrant approach (Syntetos et al. 2005, discussed in Chapter 11). The results showed a clear preference, over all target fill rates, for the modified VZ bootstrap for lumpy demand items, and for the SBA method (coupled with a gamma distribution) for erratic demand items. The results were less clear cut for the smooth and intermittent demand categories. An additional finding of this study was that the inventory control parameters should be revised monthly for the SBA method but semi-annually for the modified VZ bootstrap.

Syntetos et al. (2015a) compared the performance of the WSS method with parametric methods. The authors analysed more than 7000 demand series from two datasets: one of 52 weeks of demand from the US jewellery industry (4076 SKUs, lead time of one week), and the other of 48 months of demand from the Japanese electronics sector (3055 SKUs, lead time of three months). In addition to Croston's method, the SBA method was also used, the variance estimate being based on smoothed mean square errors, and the distribution of demand being taken to be negative binomial, thus addressing some of the concerns of Gardner and Koehler (2005), discussed earlier. A periodic review (R, S) inventory system was used, with $R = 1$. The smoothing parameter for SBA was chosen to minimise mean square error, restricting the range to be from 0.05 to 0.30. Estimates of mean square error were updated using exponential smoothing. The inventory simulations revealed some modest advantages for the WSS method for the jewellery data, with higher CSLs being achieved for the same level of inventory investment. However, this finding was reversed for the electronics data, which was noisier than the jewellery data.

Hasni et al. (2019) were the first to undertake an empirical comparison of SBA (linked to the negative binomial distribution) and both the WSS and VZ bootstrapping methods. The set-up of their experiment is summarised in Section 13.5.3. When the same initial inventory level was used for all SKUs, SBA yielded the lowest total inventory cost, taking into account both inventory holding and backordering costs. The second lowest cost was achieved by the WSS method. When different initial inventory levels were used for the SKUs, then SBA still gave the lowest cost, with the VZ method taking second place. As the penalty for backordering costs increased, the advantage of SBA over WSS and VZ reduced, but it remained the dominant method.

13.7.7 Summary

The WSS method is an advance on the simple bootstrapping method. The jittering formula has some limitations, but these can be addressed quite straightforwardly. The Markov chain modelling approach moves away from i.i.d. demand assumptions, by addressing a particular form of autocorrelation of demand intervals. The method is strong with respect to its ability to deal with non-standard demand patterns. It is more computationally demanding than parametric methods. However, this may be justifiable if it can afford greater accuracy and improved inventory performance. The empirical evidence on this matter is somewhat mixed, with some studies showing greater inventory cost savings than parametric methods, and some showing the reverse.

13.8 Chapter Summary

In this chapter, we have seen that non-parametric methods offer a viable alternative to parametric methods. The non-parametric approach is particularly useful when the demand is highly 'lumpy' and not easily characterised by a standard distribution.

Some limitations of simple bootstrapping methods have been addressed by modifications that allow the assumption of independent demand occurrences to be dropped and permit observations to be generated that have not been observed previously. The WSS method due to Willemain et al. (2004) includes these adaptations and is available in commercial software. The adoption of bootstrapping methods in forecasting and inventory management software has not been widespread, however.

Bootstrapping methods do rely on the assumption that the distribution, although unknown, has not varied over time. Demand levels may be just about to shift upwards or downwards and, if this happens during the protection interval, then the total demand distribution forecast may become inaccurate. A similar issue arises if demand levels have shifted during the period for which historical values are being used for resampling (either upwards or downwards). This problem is less pronounced for parametric methods where the parameters are re-forecasted as new data becomes available. We have already covered a number of parametric methods linked to exponential smoothing. In Chapter 14, some alternative parametric approaches are discussed.

Technical Notes

Note 13.1 Calculation of the Theta Function

The calculation is illustrated by an example. Suppose that the distribution of demand per period is as follows: $\mathbb{P}(0) = 0.7$, $\mathbb{P}(1) = 0.2$, $\mathbb{P}(2) = 0.1$. Then, over a two-period horizon ($m = 2$), for $y = 2$, the theta function for an overlap of one observation ($\Theta_1(2)$) is calculated as shown in Table 13.8.

In Table 13.8, the first two columns show the different combinations of the first two observations that will yield a total demand not exceeding two for the first block. The probabilities in the third column are found by multiplying the probabilities of the demands in the first two columns, assuming i.i.d. demand.

The second observation of the first block is taken to overlap with the first observation of the second block. For example, in the second row, we consider the possibility of a zero demand followed by a demand for one unit. Then, in the second block, the first demand is fixed as one unit, and the second demand cannot exceed one unit to ensure that the total demand in the block does not exceed two units ($y = 2$). Therefore, the second demand must be either 0 (probability of 0.7) or 1 (probability of 0.2), giving a total probability of 0.9, as shown in the fifth column of the second row of Table 13.8. The probabilities in the final column are calculated as the products of the probabilities in the third and fifth columns. The theta function, with an overlap of one period, and evaluated at $y = 2$, is the sum of the values in the final column ($\Theta_1(2) = 0.911$).

As noted earlier in this chapter, the theta function is affected by the homogeneity of the data. As a series becomes more intermittent, it also becomes more homogeneous because of the preponderance of zeroes. For example, suppose we change the distribution of demand to: $\mathbb{P}(0) = 0.8$, $\mathbb{P}(1) = 0.1$, $\mathbb{P}(2) = 0.1$. This is more intermittent than the previous example, with an 80% chance of a zero observation instead of 70%. Recalculating the theta function gives a value of 0.945, somewhat higher than the value of 0.911 shown in Table 13.8.

Table 13.8 Theta function calculation ($m = 2$, $y = 2$), overlap of one period.

Demand period 1 (block 1)	Demand period 2 (blocks 1 and 2)	Probability demands periods 1 and 2	Max. demand period 3 (block 2)	Cumulative probability period 3	Product of prob and cum prob
0	0	0.49	2	1.0	0.490
0	1	0.14	1	0.9	0.126
0	2	0.07	0	0.7	0.049
1	0	0.14	2	1.0	0.140
1	1	0.04	1	0.9	0.036
2	0	0.07	2	1.0	0.070
				$\Theta_1(2)$	0.911

Note 13.2 General Expression for the Variance of the OB Estimate

The expression for the variance of the CDF estimate using OB becomes more complicated for larger block-lengths. This complexity arises because of the inter-independence between some of the blocks. The variance expression is given in Eq. (13.7) (Boylan and Babai 2016), assuming that the number of blocks (k) is at least as great as the block-length (m).

$$\text{Var}(\hat{F}_m^{OB}(y)) = \frac{F_m(y)}{k} + \left(\frac{(k-m)(k-m+1)}{k^2} - 1 \right) F_m(y)^2$$
$$+ \frac{1}{k^2} \sum_{S=1}^{m-1} 2(k - m + S)\Theta_S(y) \tag{13.7}$$

where $\Theta_S(y)$ is given by Eq. (13.8).

$$\Theta_S(y) = \sum_{y_1=0}^{y} \cdots \sum_{y_m=0}^{y-y_1-\cdots-y_{m-1}} \sum_{y_{m+1}=0}^{y-y_{m-S+1}-\cdots-y_m} \cdots \sum_{y_{2m-S}=0}^{y-y_{m-S+1}-\cdots-y_{2m-S-1}} \prod_{j=1}^{2m-S} \mathbb{P}(y_j) \tag{13.8}$$

The theta function, $\Theta_S(y)$, in Eq. (13.8) represents the chance that two partially overlapping blocks, with S periods overlapping, both contain totals that do not exceed the value y.

Note 13.3 General Condition for OB Outperformance

The general condition for the OB approach to have a lower variance of the estimate of the CDF, for a given value of y, than the NOB approach, for block-length m, and length of history n (n a multiple of m) is given by (13.9).

$$\sum_{S=1}^{m-1} \frac{2(n-2m+S+1)}{(n-m+1)^2} \Theta_S(y) < \left(\frac{m}{n} - \frac{1}{n-m+1} \right) F_m(y)$$
$$+ \left(1 - \frac{m}{n} - \frac{(n-2m+1)(n-2m+2)}{(n-m+1)^2} \right) F_m(y)^2 \tag{13.9}$$

This result is stated and proved as Proposition 2 by Boylan and Babai (2016). The inequality in (13.5) is a special case of this general inequality, when the block-length is given by $m = 2$.

14

Model-based Methods

14.1 Introduction

In Chapter 13, we saw how simple bootstrapping can be adapted to take into account dependence between demand occurrences by using a Markov chain approach. This can be further augmented by 'jittering', to allow for the generation of demand values not previously observed.

The advantage of bootstrapping is that there is no requirement to assume that demand conforms to any of the standard distributions. However, if the demand does conform in this way, for example to the Poisson distribution, then parametric methods may be preferred. No jittering is required because these methods allow estimation of cumulative distribution functions (CDFs) across the entire range of values, including values higher than those previously observed.

So far, we have not examined how parametric methods should be used when there is correlation between successive observations, known as autocorrelation. As noted in Chapter 13, there is empirical evidence of autocorrelation of demand for some intermittent series, and so this topic is worthy of further attention.

In this chapter, we start with a general discussion on models and methods, with a particular focus on models for faster-moving demand. This is followed by five sections on integer autoregressive moving average (INARMA) models, the most well-developed models for low-volume and intermittent series. After defining the models, we move on to parameter estimation and model identification. Then, we focus on forecasting using INARMA models. A discussion of an alternative approach follows, known as state space modelling, and the chapter closes with a summary of progress that has been made in the development of model-based methods for intermittence.

14.2 Models and Methods

Firstly, we should distinguish between models and methods. Often, these terms are used interchangeably in the forecasting literature, but a clear distinction will be helpful for our discussion.

Intermittent Demand Forecasting: Context, Methods and Applications, First Edition.
John E. Boylan and Aris A. Syntetos.
© 2021 John Wiley & Sons Ltd. Published 2021 by John Wiley & Sons Ltd.
Companion Website: www.wiley.com/go/boylansyntetos/intermittentdemandforecasting

In this chapter, a 'model' will be taken to be a mathematical representation of a data generating process (DGP), with a complete specification of distributions and parameters. Although a DGP may not be able to represent all aspects of a real demand process, it should be able to capture its key features to enable better forecasting and stock control. This is in accordance with the aphorism 'All models are wrong, but some are useful', generally attributed to George Box, who was one of the world's leading forecasting experts.

A forecasting 'method' is taken to be a numerical procedure that generates forecasts of demand, based on past and present data. It may generate forecasts of mean demand or of the whole demand distribution.

Sometimes, models and methods are proposed, but the method does not produce optimal forecasts with respect to a forecast error measure (usually mean square error). For example, Croston's method (Sections 6.3–6.5) is not optimal for Croston's model (Section 6.2), although the method may work well in practice. If a method does generate optimal forecasts for a particular model, then it is said to be a 'model-based method'.

The development of model-based methods for fast-moving demand happened before any such developments for intermittent demand. Some of the concepts that are central to the former have been adapted for the latter. Therefore, it is valuable to review fast demand first, starting with single exponential smoothing (SES), before progressing to intermittent demand forecasting.

14.2.1 A Simple Model for Single Exponential Smoothing

Is SES a model-based method? The originator of this method, Robert G. Brown, posited a demand model with no trend, and for which 'all variable components are treated as noise with a zero mean' (Brown 1956, p. 3). This may be expressed in model form as a demand at time t (d_t) being composed of a constant mean (μ), unchanging through time, and a random noise term (ϵ_t), which fluctuates through time, following a normal distribution with mean zero (Brown 1963), as shown in Eq. (14.1).

$$d_t = \mu + \epsilon_t \tag{14.1}$$

To give higher weights to more recent errors and lower weights to older errors, Brown (1963) suggested that we may use a weighted (or 'discounted') least squares criterion. This is based on the idea that future accuracy is best reflected by the most recent accuracy: although all past errors are relevant, it has been argued that the most recent ones should be given the greatest weight. For a demand history of t observations, $d_1, \dots, d_t$, this would be done by identifying the estimator $\hat{\mu}_{t+1}$ of mean demand in the next period, which minimises the weighted sum of squares (WSS) of the deviations between the observations and the estimated mean, as given by Eq. (14.2).

$$\text{WSS} = \sum_{i=0}^{t-1} w^i (d_{t-i} - \hat{\mu}_{t+1})^2 \tag{14.2}$$

where w is the weighting factor. If $0 < w < 1$, then the weights decline as the data gets older. If $w = 1$, then all weights are equal (known as 'ordinary least squares'). The weighted least squares forecast of mean demand at time $t + 1$, made at the end of time t, is shown in Eq. (14.3).

$$\widehat{\mu}_{t+1} = \frac{1-w}{1-w^t} \sum_{i=0}^{t-1} w^i d_{t-i} \tag{14.3}$$

where $0 < w < 1$. The weighted least squares estimate approaches a limit as the length of history increases, as shown in Eq. (14.4).

$$\widehat{\mu}_{t+1} = (1-w) \sum_{i=0}^{\infty} w^i d_{t-i} \tag{14.4}$$

This is the same as the exponential smoothing formula given in Eq. (6.6), with the smoothing constant (α) linked to the weighting factor (w) by the equation $\alpha = 1 - w$.

Thus, it would appear that SES is a model-based method if we take Eq. (14.1) as the demand model and apply a weighted least squares criterion. Unfortunately, as we shall see in Section 14.2.2, there is a flaw in this approach to the derivation of SES.

14.2.2 Critique of Weighted Least Squares

Brown's weighted least squares approach was criticised by Chatfield et al. (2001). They pointed out that there is an inconsistency between the demand model and the weighed least squares criterion. Although lower weights on older errors seem intuitively reasonable, the intuition rests on the assumption of a mean value that changes over time. If the underlying mean is truly constant, as in Eq. (14.1), then ordinary least squares should be used, giving equal weights to all errors, rather than weighted least squares. This is because all squared deviations between observations and the estimated mean should be considered as equally important, regardless of the age of the data, if the underlying mean is unchanging.

Although SES is not the optimal method for a constant mean demand model, it will provide a forecast that is close to optimal if a low smoothing value is employed. Notwithstanding this property, the weighted least squares approach, when applied to the constant mean model, does not give a fully satisfactory basis for SES. SES does have a sound model basis for non-intermittent series in the form of an ARIMA(0,1,1) model (Box and Jenkins 1962), explained in Section 14.2.4.

The categorisation scheme proposed by Syntetos, Boylan, and Croston (2005) (see Chapter 11) is also based on a model of constant mean demand sizes and intervals. The comparison of mean square errors from SES and Croston (or SBA) is based on this assumption. Like SES, neither Croston nor SBA is optimal for constant means. Nevertheless, the categorisation rules were found to be robust when applied to real data, which may have included series for which the means were non-constant over time (Boylan et al. 2008).

14.2.3 ARIMA Models

ARIMA is an acronym for 'Auto-Regressive Integrated Moving Averages'. There are three components of ARIMA models:

1. *Auto-regressive (AR) component*, indicating the dependence of current observations on previous observations. For example, an AR(1) model is of the form $d_t = \rho_1 d_{t-1} + \epsilon_t$, and an AR(2) model is of the form $d_t = \rho_1 d_{t-1} + \rho_2 d_{t-2} + \epsilon_t$. The autoregressive (AR)

parameters (ρ_1, ρ_2) show how much the conditional expectation of demand increases if one of the lagged demand variables increases by one unit, with the other lagged variable remaining unchanged.

2. *Integrated (I) component*, indicating the degree of differencing between observations. This can be useful in modelling shifts in the mean demand level or systematic trends in demand. An I(1) model is of the form $d_t = d_{t-1} + \epsilon_t$ (also known as a random walk model), and an I(2) model is of the form $d_t - d_{t-1} = d_{t-1} - d_{t-2} + \epsilon_t$.

3. *Moving average (MA) component*, indicating the dependence of current observations on previous random noise terms (also known as 'innovation terms'). These terms can be used to represent random shocks to demand whose effect is weakened over time. An MA(1) model is of the form $d_t = \epsilon_t + \theta_1 \epsilon_{t-1}$, and an MA(2) model is of the form $d_t = \epsilon_t + \theta_1 \epsilon_{t-1} + \theta_2 \epsilon_{t-2}$. The moving average (MA) parameters (θ_1, θ_2) have a similar interpretation to the AR parameters, except that increases in the conditional expectation of demand are with respect to increases in lagged innovation terms.

Models without an 'integrated' (I) component are known as 'auto-regressive moving average' (ARMA) models. There are restrictions on the values that may be taken by the AR and MA parameters, known as stationarity and invertibility conditions. For example, in an AR(1) model, the AR parameter must be in the range $-1 < \rho < 1$, and in an MA(1) model, the MA parameter must be in the range $-1 < \theta < 1$. More complex restrictions apply for higher order models (see, for example, Hamilton 1994, Chapter 3).

14.2.4 The ARIMA(0,1,1) Model and SES

The ARIMA(0,1,1) model is of the form given in Eq. (14.5).

$$d_t = d_{t-1} + \epsilon_t + \theta_1 \epsilon_{t-1} \tag{14.5}$$

In ARIMA models, the noise term, ϵ_t, is assumed to be independent and identically distributed (i.i.d.), with a normal distribution of mean zero and constant variance.

The minimum mean square error (MMSE) forecast is equal to the conditional expectation (Box et al. 2015). Forecasting one step ahead, the conditional expectation of demand at time $t + 1$ takes into account all the information available in the model up to the end of time t. For an ARIMA(0,1,1) model, this includes d_t and $\theta_1 \epsilon_t$, but not ϵ_{t+1}, which is unknown at the end of time t. As it has a zero mean, and is independent of other model elements, the best estimate of ϵ_{t+1} is zero.

This yields a conditional expectation, and MMSE forecast, as given by Eq. (14.6).

$$\hat{d}_{t+1} = d_t + \theta_1 \epsilon_t \tag{14.6}$$

The first term on the right-hand side, d_t, is known at the end of time t and can be used directly in the calculation of the one-step-ahead forecast for time $t + 1$. The random noise term, ϵ_t, is unknown but it may be estimated by the forecast error, $d_t - \hat{d}_t$. So, for an unknown noise term but a known θ_1 parameter, the forecast may be calculated using Eq. (14.7).

$$\hat{d}_{t+1} = d_t + \theta_1 (d_t - \hat{d}_t) = \alpha d_t + (1 - \alpha)\hat{d}_t \tag{14.7}$$

where $\alpha = 1 + \theta_1$. This is the familiar form of SES. Therefore, SES can be said to be a model-based method, as it is the MMSE forecasting method for an ARIMA(0,1,1) demand model.

ARIMA models can capture a wide range of dependencies between current and previous observations, including trend (ARIMA(0,2,2)), damped trend (ARIMA(1,1,2)) and seasonal ARIMA models, although these extensions have not been adapted for intermittent demand. Interested readers may refer to Ord et al. (2017) for a discussion of these models.

14.2.5 Summary

Single exponential smoothing has sometimes been described as an 'ad hoc' method. The discussion in this section shows that this description is wrong. Although Brown's original model formulation and weighted least squares criterion are inconsistent, it has been shown that SES is underpinned by an ARIMA(0,1,1) model, for which SES is the MMSE forecasting method. As we shall see later, SES is also underpinned by state space models.

ARIMA models give the opportunity to specify forecasting methods that are rigorous and well grounded in statistical theory. Similar methods, developed for INARMA models, are suited to intermittent demand. These models will form the principal subject of discussion in the following sections of this chapter.

14.3 Integer Autoregressive Moving Average (INARMA) Models

ARIMA models were designed for higher volume data, where the innovation terms can be assumed to follow a normal distribution. It may be asked if ARIMA and ARMA models can be extended to time series with some zero observations, for which the normality assumption is not so realistic. To extend ARIMA models, there has been some research on Poisson difference models, which include first-order differencing (see, for example, Alzaid and Omair 2014). Of course, these models allow for negative values. For modelling non-negative intermittent demand, it is more natural to look for an integer equivalent to ARMA models, with no integrating component.

An ARMA(1,1) model is of the form shown in Eq. (14.8).

$$d_t = \rho d_{t-1} + \epsilon_t + \theta \epsilon_{t-1} \tag{14.8}$$

In Eq. (14.8), the random noise terms, denoted by ϵ_t, are assumed to be i.i.d., arising from a normal distribution with zero mean and constant variance.

In practical applications, demand must be non-negative (ignoring returns) and typically takes whole number values. This applies to both fast-moving and slow-moving products, including those with intermittent demand. For fast-moving demand, the normal distribution will generally yield a very low probability of negative demand, and estimates of demand percentiles can be rounded without losing much precision (e.g. rounding up 149.6 to 150). These issues are more serious for slow-moving and intermittent demand products, where the normal can give a much higher chance of negative values and rounding a percentile of 1.496 down to one or up to two can have significant inventory service implications. Therefore, to adapt ARMA models for these types of products, two issues must be addressed:

1. The normal distribution should not be used, to avoid the possibility of negative values.
2. Multiplication by scalar quantities (ρ and θ) between -1 and $+1$ should not occur. If this approach were used, there would be a possibility of negative or fractional values, which is contrary to the usual intermittent demand applications. The restriction to whole number (non-negative integer) values is fundamental to INARMA models.

These issues will be explored further in Section 14.3.1, which presents one of the simplest INARMA models and discusses its relevance to intermittent demand forecasting.

14.3.1 Integer Autoregressive Model of Order One, INAR(1)

We start with the AR model of order one, $d_t = \rho d_{t-1} + \epsilon_t$, and consider how it needs to be adapted for intermittent demand. To remove the possibility of the model generating negative demand values, we can replace the normal distribution of ϵ_t by a distribution which is guaranteed to be non-negative. However, we must also ensure that the distribution takes only whole-number values. There are many such distributions but the simplest choice is the Poisson. We proceed on that basis, whilst noting that the negative binomial distribution (NBD) has also been used in integer autoregressive models (e.g. Al-Osh and Aly 1992).

To avoid fractional values, we need to find a way of transforming one random variable (d_{t-1}) into another (d_t), in such a way that if the first takes only nonnegative whole number values, then so does the second. Two ways of achieving this have been recommended. Kachour and Yao (2009) proposed an adaptation to the standard AR(1) model which includes a rounding operation to the nearest whole number. This approach has been applied to population data (Kachour and Yao 2009) and to price change data (Kachour 2014) but has not yet been applied to intermittent demand data. An alternative approach, proposed by McKenzie (1985) and Al-Osh and Alzaid (1987), has been applied in many different domains, including guest nights in hotels (Brännäs et al. 2002), injuries in the workplace (Da Silva 2005), and statistical quality control (Weiß 2007). It has also been applied in the context of intermittent demand forecasting (Mohammadipour and Boylan 2012). The model of Al-Osh and Alzaid (1987) is an adaptation of the AR(1) model, known as the integer AR model of order one, INAR(1), and is shown in Eq. (14.9).

$$d_t = \alpha \circ d_{t-1} + z_t \tag{14.9}$$

where z_t ($t = 1, 2, 3, \ldots$) is a sequence of i.i.d. Poisson random variables with constant mean, λ. The 'thinning operator' ($\circ$) was introduced by Steutel and van Harn (1979) and is defined in Eq. (14.10).

$$\alpha \circ Y = \sum_{i=1}^{Y} X_i \tag{14.10}$$

where X_i ($i = 1, 2, 3, \ldots$) is a series of i.i.d. Bernoulli (zero-one) variables (also independent of the sequence of Poisson random variables), with a probability of α of taking the value 1, and a probability of $1 - \alpha$ of taking the value 0. Notice that, because it is a probability, α must be between 0 and 1 (unlike the autoregressive parameter in an AR(1) model, which must be between -1 and $+1$).

To visualise the 'thinning operation', imagine a hotel that has d_{t-1} rooms occupied during night $t-1$. Then, each room ($i = 1, \ldots, d_{t-1}$) has a probability (α) of still being occupied

$(X_i = 1)$ during the following night (t) by the same guests. Also, some new guests will arrive for the following night t, occupying z_t rooms. The total number of rooms occupied during night t can be represented as in Eq. (14.11).

$$d_t = \sum_{i=1}^{d_{t-1}} X_i + z_t \tag{14.11}$$

In Eq. (14.11), the first part of the expression represents the number of rooms occupied by the same guests as the previous night, and z_t, sometimes known as an 'innovation term', represents the number of rooms occupied by new guests. This is illustrated in Table 14.1, showing room occupancy over five nights, from Monday to Friday, for a small hotel with four rooms. Each room booking is denoted by a letter, with a new booking indicated in bold lettering, and a continued booking in plain lettering.

In this example, the room occupancy on the first night $(d_1 = 3)$ is composed of two rooms (3 and 4) occupied by old guests and one room (1) occupied by new guests $(z_1 = 1)$. Two of these rooms (1 and 4) remain occupied by the same guests on the second night, with no new arrivals $(z_2 = 0)$, giving a total occupancy of two rooms $(d_2 = 2)$. The remaining nights proceed in a similar way.

In this example, the probability of continued room occupation (α) was not specified. This value can be estimated from the historical data, and methods to do this will be reviewed later in the chapter. With such a short history, it would not be possible to distinguish between different models and so there is no guarantee that an INAR(1) model would be the best choice. Model identification issues will be discussed later.

In an intermittent demand setting, the hotel analogy is inexact. If customers order only one item of a stock keeping unit (SKU), then the model may be interpreted as the retention of old customers and the gaining of new customers. If customers order differing quantities, then departure and arrival of customers does not necessarily equate to the same loss and gain of demand. Nevertheless, the INAR(1) process may be interpreted more loosely as modelling the retention of previous demand, and the gaining of new demand, without reference to specific customers. The INAR(1) model can offer a good representation of real demand patterns, as we shall see later in this chapter.

Table 14.1 INAR(1) process example.

	Mon	Tues	Wed	Thurs	Fri
Room 1	**C**	C			**F**
Room 2			**E**	E	
Room 3	**B**		**D**		
Room 4	**A**	A	A		
Rooms with continuing guests	2	2	1	1	0
Rooms with new guests	1	0	2	0	1
Total rooms occupied	3	2	3	1	1

14.3.2 Integer Moving Average Model of Order One, INMA(1)

Now consider a moving average model of order one, MA(1), $d_t = \epsilon_t + \theta\epsilon_{t-1}$. To recognise dependence between the current observation and the previous innovation term for intermittent series, the MA(1) model may be adapted (Al-Osh and Alzaid 1988). This new model, an 'integer moving average model of order one', INMA(1), represents the chance of new entrants remaining for one further period but no longer. This is expressed mathematically in Eq. (14.12).

$$d_t = \beta \circ z_{t-1} + z_t \tag{14.12}$$

In Eq. (14.12), the term $\beta \circ z_{t-1}$ represents the sum of z_{t-1} Bernoulli variables, each of which has a probability β of taking the value 1.

Continuing with the case of the hotel rooms, an example of an INMA(1) process is given in Table 14.2, with bold lettering indicating new arrivals, as before.

In this example, the three rooms occupied on Monday night include one new occupancy plus two occupancies retained from the previous night. According to the INMA(1) model, it is only the room with new guests (labelled 'C') that can be retained on Tuesday, which in fact it is, with no new guests on that night. On Wednesday, there are no new guests from Tuesday to be retained. The only possible occupancy demands would be from new guests on Wednesday, of which there are none. Finally, some new guests (labelled 'D') on Thursday are retained on Friday, with no additional new guests. In this example, notice that there are no periods of stay beyond two nights because this is not possible for an INMA(1) process. Clearly, this makes an INMA(1) model an unrealistic representation of hotel occupation, unless a hotel has a policy of allowing a stay of no more than two nights.

14.3.3 Mixed Integer Autoregressive Moving Average Models

It is possible to have a mixed model for (non-negative) integer demand, containing both AR and MA terms. The simplest of these models contains one AR and one MA term; it is denoted as INARMA(1,1), and shown in Eq. (14.13).

$$d_t = \alpha \circ d_{t-1} + \beta \circ z_{t-1} + z_t \tag{14.13}$$

Table 14.2 INMA(1) process example.

	Mon	Tues	Wed	Thurs	Fri
Room 1	**C**	C			
Room 2				**D**	D
Room 3	**B**				
Room 4	**A**				
Rooms with continuing guests	2	1	0	0	1
Rooms with new guests	1	0	0	1	0
Total rooms occupied	3	1	0	1	1

The general INARMA model allows for any number of AR and MA terms and is written as shown in Eq. (14.14).

$$d_t = \sum_{i=1}^{p} \alpha_i \circ d_{t-i} + \sum_{j=1}^{q} \beta_j \circ z_{t-j} + z_t \tag{14.14}$$

This is known as the INARMA(p,q) model, with p autoregressive and q moving average terms. Researchers sometimes use this general form of model to derive properties that apply to any INARMA model, regardless of the number of AR or MA terms. However, for intermittent demand, there is a lack of empirical evidence on the accuracy of models which involve more than one AR term, or more than one MA term, and such models will not be discussed further.

14.3.4 Summary

The classic autoregressive moving average (ARMA) models were not designed for intermittent data but adaptations to these models have been developed to cater for this type of series. These INARMA models have straightforward interpretations, although these interpretations are not always natural in an intermittent demand setting.

If there is no dependence on previous observations or innovation terms, we have an INARMA(0,0) model, $d_t = z_t$, which corresponds to i.i.d. demand. This is a useful benchmark model, against which the other INARMA models may be compared to ensure that their additional complexity is justified. We return to this topic in Section 14.5.

14.4 INARMA Parameter Estimation

There are four approaches to parameter estimation that have been proposed in the time series literature: (i) Yule-Walker, (ii) conditional least squares, (iii) conditional maximum likelihood, and (iv) generalised method of moments. In this section, we focus on the Yule-Walker estimators, as these are usually of the simplest type and are available for all forms of INARMA models.

14.4.1 Parameter Estimation for INAR(1) Models

As discussed in Section 14.3 of this chapter, the INAR(1) model has two parameters, which may be interpreted as the probability of retaining previous demand (α) and the mean level of new demand (λ). The Yule-Walker estimate for α is given by the sample autocorrelation function of lag one (Al-Osh and Alzaid 1987). For a demand history $d_1, \ldots, d_n$, this function may be calculated using Eq. (14.15).

$$\hat{\alpha} = \frac{\sum_{t=2}^{n}(d_t - \bar{d})(d_{t-1} - \bar{d})}{\sum_{t=1}^{n}(d_t - \bar{d})^2} \tag{14.15}$$

where $\bar{d}$ is the sample mean of the historical demand values.

The sample autocorrelation function of lag one, shown on the right-hand side of Eq. (14.15), measures the correlation of a time series with itself, lagged by one period. The estimate for λ can be found from Eq. (14.16) (Jung and Tremayne 2006).

$$\widehat{\lambda} = \frac{1 - \widehat{\alpha}}{n} \sum_{t=1}^{n} d_t \qquad (14.16)$$

There is an alternative estimation method for λ, given by Al-Osh and Alzaid (1987). It depends on estimation of the previous innovation terms, and is not as simple as the estimator given above.

14.4.2 Parameter Estimation for INMA(1) Models

This model has two parameters, namely the probability of retaining the previous innovation (β) and the mean level of the new innovation (λ). The Yule-Walker estimates for β and λ are given by Eqs. (14.17) and (14.18) (Brännäs and Hall 2001).

$$\widehat{\beta} = \frac{r_1}{1 - r_1} \qquad (14.17)$$

$$\widehat{\lambda} = \frac{1}{(1 + \widehat{\beta})n} \sum_{t=1}^{n} d_t \qquad (14.18)$$

where r_1 is the sample autocorrelation of lag one and is calculated using the expression on the right-hand side of Eq. (14.15). Instead of using the unconditional mean, as in Eq. (14.18), the λ parameter can be estimated using the unconditional variance, recalling that these are identical for a Poisson distribution. However, this alternative estimator has been found to have higher variance than the one based on the unconditional mean (Brännäs and Hall 2001).

14.4.3 Parameter Estimation for INARMA(1,1) Models

For an INARMA(1,1) model, there are three parameters to be estimated: (i) the probability of retaining a previous demand (α), (ii) the probability of retaining a previous innovation (β), and (iii) the mean level of the new innovation (λ). The Yule-Walker estimates of these parameters are given in Eqs. (14.19) (Mohammadipour 2009).

$$\widehat{\alpha} = \frac{\sum_{t=3}^{n}(d_t - \overline{d})(d_{t-2} - \overline{d})}{\sum_{t=2}^{n}(d_t - \overline{d})(d_{t-1} - \overline{d})}$$

$$\widehat{\beta} = \frac{(1 + \widehat{\alpha})(\widehat{\alpha} - r_1)}{r_1(1 + 3\widehat{\alpha}) - 1 - \widehat{\alpha} - 2\widehat{\alpha}^2}$$

$$\widehat{\lambda} = \frac{(1 - \widehat{\alpha})\sum_{t=1}^{n} d_t}{(1 + \widehat{\beta})n} \qquad (14.19)$$

where, as before, r_1 is the sample autocorrelation of lag one.

Other estimation methods can be used for INARMA(1,1) processes, for example, conditional least squares estimates have been obtained (Mohammadipour 2009), although they are more complicated than the Yule-Walker estimates given above.

14.4.4 Summary

A variety of techniques are available to estimate the parameters of the three simplest (non-i.i.d.) INARMA models. The most straightforward is the Yule-Walker method. Closed-form formulae are available for all of the parameters for all three models, thereby simplifying the calculations.

14.5 Identification of INARMA Models

The four simplest INARMA models are shown in Table 14.3. The simplest model of all is the INARMA(0,0) model, which corresponds to i.i.d. demand. The most general model in Table 14.3 is the INARMA(1,1) model: all the other models in the table are special cases of it. The INARMA(1,0) model is the same as the INAR(1) model, with no moving average component; similarly, the INARMA(0,1) is the same as the INMA(1) model with no AR component.

For practical applications, we can use an 'order selection method' to identify which of the four models will be most appropriate for each of the intermittent demand series. This may be based on examination of the sample autocorrelation function and sample partial autocorrelation function, in a similar way to identification of ARMA models (as explained in many textbooks, e.g. Ord et al. 2017). This approach has been adopted by some integer time series researchers, for example Bu and McCabe (2008) who analysed medical injury deaths. Alternatively, we may use 'information criteria' to distinguish between models, as discussed in Section 14.5.1.

As an additional note, it is not always necessary to identify a specific INARMA model. Instead of choosing between models, we may use the most general model for all the demand series. For example, we can use an INAR(1) model to encompass both INARMA(0,0) and INARMA(1,0) models, or we can use INARMA(1,1) to encompass (0,0), (1,0), (0,1), and (1,1) INARMA models.

14.5.1 Identification Using Akaike's Information Criterion

At this point, we step back from INARMA model order selection, and see how this can be done for ARMA models, before coming back to INARMA. The standard approach for

Table 14.3 Four simplest INARMA models.

INARMA(0,1)	INARMA(1,1)
$d_t = \beta \circ z_{t-1} + z_t$	$d_t = \alpha \circ d_{t-1} + \beta \circ z_{t-1} + z_t$
INARMA(0,0)	INARMA(1,0)
$d_t = z_t$	$d_t = \alpha \circ d_{t-1} + z_t$

identifying the most appropriate ARMA model is the Akaike information criterion (Akaike 1973), also known as the AIC. A model is selected by identifying the one with the lowest AIC, which may be approximated by the expression in Eq. (14.20) for ARMA(p,q) models (Ozaki 1977).

$$\text{AIC} = n \log(\hat{\sigma}_a^2) + 2(p + q + 1) \tag{14.20}$$

where n is the number of observations and $\hat{\sigma}_a^2$ is the sample variance of the fitting errors. The lower this value, the closer the fit of the model to the historical data. The 'penalty term', $2(p + q + 1)$, penalises the total number of AR and MA terms $(p + q)$ (and one is added to take account of the estimation of the variance). This stops models becoming over-complicated, with marginal improvements of in-sample fitting errors, which can be at the expense of a deterioration of out-of-sample forecasting errors.

For short demand histories, with fewer than 40 observations, a corrected version of the AIC has been recommended (Sugiura 1978; Hurvich and Tsai 1989), as shown in Eq. (14.21).

$$\text{AICc} = n \log(\hat{\sigma}_a^2) + 2m + \frac{2m(m + 1)}{n - m - 1} \tag{14.21}$$

where $m = p + q + 1$.

The calculation of the AIC is complicated for INARMA models. Latour (1998) suggested that the ARMA expressions for AIC be used as a surrogate for identifying integer AR models, based on the similarity of the autocorrelation functions between AR and INAR models. Mohammadipour (2009), noting that the similarity extended to ARMA and INARMA models, proposed using the ARMA expressions for AIC to distinguish between the four models in Table 14.3.

14.5.2 General Models and Model Identification

Using a slightly modified identification procedure to that outlined above, Mohammadipour (2009) analysed two subsets of industrial datasets. The subsets were obtained by removing highly variable 'lumpy' demands, leaving 1943 series from 3000 automotive demand series, and 5168 from 16 000 military demand series. The identification results for Poisson INARMA models were as shown in Table 14.4.

It is immediately evident that only a small number of military SKUs have been identified as non-i.i.d. (i.e. not INARMA(0,0)), whereas a significant proportion of automotive SKUs

Table 14.4 Empirical evidence on model identification.

	Automotive (%)	Military (%)
INARMA(0,0)	54.6	98.1
INARMA(1,0)	23.9	0.7
INARMA(0,1)	18.0	1.0
INARMA(1,1)	3.6	0.2

Source: [215–217] Mohammadipour (2009).

have been identified as having a demand process other than INARMA(0,0). Further analyses showed that mis-identification of INAR(1) processes had a stronger adverse effect on forecast accuracy than mis-identification of INMA(1) processes. These considerations led to evaluation of the following approaches:

1. Treat all series as INARMA(1,1).
2. Treat all series as INAR(1) (INARMA(1,0)).
3. Identify each series individually, as summarised above.

Mohammadipour (2009) analysed the accuracy (mean square error) of these approaches on the automotive and military datasets. She found that, for both datasets, treating all series as INAR(1) produced more accurate results than treating all series as INARMA(1,1). For the military data, this may be attributed to the very low percentage of series being identified as INARMA(1,1) and those identified as INARMA(0,1) being adequately approximated by an INAR(1) model. For the automotive data, series identified as having a moving average component typically had low moving average parameters (between 0 and 0.1), indicating a relatively weak effect of the previous innovation term. A comparison of the second and third approaches was also conducted. The results were very close, with a slight advantage to treating all series as INAR(1) for the automotive dataset, and a slight advantage to the identification approach for the military dataset, which contained much longer data histories.

14.5.3 Summary

It is possible to identify an INARMA model by minimising the AIC, which has been derived for ARMA models. A corrected version of the AIC is available for short demand series.

An alternative approach is to define a set of models and to use the most general model in that set for all demand series. For example, treating all series as INARMA(1,1) encompasses all four models discussed. Greater generality does not guarantee greater forecast accuracy. The study by Mohammadipour (2009) is a case in point, where treating all series as INAR(1) led to greater accuracy than treating all series as INARMA(1,1).

Evidence on the effectiveness of INARMA identification, series by series, is still in its infancy in an intermittent demand setting. The limited empirical evidence suggests that similar accuracy is attained by treating all series as INAR(1), as would be gained from model identification from the four models analysed in this section.

14.6 Forecasting Using INARMA Models

Suppose that we have estimated the parameters of all of our candidate INARMA models, and decided that all series will be treated as INAR(1) (or as INARMA(1,1)) or, alternatively, that the most appropriate model is selected for each demand series. Now that our models are fully specified, we need to turn our attention to forecasting. As discussed in previous chapters, the forecasting of mean demand may be used to inform stock/non-stock decisions. The prediction of the whole demand distribution will be discussed in Section 14.7.

14.6.1 Forecasting INAR(1) Mean Demand

The forecasted mean demand over the next period (one-step-ahead) for an INAR(1) process is given by Eq. (14.22).

$$\hat{d}_{t+1} = \hat{\alpha}d_t + \hat{\lambda} \tag{14.22}$$

This formula makes sense. The first component, $\hat{\alpha}d_t$, represents the estimated mean demand remaining from the current period, whilst the second term $(\hat{\lambda})$ represents the estimated mean of the new demand in the next period. If there is no demand in the current period, as will often be the case for intermittent demand, then the first component is redundant and the forecasted mean demand over the next period is just $\hat{\lambda}$.

Now suppose that the protection interval is of two periods. Then, considering Eq. (14.22), the forecasted mean demand two-steps ahead is given by Eq. (14.23).

$$\hat{d}_{t+2} = \hat{\alpha}\hat{d}_{t+1} + \hat{\lambda} = \hat{\alpha}^2 d_t + (1 + \hat{\alpha})\hat{\lambda} \tag{14.23}$$

By adding the forecasts in Eqs. (14.22) and (14.23), we get the forecast for demand over a protection interval of two periods, shown in Eq. (14.24).

$$\hat{d}_{t+1} + \hat{d}_{t+2} = (\hat{\alpha} + \hat{\alpha}^2)d_t + (2 + \hat{\alpha})\hat{\lambda} \tag{14.24}$$

This can be generalised to any length of forecasting horizon, h, for which cumulative demand forecasts are required, as shown in Eq. (14.25) (Brännäs 1994).

$$\sum_{i=1}^{h} \hat{d}_{t+i} = \frac{\hat{\alpha}(1 - \hat{\alpha}^h)}{1 - \hat{\alpha}}d_t + \left(h - \sum_{i=1}^{h}\hat{\alpha}^i\right)\frac{\hat{\lambda}}{1 - \hat{\alpha}} \tag{14.25}$$

So, if the demand process is known to be INAR(1) and the parameters α and λ have been estimated, then the forecasted mean cumulative demand over the forecast horizon follows immediately from Eq. (14.25).

14.6.2 Forecasting INMA(1) Mean Demand

Returning to the simplest case of a protection interval of only one period, the forecasted mean demand over the next period for an INMA(1) process is given by Eq. (14.26).

$$\hat{d}_{t+1} = \hat{\lambda} + \hat{\beta}\,\hat{z}_t \tag{14.26}$$

The estimate of the latest residual, $\hat{z}_t$, may be found by repeated application of $\hat{z}_t = d_t - \hat{\beta}\,\hat{z}_{t-1}$ (Brännäs et al. 2002), with $\hat{z}_0$ set at, say, $\hat{\lambda}$.

For longer protection intervals, of length $h \geq 2$, the best estimate of the residuals $z_{t+1}, \ldots, z_{t+h-1}$ is simply the estimated mean, $\hat{\lambda}$. This results in a mean forecasted cumulative demand over the whole forecast horizon, as shown in Eq. (14.27), which holds for all horizons $h \geq 1$.

$$\sum_{i=1}^{h} \hat{d}_{t+i} = h\hat{\lambda} + \hat{\beta}(\hat{z}_t + (h - 1)\hat{\lambda}) \tag{14.27}$$

14.6.3 Forecasting INARMA(1,1) Mean Demand

Again, returning to the simplest case of a forecast horizon of only one period, the forecasted mean demand over the next period for an INARMA(1,1) process is given by Eq. (14.28).

$$\widehat{d}_{t+1} = \widehat{\alpha} d_t + \widehat{\lambda} + \widehat{\beta}\, \widehat{z}_t \tag{14.28}$$

The estimate of the latest residual, $\widehat{z}_t$, may be found using a similar approach to the INMA(1) model. The forecasted mean cumulative demand over the whole forecast horizon is given by Eq. (14.29).

$$\sum_{i=1}^{h} \widehat{d}_{t+i} = \frac{\widehat{\alpha}(1 - \widehat{\alpha}^h)}{1 - \widehat{\alpha}} d_t + h\widehat{\lambda} + \frac{(\widehat{\alpha} + \widehat{\beta})\widehat{\lambda}}{1 - \widehat{\alpha}}\left(h - 1 - \sum_{i=1}^{h-1} \widehat{\alpha}^i\right) + \frac{\widehat{\beta}(1 - \widehat{\alpha}^h)}{1 - \widehat{\alpha}}\widehat{z}_t \tag{14.29}$$

A derivation of this forecast function is given in Technical Note 14.1.

14.6.4 Forecasting Using Temporal Aggregation

In the previous subsections, we have produced h-step-ahead forecasts for each of the periods, $i = 1, \ldots, h$, and then added these forecasts to give the forecasted demand over the whole protection interval ($h = L + R$). An alternative approach, discussed in Section 6.8, is to use temporal aggregation. Mohammadipour and Boylan (2012) proved that overlapping temporal aggregation of an INARMA(p,q) process over a forecast horizon results in another INARMA(p,q) process. Using two empirical datasets, they compared the accuracy of mean demand forecasts produced by adding h-step-ahead forecasts with those generated by temporal aggregation. They found that the aggregation method can produce more accurate (lower mean square error) forecasts for INAR(1) demand processes, especially when the autoregressive parameter (α) is high.

14.6.5 Summary

Closed-form formulae are available for the forecasted mean demand over the forecast horizon for the three simplest non-i.i.d. INARMA processes. (The forecast for an INARMA(0,0) process is just $h\widehat{\lambda}$, where $\widehat{\lambda}$ is the average of all historical demand values.) The formulae provided in this section do not depend upon the method of estimation of the parameters. They will work just as well with other estimation methods as with the Yule-Walker method, whose parameter estimates were presented in Section 14.4.

14.7 Predicting the Whole Demand Distribution

So far, we have seen how the mean demand over an arbitrary forecast horizon may be forecasted using the four most basic INARMA models. To set order-up-to levels, we need to estimate the whole distribution of demand over the protection interval. In this section, we explain how this can be done for the INAR(1) model. This is the INARMA model that has been most commonly employed in a wide range of applications, and which is supported by empirical evidence in an intermittent demand setting.

14.7.1 Protection Interval of One Period

If demand follows an INAR(1) model with Poisson distributed innovation terms, then McKenzie (1988) obtained a result for the distribution of d_{t+1} given d_t, as given in Eq. (14.30).

$$\mathbb{P}(d_{t+1}|d_t) = \sum_{x=0}^{\min(d_t,d_{t+1})} \frac{d_t!}{x!(d_t-x)!} \alpha^x (1-\alpha)^{d_t-x} \left(\frac{e^{-\lambda}\lambda^{d_{t+1}-x}}{(d_{t+1}-x)!} \right) \tag{14.30}$$

The rationale for this formula is given in Technical Note 14.2. To see this formula being applied, consider the following time series: 1, 0, 1, 2, 1, 0, 0, 1, 2, 0, 1, 0, 1, 1, 0, 1, 0, 0, 1, 3, 2, 0, 0, 1, 1, 0, 0, 0. We suppose that this series has been identified as an INAR(1) process, or is one of a group of series, all of which are being treated as INAR(1). Using Eqs. (14.15) and (14.16), we obtain the parameter estimates, $\hat{\alpha} = 0.165$ and $\hat{\lambda} = 0.597$. Substituting these estimated parameters for the true parameters in Eq. (14.30) yields the conditional probabilities in Table 14.5 for demand values up to and including 4 (the probabilities of higher demand values are very small).

Table 14.5 shows the probabilities of demand at time $t + 1$, recorded separately in each column, conditional on demands of 0, 1, 2, 3, and 4 at time t. It is not necessary for all of these demand values to have been observed in the past (e.g. the value of 4 is not contained in the series described above). The corresponding cumulative probabilities are given in Table 14.6.

Table 14.6 shows how sensitive the cumulative probability estimates, at time $t + 1$, can be to the demand at time t. For example, the probability of demand not exceeding one unit in time $t + 1$ varies from 87.9% (if there was zero demand at time t) to 63.9% (if there was demand for four units at time t). Differences such as these can have significant implications for inventory holdings, with higher demand values signalling the need for higher order-up-to levels for INAR(1) demand with positive autocorrelation.

14.7.2 Protection Interval of More Than One Period

For an INAR(1) process, it is more challenging to predict the distribution of demand over protection intervals of two periods or longer. Two approaches that may be used for a Poisson INAR(1) demand process are (i) approximation by a normal distribution and (ii) Markov chains.

Table 14.5 Conditional probabilities of demand at time $t + 1$ (d_{t+1}) given demand at time t, (d_t), INAR(1) process.

d_{t+1}	Demand at time t, d_t				
	0	1	2	3	4
0	0.551	0.460	0.384	0.321	0.268
1	0.329	0.365	0.381	0.381	0.371
2	0.098	0.136	0.174	0.208	0.236
3	0.019	0.032	0.049	0.070	0.093
4	0.003	0.006	0.010	0.017	0.025

Table 14.6 Cumulative conditional probabilities at time $t + 1$ (d_{t+1}) given demand at time t, (d_t), INAR(1) process.

d_{t+1}	Demand at time t, d_t				
	0	1	2	3	4
0	0.551	0.460	0.384	0.321	0.268
≤ 1	0.879	0.825	0.765	0.702	0.639
≤ 2	0.977	0.961	0.939	0.910	0.876
≤ 3	0.997	0.993	0.988	0.980	0.968
≤ 4	1.000	0.999	0.998	0.997	0.993

Figure 14.1 Demand transitions from one period to the next.

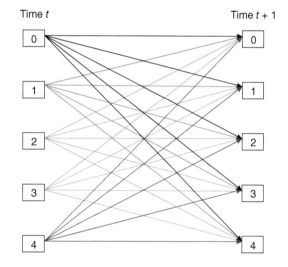

If a normal approximation is satisfactory, then order-up-to levels may be calculated based on an estimate of mean demand from Eq. (14.25) and an estimate of variance derived by Mohammadipour (2009) (see Technical Note 14.3).

As discussed earlier in this book, a normal distribution is often an inadequate approximation to data which takes very low integer values. An alternative approach, suggested by Engelmeyer (2016), is to consider the successive demands as a Markov chain, with transitions between demand at time t to demand at time $t + 1$ governed by the same conditional distributions as time moves on. The transitions are illustrated in Figure 14.1 for the case where demand per period does not exceed four units.

The probabilities of each of the 25 paths shown in Figure 14.1 can be found from Table 14.5, which gives each of the conditional probabilities of demand at time $t + 1$, given the previous demand value at time t. This table can also be used for the conditional probabilities at time $t + 2$, given the previous demand value at time $t + 1$.

The probabilities of the total demand over two periods $(t + 1, t + 2)$ can be found by identifying all the paths from an initial demand value at time t, which will give the total

Table 14.7 Cumulative probabilities of demand over two periods $(d_{t+1} + d_{t+2})$, given demand at time t, (d_t), INAR(1) process.

	Demand at time t, d_t				
$d_{t+1} + d_{t+2}$	0	1	2	3	4
0	0.303	0.253	0.212	0.177	0.148
≤ 1	0.635	0.572	0.513	0.458	0.406
≤ 2	0.847	0.803	0.756	0.708	0.659
≤ 3	0.946	0.924	0.898	0.868	0.835
≤ 4	0.983	0.974	0.963	0.948	0.931

demand required. If the demand at time t is zero, then there are two paths that will give a total demand of one unit in a diagram with three columns (time t, time $t + 1$, time $t + 2$), namely 0 – 0 – 1 and 0 – 1 – 0. Using the conditional probabilities from Table 14.5, the probability of the first path is $0.551 \times 0.329 = 0.181$, and the probability of the second path is $0.329 \times 0.460 = 0.151$, giving an overall probability of total demand of one unit of 0.332. For a protection interval of two periods, the formula is given by Eq. (14.31).

$$\mathbb{P}(d_{t+1} + d_{t+2} = D | d_t) = \sum_{d_{t+1}=0}^{D} \mathbb{P}(d_{t+1} | d_t) \mathbb{P}(d_{t+2} = D - d_{t+1} | d_{t+1}) \tag{14.31}$$

In our example, employing Eq. (14.31) gives the results shown in Table 14.7 for the cumulative probability of demand over the two periods $t + 1$ and $t + 2$. This set of results would lead, for a target cycle service level of 90%, to order-up-to levels of 3, 3, 4, 4, and 4 for demands at time t of 0, 1, 2, 3, and 4, respectively.

This approach can be generalised to any length of protection interval, although the number of combinations of demand transitions may become very large.

14.7.3 Summary

For an INAR(1) demand process, the key to calculating the cumulative distribution of demand over the protection interval lies in finding the conditional distribution of demand at time $t + 1$, given demand at time t. This then immediately yields the cumulative distribution of demand at time $t + 1$, and may be used directly for a protection interval of one period. For longer protection intervals, the conditional distribution is used repeatedly, over all paths in the Markov chain that yield the required total demand.

14.8 State Space Models for Intermittence

For non-intermittent demand, an alternative to the ARIMA framework is the state space modelling approach. State space models are not generally expressed as one equation but in the form of two equations, with a 'measurement equation' being followed by a 'transition equation'. (In fact, there may be more than one transition equation, but they can be expressed as a single equation with appropriate use of vectors and matrices.) An example of a state space model is given in Eq. (14.32).

$$d_t = \mu_{t-1} + \epsilon_t$$
$$\mu_t = \mu_{t-1} + \alpha\epsilon_t \qquad (14.32)$$

where, as previously, the innovation terms (ϵ_t) are i.i.d. and normally distributed with mean zero and a constant variance. The model, with parameter α, underpins the SES method, with smoothing constant α. This particular form of state space model is sometimes known as a 'local level model'. It is a special case of a more general state space formulation, as described by Ord et al. (1997).

It is worth noting that a changing mean value (μ_t) is explicit in the model, and that the same innovation term is used in both the measurement and transition equations, as proposed by Snyder (1985). For this reason, models such as these are described as 'single source of error' (SSOE) models. An alternative formulation, discussed in Chapter 7, assumes mutually independent error terms, and is known as the 'multiple source of error' (MSOE) model (see, for example, Durbin and Koopman 2012). The two forms of model also differ in their treatment of the dependence of the current demand observation (d_t) on the current mean demand (MSOE) and the previous mean demand (SSOE).

State space models are very flexible and can allow for changing levels, trends, and seasonal factors and can incorporate explanatory variables. The flexibility to allow for changing mean levels is of particular interest for intermittent demand forecasting, as reflected by Croston's method and Syntetos–Boylan approximation (Chapter 6), as well as the Teunter–Syntetos–Babai method (Chapter 12). INARMA models, on the other hand, are based on the stationarity assumption of unchanging unconditional mean demand.

14.8.1 Croston's Demand Model

Croston (1972) postulated an intermittent demand model in Appendix B of his paper, as shown (with minor changes in notation) in Eq. (14.33).

$$d_t = o_t(\bar{z}_{\eta-1} + \epsilon_\eta)$$
$$\bar{z}_{\eta-1} = \lambda \sum_{j=1}^{\infty} (1-\lambda)^{j-1} z_{\eta-j} \qquad (14.33)$$

where t is the time index and η is a serial number of the non-zero demands (z_η), with η increasing by 1 each time $o_t = 1$, and o_t is a binary variable representing demand occurrence at time t, taking a value of 1 when demand occurs and zero when it does not. In Croston's model, the probability of demand occurrence is assumed to be constant and unchanging over time. The demand sizes, z_η, are assumed to follow an ARIMA(0,1,1) model that applies only in those periods when demand occurs. Therefore, the mean demand size $\bar{z}_{\eta-1}$ is an exponentially weighted moving average of all past observations. The innovation terms, ϵ_η, are assumed to be i.i.d. normal with zero mean and constant variance.

Snyder (2002) remarked on inconsistencies between Croston's model and method. If the occurrence probability is constant over time, then exponential smoothing is not the optimal estimator of the mean demand interval. Instead, the best estimator is the average of all the observed demand intervals.

In our earlier discussion, we found that there was an inconsistency in Brown's model of demand to underpin SES. In that case, it was due to an application of weighted least squares when weighting is inappropriate. In the case of Croston's model, there is an inconsistency between a demand occurrence process that does not require exponentially weighted estimates and a forecasting method that does.

14.8.2 Proposed State Space Models

A further problem with Croston's model, as pointed out by Snyder (2002), is that an ARIMA(0,1,1) process can generate negative values, which is contrary to any sensible notion of demand size. To overcome this problem, Snyder proposed a log-space adaptation model, in which demand at time t, denoted by d_t^+, is generated by Eq. (14.34).

$$d_t^+ = o_t \exp(d_t) \tag{14.34}$$

where exp denotes natural exponentiation ($\exp(x) = e^x$).

In Eq. (14.34), o_t is a zero-one demand occurrence variable, as in Eq. (14.33), with constant probability p of taking the value 1, representing occurrence. The variable d_t does not represent demand itself but the natural logarithm of demand size, when $o_t = 1$, thereby ensuring that demand, represented by d_t^+, is never negative. (If $o_t = 0$, then d_t can take any value, as Eq. (14.34) will always give $d_t^+ = 0$.) This is a more appropriate representation of intermittent demand with an ARIMA(0,1,1) process for demand sizes. However, the log-space adaptation model does not underpin Croston's method but a variant of it, according to which:

1. The probability of demand occurrence is estimated as the proportion of all periods with non-zero demand, and not by exponential smoothing.
2. Demand size is not smoothed; instead, the logarithm of demand size is predicted by exponential smoothing.

Shenstone and Hyndman (2005) investigated the properties of models that could underpin Croston's method and concluded that there is no such model unless we allow for active demand periods that can take negative or positive values. Svetunkov and Boylan (2019) pointed out that this conclusion depends on the assumption that the error term (ϵ_t) is additive, and does not necessarily hold for models with other error term formulations.

Hyndman et al. (2008, Chapter 16) proposed a basis for a modified Croston method (the 'hurdle shifted Poisson' model; HSP). The time-gaps between active demand periods are assumed to follow a geometric distribution (starting at 1, rather than 0) and the positive demands are taken to follow a Poisson distribution, shifted up by 1 (to avoid zeroes). The time gaps and the positive demand sizes are assumed to be governed by local distributions, allowing variation of the geometric and Poisson parameters over time. This approach to modelling gives one-step-ahead forecasts equivalent to Croston's method, but does not give equivalent forecasts for longer horizons.

Snyder et al. (2012) compared predictions based on three distributions, namely Poisson, negative binomial, and HSP. The authors assessed the ability of each of the three approaches to predict the one-step, multiple-step, and lead time distribution of demands of 1046 auto parts, with 51 months of data history. The results showed the HSP to perform better than the Poisson, but not as well as the NBD. Further development of time-varying NBD models would appear to be a promising direction for future research.

14.8.3 Summary

State space models have an advantage over INARMA models in so far as they can cater for changing mean demand sizes and changing probabilities of demand occurrence. However, this flexibility introduces significant difficulties in state space models representing non-negative integer demand values. A number of suggestions have been made but, as yet, no state space model has been established for which Croston's method gives optimal forecasts for all horizons.

14.9 Chapter Summary

In this chapter, we have seen that a fully specified statistical model can yield the following potential benefits for demand forecasting:

1. Coherent approach to model selection.
2. Rigorous parameter estimation methods.
3. Complete specification of the prediction distribution.

These benefits have been fully realised for faster moving demand, using the ARIMA approach and the state space framework for exponential smoothing models. For intermittent demand, the benefits have been partially realised using INARMA models. Model-based estimation methods have been proposed for INARMA models. In this chapter, we have focused on Yule-Walker estimates, to avoid excessive complexity, but alternative estimation methods may be considered.

The distribution of demand over the protection interval, required for determination of order-up-to levels, can be found for an INAR(1) process. It depends on an analytical result showing the conditional distribution of demand in one period, given the demand in the previous period.

There has been some progress in state space models but we still lack a fully coherent state space model based approach for Croston's method for intermittent demand forecasting. Nevertheless, this remains a promising route of enquiry, as such models allow for changing mean demands over time, unlike the INARMA approach.

Technical Notes

Note 14.1 INARMA(1,1) Cumulative Forecasts

We suppose that demand follows an INARMA(1,1) process, as shown in Eq. (14.35).

$$d_{t+1} = \alpha \circ d_t + \beta \circ z_t + z_{t+1} \tag{14.35}$$

Repeated application of Eq. (14.35) gives Eq. (14.36), for $i = 1$ to $i = h$.

$$d_{t+i} = \alpha^i \circ d_t + \alpha^{i-1}\beta \circ z_t + \alpha^{i-1}\circ z_{t+1} + \alpha^{i-2}\beta \circ z_{t+1} + \cdots + \alpha \circ z_{t+i-1} + \beta \circ z_{t+i-1} + z_{t+i}$$

$$(14.36)$$

This yields the i-step-ahead forecast given by Eq. (14.37).

$$\widehat{d}_{t+i} = \widehat{\alpha}^i d_t + \widehat{\alpha}^{i-1}\widehat{\beta}\,\widehat{z}_t + \widehat{\alpha}^{i-2}(\widehat{\alpha}+\widehat{\beta})\widehat{\lambda} + \cdots + (\widehat{\alpha}+\widehat{\beta})\widehat{\lambda} + \widehat{\lambda}$$

$$(14.37)$$

Adding the forecasts over the whole horizon, h, we obtain the cumulative demand forecast shown in Eq. (14.38).

$$\sum_{i=1}^{h}\widehat{d}_{t+i} = \frac{\widehat{\alpha}(1-\widehat{\alpha}^h)}{1-\widehat{\alpha}}d_t + \frac{\widehat{\beta}(1-\widehat{\alpha}^h)}{1-\widehat{\alpha}}\widehat{z}_t +$$

$$\widehat{\alpha}^{h-2}(\widehat{\alpha}+\widehat{\beta})\widehat{\lambda} + 2\widehat{\alpha}^{h-3}(\widehat{\alpha}+\widehat{\beta})\widehat{\lambda} + \cdots + (h-1)(\widehat{\alpha}+\widehat{\beta})\widehat{\lambda} + h\widehat{\lambda} \qquad (14.38)$$

The terms on the second line of Eq. (14.38), except for the last term, $h\widehat{\lambda}$, form an arithmetico-geometric progression with its total given by Eq. (14.39).

$$(\widehat{\alpha}+\widehat{\beta})\widehat{\lambda}(h-1+(h-2)\widehat{\alpha}+\cdots+\widehat{\alpha}^{h-2}) = \frac{(\widehat{\alpha}+\widehat{\beta})\widehat{\lambda}}{1-\widehat{\alpha}}\left(h-1-\sum_{i=1}^{h-1}\widehat{\alpha}^i\right) \qquad (14.39)$$

This establishes the forecast function given in Eq. (14.29) for an INARMA(1,1) process. The result for INMA(1) processes, given in Eq. (14.27), follows immediately from Eq. (14.29) by setting $\widehat{\alpha} = 0$. The forecast function for an INAR(1) process, given in Eq. (14.25), follows from Eq. (14.29) by setting $\widehat{\beta} = 0$ and noting the identity in Eq. (14.40).

$$h\widehat{\lambda} + \frac{\widehat{\alpha}\widehat{\lambda}}{1-\widehat{\alpha}}\left(h-1-\sum_{i=1}^{h-1}\widehat{\alpha}^i\right) = h\widehat{\lambda} + \frac{\widehat{\lambda}}{1-\widehat{\alpha}}\left(\widehat{\alpha}h - \sum_{i=1}^{h}\widehat{\alpha}^i\right) = \frac{\widehat{\lambda}}{1-\widehat{\alpha}}\left(h-\sum_{i=1}^{h}\widehat{\alpha}^i\right)$$

$$(14.40)$$

Note 14.2 INAR(1) Conditional Probabilities

The demand at time $t + 1$, denoted by d_{t+1}, is Poisson distributed, with two components:

1. Demand retained from time t (denoted by $\alpha \circ d_t$).
2. New demand generated at time $t + 1$ (denoted by z_{t+1}).

Each of the d_t elements of demand at time t may be retained with probability α or not retained with probability $1 - \alpha$. The number of combinations of x elements from d_t elements is $d_t!/(x!(d_t - x)!)$. Hence, the probability of x elements being retained and $d_t - x$ elements not being retained is given by the binomial formula, as shown in Eq. (14.41).

$$\mathbb{P}(\alpha \circ d_t = x|d_t) = \frac{d_t!}{x!(d_t - x)!}\alpha^x(1-\alpha)^{d_t-x} \qquad (14.41)$$

The probability of observing $d_{t+1} - x$ new elements is given by the standard Poisson formula with mean λ, given by Eq. (14.42).

$$\mathbb{P}(z_{t+1} = d_{t+1} - x|x) = \frac{\lambda^{d_{t+1}-x}e^{-\lambda}}{(d_{t+1}-x)!} \qquad (14.42)$$

By definition, x cannot exceed either d_t or d_{t+1}. Therefore, the possible values of x range from 0 to min (d_t, d_{t+1}) (minimum of d_t and d_{t+1}). The formula given earlier in the chapter (Eq. (14.30)) now follows because of the identity in Eq. (14.43).

$$\mathbb{P}(d_{t+1}|d_t) = \sum_{x=0}^{\min(d_t,d_{t+1})} \mathbb{P}(z_{t+1} = d_{t+1} - x|x)\mathbb{P}(\alpha \circ d_t = x|d_t) \tag{14.43}$$

Note 14.3 Normal Approximation to Order-up-to Level for an INAR(1) Process

The mean demand over the protection interval, conditional on the last observed demand d_t, can be calculated using Eq. (14.25). Mohammadipour (2009) derived the conditional variance expression for the total demand over a horizon h, for an INAR(1) process, as shown in Eq. (14.44).

$$\text{Var}\left(\sum_{i=1}^{h} d_{t+i}|d_t\right) = d_t \sum_{i=1}^{h} \alpha^i(1 - \alpha^i) + \frac{\lambda}{1 - \alpha}\left(h - \sum_{i=1}^{h} \alpha^i\right)$$

$$+ \frac{2\lambda}{1 - \alpha} \sum_{i=1}^{h-1} \alpha^{2i-1}\left(h - i - \frac{\alpha(1 - \alpha^{h-i})}{1 - \alpha}\right) \tag{14.44}$$

This result hold for all horizons $h \geq 1$; in the case of $h = 1$, the final summation does not apply. Note: Equation (14.44) was also reported by Mohammadipour and Boylan (2012), but with a typographical error in the formula, with the final summation being shown as from $i = 1$ to h (incorrect) instead of from $i = 1$ to $h - 1$ (correct).

15

Software for Intermittent Demand

15.1   Introduction

The methods discussed so far in this book are analytical in nature, thus lending themselves to algorithmic implementation. Indeed, all procedures previously considered (e.g. for forecasting the mean and variance of demand, appropriately classifying demand patterns, deciding on the most appropriate distributional assumptions, or building empirical demand distributions) constitute, potentially, key features of a forecasting software package. In this chapter, we discuss progress in implementing the procedures covered in this book, and what remains to be done to enable the full utilisation of the knowledge available in intermittent demand inventory forecasting.

   To put the above in context, we start with a discussion of alternative types of software packages. We distinguish between proprietary software (including in-house developed solutions), open source software, and hybrid solutions that seem to be gaining momentum in industry at the present time.

   Subsequently, previous work in forecasting software evaluation is reviewed, and some important generic features are identified, to enable a comprehensive assessment of software capabilities. We extend the discussion to the context of intermittent demand forecasting and present some features, over and above the generic ones, for evaluating software solutions. This is followed by an assessment of what is currently available in terms of the methods and approaches advocated in this book.

   We argue for the importance of the human factor in software implementation, in terms of (i) appropriate training that allows users to learn and engage fully with the software's functionality, which then leads to (ii) the effective incorporation of judgement into, otherwise, algorithmically derived decisions. Facilitating value-adding judgemental interventions requires some appropriate features which, if available, lead to the notion of a forecast support system (FSS). FSSs include forecasting software but constitute a wider class of solutions, discussed later in this chapter.

   We then discuss two alternative perspectives on intermittent demand forecasting, not previously considered in the book: Bayesian and neural network (NN) methods. Although not so well established in practice as the approaches discussed in earlier chapters, ongoing computational advances are making their implementation more viable. This then leads to a discussion of how things could develop in the future to allow companies to benefit

Intermittent Demand Forecasting: Context, Methods and Applications, First Edition.
John E. Boylan and Aris A. Syntetos.
© 2021 John Wiley & Sons Ltd. Published 2021 by John Wiley & Sons Ltd.
Companion Website: www.wiley.com/go/boylansyntetos/intermittentdemandforecasting

further from the knowledge available in the area of intermittent demand forecasting, and which areas of academic research could generate fruitful additions to the current body of knowledge.

15.2 Taxonomy of Software

The global retail analytics market attained a market size of around $3 billion in 2016 and was expected to reach $10.5 billion by 2023 by growing at a compound annual growth rate of 19.6% during 2017–2023 (KBV Research 2017). The analytics market consists of both software and associated services. The key analytical software for supply chains in the retail sector is built with a focus on inventory management, supply and demand forecasting, and vendor management (KBV Research 2017). It has been reported that US and European retailers spend 1% of annual sales on automated decision support tools that use recorded inventory quantities to forecast demand, plan product assortments, and replenish store shelves (DeHoratius and Raman 2008; Rekik et al. 2019). Put simply, for a 'typical' European grocery retailer (with turnovers being around € 10 billion) this would translate, collectively, across all solutions employed, to about € 100 million investment. This indicates the importance of software packages and the need to appreciate the scope of their functionality.

Not all solutions are equally expensive and, indeed, some of them may come absolutely free. (We refer only to the cost of acquiring a new solution, and not to any costs of their installation or for tying them to the existing systems.) The wider their scope, and the more business functions they are designed to coordinate, the more expensive these solutions are. Conversely, the more specialist a solution is, the less expensive it is (with an academic license of a well-known specialised forecasting software package being about £15 000, at the time of writing). So, an important question is, what are the main types of software? Leaving aside specific brands, what do these various types of solutions try to achieve? And how do they link to specific business needs? One linkage, for example, is facilitating the sales and operations planning (S&OP) process of an organisation. Other linkages may target more specific objectives, such as trading off inventory cost versus achieved service.

In this section, we discuss the various types of software packages and how they link to business needs. In doing so, we also consider the type of users of these solutions, as this affects their degree of utilisation.

15.2.1 Proprietary Software

An important distinction needs to be drawn between proprietary software and software that is free to use (open source). We consider the former here, and return to open source software in Section 15.2.2.

Proprietary software varies in scope and organisational coverage, from (i) enterprise-wide software, to (ii) software covering major organisational functions (e.g. manufacturing and/or supply chain management), to (iii) specialised solutions that address some specific business needs (e.g. forecasting and inventory optimisation). Software vendors may target any of these 'levels'. SAP, for example, produce software that is enterprise-wide (enterprise resource planning, ERP); Blue Yonder (formerly JDA) produce software that covers the entire supply chain function of an organisation; and Smart Forecasts produce specialised software for forecasting and inventory control. Based on a component-based (modular) structure, Blue Yonder has an inventory forecasting module, just as SAP has a supply chain module (SAP Advanced Planning and Optimisation - APO). Let us discuss these differences in some more detail.

At the higher level, ERP systems are enterprise-wide software applications that integrate data across, and support, all the major functions of an organisation (Motiwalla and Thompson 2014) (Technical Note 15.1). Given the considerable size differences of organisations, various vendors target alternative organisational sizes, from large to medium to small organisations (tier 1, 2, and 3 vendors, respectively). Modern ERP systems have expanded to integration of inter-organisational systems for e-business operations, and they are more process than function oriented. SAP R/3, for example, has been replaced by SAP S/4HANA to reflect exactly these priorities. Januschowski and Kolassa (2019) commented that the degree to which new forecasting solutions integrate with an existing ERP system is as important in its selection as the methods it supports.

At the next level, supply chain (or, more generally, functional) specific software solutions are available either in a 'component' form, being part of a wider ERP infrastructure, or independently developed by other companies. In the former case, for example, SAP APO (succeeded by SAP Digital Manufacturing) is the function-oriented supply chain solution provided by SAP in relation to their SAP R/3 backbone operation (succeeded by SAP HANA cloud). Alternatively, organisations may opt for supply chain solutions, such as Blue Yonder. In any case, such solutions modularly consist of lower-level functional solutions, such as S&OP, supply chain and inventory planning, and warehouse management. Forecasting would typically fall under S&OP processes or demand planning modules.

Finally, specialised statistical forecasting software packages are also available, such as Forecast Pro or Smart Forecasts. In that case, forecasting functions may or may not be linked to inventory optimisation. Also, such packages may or may not be compatible with higher level software, something that determines their degree of connectivity with other solutions employed by a company. In any case, forecasting constitutes an important 'module' of generic software, or a specialised software solution, with intermittent demand forecasting being an indispensable part within it.

Forecasting modules may also be present in standard statistical software such as SAS. Further, companies also develop their own in-house solutions, upon which they rely to perform their forecasting tasks. This is common in industry, particularly in smaller organisations, or small divisions/departments of (not-particularly well integrated) larger organisations. They are usually Excel based, with or without Visual Basic functionality, and they are generally designed to meet the particular forecasting needs faced by the company under concern. Their effectiveness varies considerably, depending on the knowledge and experience of those involved in their development. We are aware, for example, of in-house developed solutions in the spare parts industry that are well informed but we have also come across solutions with very basic functionality. In any case, these Excel-based solutions are often poorly documented and not well understood when the designer moves on to another company. Further, a major problem associated with such solutions is scaling them up to accommodate calculations across hundreds or even thousands of stock keeping units (SKUs) and handling large amounts of data. We return to this issue in Section 15.2.2.

15.2.2 Open Source Software

In contrast to proprietary solutions, open source software is freely available for anyone to use. In this case, the source code is released so that the users are granted the rights to study, use, change, and distribute the software to anyone and for any purpose. This is the fundamental difference from proprietary (or closed source) software where licenses are purchased and the source code is not open to 'play with'. The publicly available nature of open source software (being reflective of the very nature of scientific research) has made it very popular with academics. The rigour with which such software is often (but not always) prepared, its transparency and free use has made it very popular with industry too. This is also because open source solutions can be 'called' and integrated with other proprietary solutions.

A most popular open source software is R. It runs on a large number of platforms, from Microsoft Windows and MacOS to Linux, with new versions being released very frequently. Other advantages of R (aside from its zero cost of course) include the large number of user-contributed packages, its production-quality graphics, and the capability to extend its functionality by linking fast-compiled C/C++/Fortran code. It has been claimed that, overall, 'it compares favourably to professionally produced and quality controlled commercial software' (Kolassa and Hyndman 2010). Further, and since R is open source, users may look at the source code, if they are unsure whether functionality is implemented correctly, and change things accordingly.

Unfortunately, R is mainly command line based, and although graphical user interfaces (GUIs) such as R Studio and R Commander (Rcmdr) exist to make life easier for beginners, it does require a steep learning curve. Another disadvantage is the lack of speed when dealing with truly massive amounts of data.

User contributed packages for time-series forecasting extend the native R forecasting capabilities. As will be discussed later in the chapter, many of the methods presented in this book have actually been implemented in R. However, R's general purpose means that users must write their own code if, for example, forecasts will be used for subsequent decisions, such as inventory optimisation. Such specific requirements may ultimately demand specific software – or a lot of work in R (Kolassa and Hyndman 2010) or any other open source software, such as Python. This point was reinforced by Fildes et al. (2020), who warned of the potential expense of programming a feature into a standard package.

This raises an important issue about the expertise levels of those using software. Proprietary software is designed *for* the (average) user, whereas open source software is designed (at least in part) *by* the user. As such, proprietary software has an advantage over open source software because it offers accessible solutions to a wide range of users. Users are only required to possess a minimum understanding of the software's functions (in our case, some understanding of what forecasting is about), but not how it is designed (i.e. where the forecasts come from). This advantage, however, is also a disadvantage as proprietary software does not require any engagement by the user with the underlying principles upon which the software is built. Therefore, there is no guarantee that the software will be used either extensively or effectively. If users do not understand where the forecasts come from, then the software is essentially a black box. In this case, the software may not be extensively used, or there may be unnecessary judgemental intervention, as discussed in Chapter 10.

In cases where the functions of the software are used more extensively, these functions may be less effective if users do not possess sufficient knowledge to exploit them fully.

15.2.3 Hybrid Solutions

Interestingly, the widespread application of open source software makes it feasible to integrate, say, R routines in in-house developed solutions. Also, it makes it possible to call such routines and integrate them with proprietary software. Currently, there is a more general emphasis by software designers on enabling extensions of software through additional programming. The new SAP APO, for example, is an open system, with additional functionality being possible with macro programming and ABAP (advanced business application programming).

Proprietary systems have been extensively tested, will not 'fall over' and do come with (extensive) ongoing technical support. However, their customisation potential, in terms of functionality, is limited and they may be very expensive. Another issue is that they often contain their own proprietary methods, which may not have been tested in publicly available research. Open source software, by contrast, is free to use and increasingly popular with industry and academia alike. It needs to be tested though, and appropriately linked to subsequent decisions. Also, only forecasters with a technical background and who are comfortable with the command line can benefit fully from open source software.

In our view, the strengths of open source and proprietary software are complementary. Moreover, there seem to be excellent opportunities for software companies to embed open source solutions in their products. The same is true for companies that employ data science, analytics, or operational research teams who could amend their proprietary software on the basis of what is available in R, Python, or other solutions.

15.2.4 Summary

A taxonomy of software solutions was discussed in this section, to allow a better understanding of how (inventory) forecasting features within these solutions: from stand-alone algorithms that execute specific forecasting methods in open source software, to specialist forecasting software packages, to higher level (supply chain) modular packages that contain forecasting algorithms in a component-based fashion, and to ERP packages. This classification allows us to evaluate software packages against their intended use, and in relation to the business needs they serve. We discuss evaluation in the next section, where we also consider how to foster greater utilisation.

15.3 Framework for Software Evaluation

An intuitively appealing way of addressing forecasting software requirements was proposed by Tashman and Hoover (2001), in their review of software features. This constitutes a framework that can be used to evaluate and assess various aspects of forecasting software solutions. We should note that this framework emphasises forecasting rather than inventory forecasting, which is the focus of this book. This section concentrates on general requirements. In the following section, we turn to the particular requirements for intermittent demand.

15.3.1 Key Aspects of Software Evaluation

The framework put forward by Tashman and Hoover (2001) encompasses the following elements: (i) preparation of data; (ii) method selection; (iii) method implementation; (iv) method evaluation; (v) assessment of uncertainty; (vi) forecast presentation; and (vii) forecasting across a product hierarchy. These topics were also covered by Fildes et al. (2018) in their review of forecast software commissioned by *ORMS Today* (published by the Institute for Operations Research & Management Science, INFORMS). The elements of the framework are discussed below.

Preparation of data: The quality of the output of a process is typically conditioned by the quality of the data inputted. This is certainly the case with forecasting software, where method selection and forecast calculations are dependent upon the quality of the data. In an inventory forecasting context, demand data and stock levels are the most important issues. With regard to the former, it is known that sales are often used as a proxy for demand – which is what should drive calculations. As discussed in the first chapter of this book, demand information may often not be available, especially in retail operations where lost sales are not known. Are there any functions to allow demand to be better approximated by sales? This is a highly desirable feature of software packages. Also, it is well known that inventory record inaccuracy is a major problem in industry, whereby what we think we have in stock (as recorded by the information system) differs from what we actually have in stock (due to a wide range of reasons, such as theft, misplacement, damage, and scanning errors) (Rekik et al. 2019). The extent to which this discrepancy is addressed determines the validity of the inventory calculations performed in the system.

Method selection: Methods are selected on the basis of the features present in the data. Automatic identification of time series components is crucial in this process. However, enabling some visual identification of what may drive the time series evolution (say trend and/or seasonality) may be equally important. There has been some research showing that judgemental forecast model selection may be effective (Petropoulos et al. 2018).

Method implementation refers to decisions and functionality related to implementing a method. There are two critical aspects of method implementation:

1. The first refers to the difference between what is available for implementation and what is actually utilised. Utilisation rates of software systems are very low and, in that respect, it is important not only to enrich functionality with new features but also to appropriately motivate users to fully understand and take advantage of that functionality. Further, it is the right functionality we should care about. A wide range of inappropriate methods is not necessarily helpful. This equally applies to method selection, implementation, and evaluation.

2. The second relates to the difference between live (real-time) implementation and simulation capabilities that enable what-if analysis and learning by using the system. These are not the same thing. The former is what one may use for real-time inventory forecasting. The latter enables the user to see what would have happened if a particular method or approach had been implemented in a particular way (see Chapter 9).

This enables experimentation, engagement with the system, and ultimately increased understanding and learning about forecasting.

Method evaluation and assessment of uncertainty: Forecast error metrics are useful both for selecting (optimising) a method and for reporting forecast accuracy results. It has been argued that the selection of forecast error metrics is as important as that of the forecast methods themselves (Kolassa 2020). Further, forecast-implication metrics may also be used to inform an appropriate assessment of the implications of forecasting for decision-making, as discussed in Chapter 9.

Forecast presentation: Good forecast presentation will help to demystify the forecasts and reveal the foundations on which they are built. This is essential for an understanding of the soundness (or otherwise) of these foundations and the plausibility of the forecasts. It should include a description of assumptions, an explanation of and justification for the method selected, a graphical demonstration of the forecasts and their progression from historical patterns, a description and illustration of how the forecasts are generated, and a presentation of the uncertainty surrounding the forecasts.

Intelligent forecast presentation can help not only demand planners' appreciation of forecasts but also more senior colleagues who are responsible for strategic inventory decisions. We concur with the following statement by Tashman and Hoover (2001, p. 667): 'Gaining acceptance for forecasts is partly an educational process: the more decision makers learn about forecasting and statistical methodology, the better they will be able to recognize effective forecasting efforts'.

Forecasting across a product hierarchy (cross-sectional forecasting): Given its importance, this topic is treated separately from method implementation by Tashman and Hoover in their framework. Hierarchical forecasting offers interesting method implementation opportunities: bottom-up, top-down and optimal reconciliation (Hyndman et al. 2011). In addition to cross-sectional aggregation, temporal aggregation is also crucial as it may act as a method's self-improving mechanism, as previously discussed. Moreover, aggregation across both cross-sections and time (e.g. planning horizons) can prove beneficial (Kourentzes and Athanasopoulos 2019).

15.3.2 Additional Criteria

We discuss now a number of additional criteria that are not addressed in previous evaluation frameworks but arguably are equally important. Tashman and Hoover (2001) state explicitly that they do not address the following in their framework: interface, price, and technical support. These issues are discussed below.

The (design of the) interface is a very important issue as it determines the extent to which users can or cannot engage at a first level with the software. Some software packages are easier to use than others and an intuitively appealing interface is likely to result in the software being perceived as less of a 'black box'.

Although price may not always be the most important selection criterion for large organisations, it will surely influence the choice of software packages in smaller companies. It would also be important when universities or research institutes buy software for research and educational purposes.

The technical support offered to software users is as important as the software itself. Software companies complement their offering with the provision of support in terms of installation and integration within existing systems, and with training. The latter typically takes the form of familiarisation with the system and its functionality. But if training were to go beyond the 'help' functions, to actually enable the users to learn about the methods they are using, then this would be a very desirable feature. This is a key issue and we dedicate a separate section to this topic later in the chapter.

15.3.3 Summary

The extent to which software programs facilitate good practices in the selection, evaluation, and presentation of appropriate forecasting methods varies. A set of guiding principles to enable the assessment of forecasting software was discussed in this section. This should be a helpful starting point for organisations wishing to invest in new software packages or evaluate the capabilities of existing ones.

15.4 Software Features and Their Availability

In this section, we extend the discussion on software evaluation to consider some features specifically related to intermittent demand forecasting. Following that, we summarise the key methods and approaches we have advocated in this book and assess the extent to which they are currently implemented in software solutions.

15.4.1 Software Features for Intermittent Demand

Although the basic principles applying to demand forecasting in general are also applicable to the case of intermittent demand forecasting in particular, the latter calls for some additional considerations. These stem from the very structure of the time series.

Preparation of data: The detection of outliers in intermittent demand time series is not an easy task. Because of their occasional lumpy behaviour, it is very difficult to distinguish between particularly erratic demand sizes and observations that are genuine outliers. Nevertheless, the facility to include 'exception rules' to flag very large orders is a useful feature in software, as it enables such orders to be handled differently from other orders.

Method selection: Operationalised rules are available to distinguish between intermittent and non-intermittent demand patterns, as previously discussed in this book. Although these rules have empirical support and are used by both proprietary and open source software packages, an effective graphical display of the series' characteristics should facilitate further judgemental selection of appropriate forecast methods.

Method implementation: Temporal aggregation is a natural consideration for intermittent demand forecasting, and there is empirical evidence to suggest that it may offer forecast accuracy benefits. However, temporal aggregation is seldom supported by proprietary software packages and, when it is, this support may be erroneous. For example, the default time bucket may be a week (e.g. refer to the forecasting engine of SAP R/3 when daily forecasts are actually needed. As it stands, the weekly forecasts provided must be disaggregated in order to obtain daily forecasts using this software. This disaggregation is a form of obligatory temporal manipulation, as opposed to an elective one that is driven by forecast accuracy comparisons.

Method evaluation: We have argued against the use of a single error measure, based on absolute errors, for intermittent demand. Such measures are considered as 'standard' and therefore are expected to be present in most forecasting software packages. For intermittent demand, the mean absolute percentage error (MAPE) should not be reported at all. For other absolute measures (e.g. mean absolute error, MAE), it is important that they are reported alongside equivalent signed errors (e.g. mean error, ME) in dashboards that facilitate their joint reading and collective interpretation. The inclusion of more recently developed measures, which can be read on their own (e.g. scaled mean square error, sMSE) would be desirable. Development of more intelligent error measure dashboards for intermittence would make performance management easier and more effective.

Forecast presentation: The importance of graphical display of intermittent demand (forecasts) has been highlighted in the literature (Boylan and Syntetos 2010), but currently there is nothing available, as far as we are aware, over and above the standard presentation of such information for fast demand items, to recognise the size-interval structure of the time series.

15.4.2 Availability of Software Features

We now consider what distributions, methods, and error metrics are available for implementation in practice, focussing on those that have been advocated in this book.

Distributional assumptions: Empirical evidence (and intuitive appeal) supports the use of the negative binomial distribution (NBD) or stuttering Poisson to represent intermittent demand patterns. The former is available in much inventory forecasting software; the latter is not. The normal distribution still dominates software applications. Relevant as it may be for long lead times, its value diminishes for modelling per-period intermittent demand.

Forecasting methods: We advocate the use of SBA. If not available, the minimum requirement is Croston's method (in conjunction with appropriate variance estimation). Croston's method is incorporated in statistical forecasting software packages (e.g. Forecast Pro), and demand planning modules of component based enterprise and manufacturing solutions (e.g. Industrial and Financial Systems, IFS AB). It is also included in integrated real-time S&OP processes (e.g. SAP APO 4.0). SBA is available in iqast and Vanguard Software. SBA and Croston are coded in R software, and both are utilised by in-house developed solutions we are familiar with. Model-based methods, discussed in Chapter 14, have yet to achieve any significant adoption for intermittent demand forecasting. Further empirical validation is needed for these methods, and this should facilitate their adoption more widely. More advanced methods, based on general linear models, are available in R (Liboschik et al. 2017).

Empirical methods: We also advocate the use of bootstrapping for directly estimating percentiles of the demand distribution; this is incorporated in Smart Forecasts.

Aggregation approaches: We have discussed the importance of cross-sectional and temporal aggregation for forecasting. The former is supported by inventory forecasting packages, but the latter rarely is. However, temporal aggregation is supported by SAS and algorithms are available in R software (Hyndman and Kourentzes 2018).

Classification for forecasting: The four-quadrant type (SBC) method we have discussed, and provided evidence for, is becoming more commonly implemented in software, including Blue Yonder and LLamasoft.

Forecast error metrics: We have advocated the concurrent use of two scaled error metrics towards a more constructive evaluation of forecast accuracy and a better diagnosis of the forecasting system. As yet, there are no systems that provide the user with a cross-cutting view across scaled error metrics; instead, these metrics can only be consulted individually. More recently developed error metrics, which can be read on their own, such as the sMSE, are not yet available in commercial software, although sMSE is available in the *Greybox* R package (Svetunkov and Sagaert 2020).

Table 15.1 summarises the key methods, distributions, and approaches we have advocated in this book, accompanied by an assessment of the extent to which they are implemented in software solutions. We distinguish between proprietary and open source software, and we present in-house developed solutions separately.

Table 15.1 offers some encouragement, as there are few blank spaces. However, there is limited implementation of some key methods and approaches in proprietary software, indicating that there is still some way to go before the state of the art in intermittent demand forecasting is reflected in practice.

15.4.3 Summary

The trend over the last decade towards 'big data', which is facilitated by new developments in database technology, has major implications for forecasting in supply chains (Syntetos

Table 15.1 Software implementation.

Approaches	Type of software		
	Proprietary	Open source	In-house
Negative binomial	★ ★	☆	☆
Stuttering Poisson		☆	☆
Croston	★ ★	☆	☆
SBA	★	☆	☆
Empirical methods	★		☆
Temporal aggregation	★	☆	☆
Four quadrants	★ ★	☆	☆
Error metrics	★	☆	☆

Notes: ★ ★ wide implementation; ★ limited implementation; and ☆ implementation.

et al. 2016a). Data are kept at finer and finer granularities. For example, whereas in the past, retailers would store aggregated sales on an SKU by outlet on a weekly basis, today they commonly keep far more disaggregated data, at least on a daily level. Highly granular data raise the question of what aggregation level to forecast on and leads to the problem of forecasting intermittent time series. It is only natural to expect that intermittent demand forecasting will become even more relevant as time goes by and, in this section, we discussed: (i) some important features that software packages must contain to support intermittent demand forecasting and (ii) what methods and approaches advocated in this book are, or are not, being used in software applications.

15.5 Training

Let us now focus on the issue of training and whether this could foster higher and more effective utilisation of forecasting software. Forecasting software packages have statistical foundations but are being used by people who may or may not have a statistical background. How to balance, then, functionality and its comprehension?

As previously discussed, if users do not understand how the forecasts are produced, then it is likely that the software will be perceived as a black box. In this case, the software will not be used extensively or, if it is, it will be not be exploited fully and may be subject to unnecessary judgemental intervention.

Training can allow users to engage more deeply with a software package, but there is a great variation as to what may constitute training. Is this about clicking the right buttons, or understanding enough to be able to 'play' with methods and produce alternative forecasts, or specifying parameters for the methods themselves, or understanding fully what these methods are about and thus making informed decisions as to what should be used when? Forecasting software manufacturers can (and very often do) provide training in terms of how to use their software. However, this does not ensure understanding of the fundamentals of forecasting or, even further, the statistical principles underlying the development of forecasting methods. Companies should supplement the introduction of forecast software packages with training courses that would allow users to make the most of those packages. Given time and resource constraints, though, it is not always feasible to introduce an extensive coverage of all that a forecast software package does. This prompts the question as to how extensive the forecasting functionality should be. Few robust methods that are likely to perform well in a wide range of situations, and are simple enough to be taught to the users, may compare favourably to a wide range of methods that may incrementally advance accuracy at the expense of hindering understanding. This is an important argument and, from that perspective, less may sometimes be more.

Further, and as already discussed in this chapter, there is an important distinction between using software packages for real time decision-making, and using them as simulation tools and what-if scenario planners. The latter allow users to appreciate the implications of their decisions, and better engage with what the software has to offer. Not all forecast software packages offer this feature. In fact, this is a more popular feature in inventory packages than in forecasting software. Take, as an example, the Inventory Strategist function of RightStock, presented in Chapter 3 (Figure 3.3). This software estimates the effects on inventories of altering a number of quantities, including the target service level and the lead times. This allows managers to experiment with these variables and identify the 'best' target cycle service levels for different lead time settings.

Ideally, being able to monitor and track the inventory implications of alternative forecasting choices is what ultimately should be promoted in software. Allowing users to evaluate what different forecasts may imply in terms of inventory investments (and service levels) should lead to the most effective use of software packages. This enables forecasting choices to be linked to their inventory performance implications, as discussed in Chapter 9.

15.5.1 Summary

Training users of forecasting software on the software's functionality is an important enabler of its utilisation. The deeper the user's knowledge is, the higher and more effective the software's utilisation will be. Software packages are only facilitators of the forecasting task, which ultimately will involve human beings too. No matter the degree of automation associated with a software package, there is an array of decisions that need to be made, all of which involve human judgement. These include the very basic decision as to which software to choose, what functionality is activated and what is not, accepting (or not) default options and (re-)setting model selection and method parameter calculations, selecting what error metrics to use to report accuracy, and superimposing judgement on the forecasts produced by the software. The deeper the knowledge of forecasting, the more informed (and thus more effective) the above decisions will be. No matter how good or advanced a software's capabilities are, judgement is an indispensable part of the forecasting process. But is it possible that the software package itself may support, in an interactive way, the process of exercising judgement? This would lead to an elevated concept of software packages: systems that support the forecasting process. We discuss this in Section 15.6.

15.6 Forecast Support Systems

Forecast Support Systems (FSS) are systems designed on the premise that the human factor is an indispensable part of the forecasting process, thereby emphasising both the capabilities and limitations of humans. They bring the human element to the forefront of the forecasting process by highlighting the importance of 'soft' factors and their interaction with an, otherwise, automated system. Apart from general user experience and user interface requirements, FSS features reflect the following important issues that differentiate them from software packages (Fildes et al. 2006; see also Fildes and Goodwin 2012):

Taking account of the organisational context: This will determine the qualitative information that needs to be stored to enable forecasters to produce judgemental forecasts or judgementally adjust statistical forecasts.

Assigning responsibilities for the forecasting task: Clear responsibilities about the forecasting task lead to removing system inadequacies as a source of blame for failure to meet targets.

Fostering ease of use and ease of understanding of the system: The easier the system is to use and understand, the higher its effective utilisation will be.

Taking known cognitive and behavioural biases into account: This would include display-ing statistical and business information about a time series to be forecast, allowing for judgemental adjustments, providing for, or even requiring, the user to give reasons for adjustments, tracking, monitoring, and evaluating adjustments, providing feedback and enabling users to share information within the system. Ultimately, this leads to a system that emphasises user guidance and fosters learning.

Linking forecast accuracy to business performance: Enabling forecasters to see the implica-tions of their forecasts (for inventory control, in the context of this book) ensures that such forecasts are used effectively for decision-making.

In principle, addressing the above issues, collectively, should lead to a system that may support forecasting more effectively than current software packages. There is some evi-dence to suggest that when forecasters are guided along the lines discussed above, per-formance improves (Petropoulos et al. 2016). Some of the FSS features have already been addressed by software packages, either fully (e.g. in terms of pertinent information storage and retrieval) or partly (e.g. in terms of linking accuracy to business performance), whereas others constitute work in progress. Admittedly, the operationalisation and implementation of such features in not always an easy task and we are yet to see how FSSs will be adopted by industry.

15.6.1 Summary

There is often an unfortunate interchangeable use of terms 'FSS' and 'forecast software', when the latter is only a part of the former. FSSs emphasise both understanding of the algorithms and interpreting the results provided by forecast software.

There has been a considerable amount of theoretical and empirical work in this area, and it is due to that work that we now have a clear idea of what an FSS may include and how advantageous the constructive incorporation of human judgement can be. At the time of writing, better understanding is needed on how judgement should be aided (De Baets and Harvey 2018) and how to operationalise some of the FSS features advocated in the literature.

15.7 Alternative Perspectives

At this point, we wish to discuss two other perspectives on intermittent demand fore-casting, not previously considered in the book. They are both methodologically different to the approaches discussed in the preceding chapters. The first, Bayesian methods, rely upon a different statistical paradigm than that underlying all discussions that have been undertaken so far. The second, neural network methods, are data-driven. We touched on this issue in Chapter 12, when we discussed explanatory/causal methods. Both approaches are computationally intensive, but it is worthwhile considering them here, given ongoing computational advancements, the lack of which has hindered their implementation in the past.

15.7.1 Bayesian Methods

Unlike the methods discussed in Chapter 6, Bayesian methods provide a formal way to incorporate into the forecasting task some prior information we often possess about the data, before seeing such data. They use Bayes' Theorem to update a prior distribution (probabilities specified prior to data collection) into a posterior distribution (the probabilities following data analysis), by incorporating information (likelihoods) provided by the observed data.

The Bayesian approach, with its own statistical theory, has been applied successfully in many areas and forecasting contexts. Its major strength is that it provides practitioners with an opportunity to incorporate intuition and previous experience in a quantifiable form by making an appropriate choice of the prior distribution. Practitioners can select a prior with a value for the variance that reflects their perceived level of uncertainty about the distribution of demand. As demand evolves, the observed data are used to update the likelihood function and, as a result, the posterior distribution of demand. The ability to combine such diverse information and sources of uncertainty, and revise and update it as more data are acquired is particularly appealing when data are scarce, or there are considerable changes in the data.

Aronis et al. (2004), based on the work of Popovic (1987), proposed a Bayesian method in which demand has a Poisson distribution and the prior distribution is gamma. This leads to a posterior distribution equivalent to the NBD. In addition to its intuitive appeal, the proposed method has the advantage of offering a closed form expression of the lead time demand distribution that can be used in a straightforward way to calculate the order-up-to level. However, to the best of our knowledge, the performance of this method has not yet been empirically evaluated. Dolgui and Pashkevich (2008) proposed a Bayesian method assuming the demand to follow the binomial distribution and using the beta distribution as the prior. This results in a beta-binomial posterior distribution, which has some challenges with respect to the estimation of its parameters, and empirical evidence is yet to be provided in support of the beta-binomial for intermittent demands.

An important problem associated with Bayesian methods relates to the analytically intractable posterior distributions that often result from them. Simulation methods (Markov chain Monte Carlo, MCMC, in particular) may be used in such cases to estimate the parameters of interest (see, for example, Neal and Rao 2007). However, we still know relatively little about the viability and performance of Bayesian methods in intermittent demand forecasting contexts.

15.7.2 Neural Networks

The continued growth in computing power has facilitated the implementation of computationally intensive methods. Neural networks (NN), in particular, have attracted considerable attention as a plausible way to forecast demand. NNs are data driven machine learning algorithms; the idea behind them is to mimic the functionality of the human brain for solving problems. In a time series context, input information (demand time series characteristics) is linked to output information (demand forecasts) through a network of 'neurons'. These operate in a number of (hidden) layers, and neurons in each layer are functions of neurons in previous layers. In an intermittent demand context, NNs allow for interactions between the demand size and the inter-demand intervals of demand events, or their lags, if such can be identified from the data.

Early research that used NNs to forecast intermittent demand was presented by Gutierrez et al. (2008). The researchers proposed a NN method that outperformed, in their experiments, SES, Croston's method, and the SBA on the basis of the MAD : Mean ratio (described as the 'MAPE', following Gilliland 2002), the relative geometric root mean square error (RGRMSE), and percentage best (based on absolute errors). In a follow-up work, the same researchers (Mukhopadhyay et al. 2012) showed empirically the outperformance of a simple (three-layer) NN method, based on the same data set, error measures, and benchmark forecast methods used by Gutierrez et al. (2008). Kourentzes (2013) replicated the method of Gutierrez et al. (2008) and evaluated a new NN method. This method adopted a more flexible modelling framework, allowing for interaction between demand sizes and intervals. The accuracy results, based on the mean error (ME) and mean absolute error (MAE), showed little benefit in using NNs over parametric methods. However, an evaluation of the impact of the NN forecasts on an (R, S) inventory system (with $R = 1$) showed improvements in cycle service levels and fill rates, albeit at some cost from increased stock holding.

Lolli et al. (2017) considered a set of NN methods (associated with different input patterns, architectures, and 'training'), comparing their empirical performance with SBA and Croston on 24 real time series. Performance was evaluated by means of a 'MAPE' (MAD : Mean ratio) and the ratio of the ME to the average demand (ME/A). The results indicated a superior performance of one of the NN alternatives in terms of the 'MAPE'. The ME/A results did not indicate any performance differences. Finally, some good inventory efficiency was reported by Babai et al. (2020) who compared a new NN method with SES, Croston, and SBA, and also two bootstrapping methods (Willemain et al. 2004; Zhou and Viswanathan 2011). Their results were obtained by means of experimentation on more than 5000 spare parts demand series from an airline company.

For intermittent demand, caution is needed in putting too much emphasis on findings based on absolute errors, as discussed in Chapter 9. Those studies including inventory evaluations should prove more robust although, even then, care is needed in extrapolating from one inventory system to another.

15.7.3 Summary

In this section, we discussed developments in Bayesian and NN methods, made feasible for large collections of SKUs by increased computing power. It is too early to predict the uptake of such methods in industry, but we anticipate more research into their empirical performance in the near future.

15.8 Way Forward

So, what is the way forward? There is much that remains to be done in terms of (i) theory development, (ii) empirical validation of what is already available, and (iii) enhancing the communication between industry and academia to bridge the gap between theory and practice. Let us start with a summary of the key theoretical gaps identified in previous chapters, followed by various areas where further empirical knowledge is needed. We then discuss how to foster tighter links between academic researchers and practitioner-users of academic research.

In terms of further theoretical developments, the following issues have been highlighted in this book:

- Forecasting of demand variance is as important as forecasting mean demand (Chapter 7). However, less is known about the former despite its relevance for determining inventory requirements.
- Linking forecast accuracy to inventory performance or, more generally, understanding the interface between forecasting and inventory control is perhaps the most important and promising area for future developments (see Chapters 9 and 12).
- Predicting entire distributions (rather than producing point forecasts) is more compatible with the requirements of inventory control; there is more that needs to be done in this area, as discussed in Chapters 9, 13, and 14.

The above are very promising areas for future research, and addressing these gaps should enable important theoretical developments in intermittent demand inventory forecasting. Similarly, there are a number of areas that would benefit from empirical knowledge and insights.

- There is some evidence to suggest that temporal aggregation may be particularly helpful for forecasting mean demand. However, less is known about the effects of cross-sectional aggregation, both when considered over a single time period, or over multiple (temporally aggregated) periods (please refer to Chapter 6).
- Measuring forecast accuracy in an intermittent demand context is not a straightforward exercise, as discussed in Chapter 9. Understanding the behaviour of the (combination of the) metrics we have advocated, in real-world applications, requires further testing and experimentation.
- There is a lack of empirical evidence on the performance of the model based methods discussed in Chapter 14. Understanding when accuracy improvements are achievable should offer a valuable guide towards their implementation.
- Computationally intensive (machine learning) methods are currently attracting a lot of attention both in academic research and industry. We are yet to understand fully how these methods should be best utilised in practice. The same applies to the use of Bayesian methods, that were discussed earlier in this chapter.

Whilst developments in these areas would be very desirable, they remain only of academic interest if they are not used in practice. It is crucially important that theory development, empirically tested, is operationalised in software packages. We have commented previously on the need for improved communication between academia and practice (Boylan and Syntetos 2016) and software packages can facilitate that communication and help to bridge the gap between them.

Academics should pay greater attention to forecasting in organisations to complement the more theoretical work they are conducting on method development. Further, they should undertake more academic and case-oriented research to offer frameworks for evaluating forecasting and its impact on business performance. Companies can help by sharing data more readily with universities, and academics should put greater emphasis on the empirical testing of methods (claimed to work well) in industry. Finally, software providers should be more proactive in collaborating with universities on the implementation of new methods, particularly those that have performed well in empirical tests.

In summary, there are some promising avenues for further research and empirical testing put forward in this book, and addressing these issues should be of great value for the theory and practice of intermittent demand inventory forecasting. For this value to be realised, it is vital for universities and companies to work more closely together, and for software providers to facilitate the transition of knowledge and information between them.

15.9 Chapter Summary

In this chapter, we have discussed the extent to which the methods and approaches previously considered in the book are actually implemented in practice. To do so, some alternative types of software packages were considered, enabling us to determine what is currently available for implementation and what is yet to be done to enable the full utilisation of the knowledge available in intermittent demand inventory forecasting.

We have argued for the importance of training for software users; this could help narrow the gap between academia and industry, a gap we are particularly concerned with. Academics are often accused of not researching issues of practical relevance, resulting in forecasting theory lagging behind real-world practices. Although this is often true, the converse is also frequently the case. Practitioners and software developers do not often employ methods or approaches that have been shown in empirical studies to be both effective and easy to implement, thus leading to real-world practices lagging behind theoretical developments. Closing the gap between industry and academia is absolutely vital and we hope that this book is a good step in that direction.

Technical Note

Note 15.1: Evolution of ERP Systems

ERP systems evolved from attempts to streamline inventory management through material requirements planning (MRP) systems (see Chapter 2) in the 1960s and 1970s. Such systems integrated data across three organisational functions: engineering/design, inventory (control), and purchasing. Integrating information related to the bill of materials (from Engineering) with information on what is available in stock (from Inventory) and the lead times for purchasing raw materials from suppliers (from Purchasing) enabled (as it still does) job shop scheduling and production planning. Built on the technological foundations of MRP (and extensions thereafter, through MRP II), ERP systems integrate business processes across activities of the organisation's value chain.

References

Adelson, R.M. (1966). Compound Poisson distributions. *Operational Research Quarterly* 17: 73–75.

Akaike, H. (1973). Information theory and an extension of the maximum likelihood principle. In: *Proceedings of the 2nd International Symposium on Information Theory* (ed. B.N. Petrov and F. Csáki). Budapest: Akadémiai Kiadó. Republished in: (1992). *Breakthroughs in Statistics*, vol. 1 (ed. S. Kotz and N.L. Johnson). New York, NY: Springer-Verlag.

Al-Osh, M.A. and Aly, E.-E. (1992). First order autoregressive time series with negative binomial and geometric marginals. *Communications in Statistics - Theory and Methods* 21: 2483–2492.

Al-Osh, M.A. and Alzaid, A.A. (1987). First-order integer-valued autoregressive (INAR(1)) process. *Journal of Time Series Analysis* 8: 261–275.

Al-Osh, M.A. and Alzaid, A.A. (1988). Integer-valued moving average (INMA) process. *Statistical Papers* 29: 281–300.

Altay, N., Litteral, L.A., and Rudisill, F. (2012). Effects of correlation on intermittent demand forecasting and stock control. *International Journal of Production Economics* 135: 275–283.

Altay, N., Rudisill, F., and Litteral, L.A. (2008). Adapting Wright's modification of Holt's method to forecasting intermittent demand. *International Journal of Production Economics* 111: 389–408.

Alzaid, A.A. and Omair, M.A. (2014). Poisson difference integer valued autoregressive model of order one. *Bulletin of the Malaysian Mathematical Sciences Society* 37: 465–485.

Armstrong, J.S. (1985). *Long-Range Forecasting: From Crystal Ball to Computer*, 2e. New York, NY: Wiley-Interscience.

Aronis, K.-P., Magou, L., Dekker, R., and Tagaras, G. (2004). Inventory control of spare parts using a Bayesian approach: a case study. *European Journal of Operational Research* 154: 730–739.

Athanasopoulos, G., Hyndman, R.J., Kourentzes, N., and Petropoulos, F. (2017). Forecasting with temporal hierarchies. *European Journal of Operational Research* 262: 60–74.

Aucamp, D.C. and Barringer, R.L. (1987). A table for the calculation of safety stock. *Journal of Operations Management* 7: 153–163.

Axsäter, S. (2015). *Inventory Control*, 3e. Switzerland: Springer International.

Babai, M.Z., Ali, M.M., and Nikolopoulos, K. (2012). Impact of temporal aggregation on stock control performance of intermittent demand estimators: empirical analysis. *Omega* 40: 713–721.

Babai, M.Z., Dallery, Y., Boubaker, S., and Kalai, R. (2019). A new method to forecast intermittent demand in the presence of inventory obsolescence. *International Journal of Production Economics* 209: 30–41.

Babai, M.Z., Syntetos, A.A., and Teunter, R. (2010). On the empirical performance of (*T,s,S*) heuristics. *European Journal of Operational Research* 202: 466–472.

Babai, M.Z., Syntetos, A.A., and Teunter, R. (2014). Intermittent demand forecasting: an empirical study on accuracy and the risk of obsolescence. *International Journal of Production Economics* 157: 212–219.

Babai, M.Z., Tsadiras, A., and Papadopoulos, C. (2020). On the empirical performance of some new neural network methods for forecasting intermittent demand. *IMA Journal of Management Mathematics* 31: 281–305.

Badkook, B. (2016). Study to determine the aircraft on ground (AOG) cost of the Boeing 777 fleet at X airline. *American Scientific Research Journal for Engineering, Technology, and Sciences* 25: 51–71.

Bagchi, U. (1983). Compound distributions for slow-moving items. Paper presented at the 15th Annual Meeting, *American Institute of Decision Sciences*.

Bagchi, U. (1987). Modeling lead-time demand for lumpy demand and variable lead time. *Naval Research Logistics* 34: 687–704.

Bagchi, U., Hayya, J.C., and Chu, C.-H. (1986). The effect of lead-time variability: the case of independent demand. *Journal of Operations Management* 6: 159–177.

Bartezzaghi, E. and Verganti, R. (1995). Managing demand uncertainty through order overplanning. *International Journal of Production Economics* 40: 107–120.

Bartezzaghi, E., Verganti, R., and Zotteri, G. (1999). A simulation framework for forecasting uncertain lumpy demand. *International Journal of Production Economics* 59: 499–510.

Bijvank, M., Huh, W.T., Janakiraman, G., and Kang, W. (2014). Robustness of order-up-to policies in lost-sales inventory systems. *Operations Research* 62: 1040–1047.

Blattberg, R.C. and Hoch, S.J. (1990). Database models and managerial intuition: 50% model + 50% manager. *Management Science* 36: 887–899.

Bolger, F. and Önkal-Atay, D. (2004). The effects of feedback on judgmental interval predictions. *International Journal of Forecasting* 20: 29–39.

Boone, T., Ganeshan, R., Jain, A., and Sanders, N.R. (2019). Forecasting sales in the supply chain: consumer analytics in the big data era. *International Journal of Forecasting* 35: 170–180.

Boothroyd, H. and Tomlinson, R.C. (1963). The stock control of engineering spares - a case study. *Operational Research Quarterly* 14: 317–332.

Box, G.E.P. and Jenkins, G.M. (1962). Some statistical aspects of adaptive optimization and control. *Journal of the Royal Statistical Society: Series B (Methodological)* 24: 297–343.

Box, G.E.P., Jenkins, G.M., Reinsel, G.C., and Ljung, G.M. (2015). *Time Series Analysis: Forecasting and Control*, 5e. Hoboken, NJ: Wiley.

Boylan, J.E. (1997). *The centralisation of inventory and the modelling of demand*. PhD thesis. University of Warwick, UK.

Boylan, J.E. (2005). Intermittent and lumpy demand: a forecasting challenge. *Foresight: The International Journal of Applied Forecasting* 1: 36–42.

Boylan, J.E. (2016). Reproducibility. *IMA Journal of Management Mathematics* 27: 107–108.

Boylan, J.E. (2018). Commentary on retail forecasting. *International Journal of Forecasting* 34: 832–834.

Boylan, J.E. and Babai, M.Z. (2016). On the performance of overlapping and non-overlapping temporal demand aggregation approaches. *International Journal of Production Economics* 181: 136–144.

Boylan, J.E. and Johnston, F.R. (1994). Relationships between service level measures for inventory systems. *Journal of the Operational Research Society* 45: 838–844.

Boylan, J.E. and Johnston, F.R. (1996). Variance laws for inventory management. *International Journal of Production Economics* 45: 343–352.

Boylan, J.E. and Syntetos, A.A. (2003). Intermittent demand forecasting: size-interval methods based on averaging and smoothing. In: *Proceedings of the International Conference on Quantitative Methods in Industry and Commerce* (ed. C.C. Frangos). Athens: Technological Educational Institute. 87–96. https://www.researchgate.net/publication/342178473_Boylan_Syntetos_QMIC_2003.

Boylan, J.E. and Syntetos, A.A. (2006). Accuracy and accuracy-implication metrics for intermittent demand. *Foresight: The International Journal of Applied Forecasting* 4: 39–42.

Boylan, J.E. and Syntetos, A.A. (2007). The accuracy of a modified Croston procedure. *International Journal of Production Economics* 107: 511–517.

Boylan, J.E. and Syntetos, A.A. (2008). Forecasting for inventory management of service parts. In: *Complex System Maintenance Handbook* (ed. K.A.H. Kobbacy and D.N.P. Murthy). London: Springer-Verlag. 479–506.

Boylan, J.E. and Syntetos, A.A. (2010). Spare parts management: a review of forecasting research and extensions. *IMA Journal of Management Mathematics* 21: 227–237.

Boylan, J.E. and Syntetos, A.A. (2016). Commentary: it takes two to tango. *Foresight: The International Journal of Applied Forecasting* 42: 26–29.

Boylan, J.E., Chen, H., Mohammadipour, M., and Syntetos, A.A. (2014). Formation of seasonal groups and application of seasonal indices. *Journal of the Operational Research Society* 65: 227–241.

Boylan, J.E., Goodwin, P., Mohammadipour, M., and Syntetos, A.A. (2015). Reproducibility in forecasting research. *International Journal of Forecasting* 31: 79–90.

Boylan, J.E., Syntetos, A.A., and Karakostas, G.C. (2008). Classification for forecasting and stock control: a case study. *Journal of the Operational Research Society* 59: 473–481.

Brännäs, K. (1994). Estimation and testing in integer-valued AR(1) models. *Umea Economic Studies 335, 1994 (revised).* https://www.researchgate.net/publication/262150820_Estimation_and_Testing_in_Integer-valued_AR1_Models.

Brännäs, K. and Hall, A. (2001). Estimation in integer-valued moving average models. *Applied Stochastic Models in Business and Industry* 17: 277–291.

Brännäs, K., Hellström, J., and Nordström, J. (2002). A new approach to modelling and forecasting monthly guest nights in hotels. *International Journal of Forecasting* 18: 19–30.

Bretschneider, S. (1986). Estimating forecast variance with exponential smoothing. Some new results. *International Journal of Forecasting* 2: 349–355.

Brighton, H. and Gigerenzer, G. (2015). The bias bias. *Journal of Business Research* 68: 1772–1784.

Brown, R.G. (1956). *Exponential Smoothing for Predicting Demand*. Cambridge, MA: Arthur D. Little Inc. http://legacy.library.ucsf.edu/tid/dae94e00.

Brown, R.G. (1959). *Statistical Forecasting for Inventory Control*. New York, NY: McGraw-Hill.

Brown, R.G. (1963). *Smoothing, Forecasting and Prediction of Discrete Time Series*. Englewood Cliffs, NJ: Prentice Hall.

Brown, R.G. (1967). *Decision Rules for Inventory Management*. New York, NY: Holt, Rinehart and Winston.

Brown, R.G. (1982). *Advanced Service Parts Inventory Control*, 2e. Norwich, VT: Materials Management Systems.

Bu, R. and McCabe, B.P.M. (2008). Model selection, estimation and forecasting in INAR(p) models: a likelihood-based Markov chain approach. *International Journal of Forecasting* 24: 151–162.

Burgin, T.A. (1972). Inventory control with normal demand and gamma lead times. *Operational Research Quarterly* 23: 73–80.

Burgin, T.A. (1975). The gamma distribution and inventory control. *Operational Research Quarterly* 26: 507–525.

Burgin, T.A. and Wild, A.R. (1967). Stock control - experience and usable theory. *Operational Research Quarterly* 18: 35–52.

Cardós, M. and Babiloni, E. (2011). Exact and approximate calculation of the cycle service level in periodic review inventory policies. *International Journal of Production Economics* 131: 63–68.

Cardós, M., Miralles, C., and Ros, L. (2006). An exact calculation of the cycle service level in a generalized periodic review system. *Journal of the Operational Research Society* 57: 1252–1255.

Cattani, K.D., Jacobs, F.R., and Schoenfelder, J. (2011). Common inventory modeling assumptions that fall short: arborescent networks, Poisson demand, and single-echelon approximations. *Journal of Operations Management* 29: 488–499.

Çetinkaya, S. and Lee, C.-Y. (2000). Stock replenishment and shipment scheduling for vendor-managed inventory systems. *Management Science* 46: 217–232.

Chase, R.B., Jacobs, F.R., and Aquilano, N.J. (2006). *Operations Management for Competitive Advantage*, 11e. New York, NY: McGraw-Hill/Irwin.

Chatfield, C. (1988). Apples, oranges and mean square error. *International Journal of Forecasting* 4: 515–518.

Chatfield, C. and Goodhardt, G.J. (1973). A consumer purchasing model with Erlang inter-purchase times. *Journal of the American Statistical Association* 68: 828–835.

Chatfield, C., Koehler, A.B., Ord, J.K., and Snyder, R.D. (2001). A new look at models for exponential smoothing. *Journal of the Royal Statistical Society: Series D (The Statistician)* 50: 147–159.

Chen, H. and Boylan, J.E. (2007). Use of individual and group seasonal indices in subaggregate demand forecasting. *Journal of the Operational Research Society* 58: 1660–1671.

Chen, H. and Boylan, J.E. (2008). Empirical evidence on individual, group and shrinkage seasonal indices. *International Journal of Forecasting* 24: 525–534.

Chen, Z. and Yang, Y. (2004). *Assessing Forecast Accuracy Measures*. https://www.researchgate.net/publication/228774888.

Clark, C.E. (1957). Mathematical analysis of an inventory case. *Operations Research* 5: 627–643.

Council of Supply Chain Management Professionals (CSCMP) (Wilson, R.) (2015). *The 26th Annual State of Logistics Report*. http://rightplace.org/assets/img/uploads/resources/State-of-Logistics_Rosalyn-Wilson.pdf.

Council of Supply Chain Management Professionals (CSCMP) (Zimmerman, M.) (2019). *The 30th Annual State of Logistics Report*. Available (for purchase) at http://cscmp.org/store/detail.aspx?id=SOL-19

Croston, J.D. (1972). Forecasting and stock control for intermittent demands. *Operational Research Quarterly* 23: 289–303.

Croston, J.D. (1974). Stock levels for slow-moving items. *Operational Research Quarterly* 25: 123–130.

Da Silva, I.M.M. (2005). *Contributions to the analysis of discrete-valued time series*. PhD thesis. University of Porto, Portugal.

Davydenko, A. and Fildes, R. (2013). Measuring forecasting accuracy: the case of judgmental adjustments to SKU-level demand forecasts. *International Journal of Forecasting* 29: 510–522.

De Baets, S. and Harvey, N. (2018). Forecasting from time series subject to sporadic perturbations: effectiveness of different types of forecasting support. *International Journal of Forecasting* 34: 163–180.

DeHoratius, N. and Raman, A. (2008). Inventory record inaccuracy: an empirical analysis. *Management Science* 54: 627–641.

Deloitte Research (2006). *The Service Revolution in Global Manufacturing Industries*. New York, NY: Deloitte. https://www.researchgate.net/publication/267268075

Department of Defense (1980). *Procedures for Performing a Failure Mode, Effects and Criticality Analysis*. Military Standard, MIL-STD-1629A. Washington, DC: Department of Defense, USA. https://elsmar.com/pdf_files/Military%20Standards/mil-std-1629.pdf

Diamantopoulos, A. and Mathews, B. (1989). Factors affecting the nature and effectiveness of subjective revision in sales forecasting: an empirical study. *Managerial and Decision Economics* 10: 51–59.

Disney, S.M., Gaalman, G.J.C., Hedenstierna, C.P.T., and Hosoda, T. (2015). Fill rate in a periodic review order-up-to policy under auto-correlated normally distributed, possibly negative, demand. *International Journal of Production Economics* 170: 501–512.

Dolgui, A. and Pashkevich, M. (2008). On the performance of binomial and beta-binomial models of demand forecasting for multiple slow-moving inventory items. *Computers and Operations Research* 35: 893–905.

Donnelly, J.M. (2013). The case for managing MRO inventory. *Supply Chain Management Review* 17: 18–22, 24.

Dunn, R., Reader, S., and Wrigley, N. (1983). An investigation of the assumptions of the NBD model as applied to purchasing at individual stores. *Journal of the Royal Statistical Society: Series C (Applied Statistics)* 32: 249–259.

Dunsmuir, W.T.M. and Snyder, R.D. (1989). Control of inventories with intermittent demand. *European Journal of Operational Research* 40: 16–21.

Durbin, J. and Koopman, S.J. (2012). *Time Series Analysis by State Space Methods*, 2e. Oxford: Oxford University Press.

Eaves, A.H.C. (2002). *Forecasting for the ordering and stock-holding of consumable spare parts.* PhD thesis. University of Lancaster, UK.

Eaves, A.H.C. and Kingsman, B.G. (2004). Forecasting for the ordering and stock-holding of spare parts. *Journal of the Operational Research Society* 55: 431–437.

Ehrhardt, R. (1979). The power approximation for computing (s,S) inventory policies. *Management Science* 25: 777–786.

Ehrhardt, R. and Mosier, C. (1984). A revision of the power approximation for computing (s,S) policies. *Management Science* 30: 618–622.

Engelmeyer, T. (2016). *Managing Intermittent Demand.* Wiesbaden: Springer (PhD thesis. University of Wuppertal, Germany).

Fildes, R. (1992). The evaluation of extrapolative forecasting methods. *International Journal of Forecasting* 8: 81–98.

Fildes, R. and Goodwin, P. (2007). Against your better judgment? How organizations can improve their use of management judgment in forecasting. *Interfaces* 37: 570–576.

Fildes, R. and Goodwin, P. (2012). Guiding principles for the forecasting support system. *Foresight: The International Journal of Applied Forecasting* 25: 10–15.

Fildes, R. and Petropoulos, F. (2015). Improving forecast quality in practice. *Foresight: The International Journal of Applied Forecasting* 36: 5–12.

Fildes, R., Goodwin, P., and Lawrence, M. (2006). The design features of forecasting support systems and their effectiveness. *Decision Support Systems* 42: 351–361.

Fildes, R., Goodwin, P., Lawrence, M., and Nikolopoulos, K. (2009). Effective forecasting and judgmental adjustments: an empirical evaluation and strategies for improvement in supply-chain planning. *International Journal of Forecasting* 25: 3–23.

Fildes, R., Schaer, O., and Svetunkov, I. (2018). Software survey: forecasting 2018. *ORMS Today* 45 (3). Available (open access) at: https://www.informs.org/ORMS-Today/Public-Articles/June-Volume-45-Number-3/Software-Survey-Forecasting-2018.

Fildes, R., Schaer, O., Svetunkov, I., and Yusupova, A. (2020). Survey: what's new in forecasting software? *ORMS Today* 47 (4): 54–58.

Fortuin, L. and Martin, H. (1999). Control of service parts. *International Journal of Operations and Production Management* 19: 950–971.

Franses, P.H. (2014). *Expert Adjustments of Model Forecasts: Theory, Practice and Strategies for Improvement.* Cambridge: Cambridge University Press.

Gaiardelli, P., Saccani, N., and Songini, L. (2007). Performance measurement of the after-sales service network - evidence from the automotive industry. *Computers in Industry* 58: 698–708.

Galliher, H.P., Morse, P.M., and Simond, M. (1959). Dynamics of two classes of continuous-review inventory systems. *Operations Research* 7: 362–384.

GAO (1999). *Defense Inventory: Continuing Challenges in Managing Inventories and Avoiding Adverse Operational Effects*, GAO/T-NSIAD-99-83. Washington, DC: United States General Accounting Office. https://www.gao.gov/assets/t-nsiad-99-83.pdf.

GAO (2011). *DOD's 2010 Comprehensive Inventory Management Improvement Plan Addressed Statutory Requirements, but Faces Implementation Challenges*, GAO-11-240R. Washington, DC: United States Government Accountability Office. http://www.gao.gov/products/GAO-11-240R.

GAO (2012). *Defense Inventory: Actions Underway to Implement Improvement Plan, but Steps Needed to Enhance Efforts*, GAO-12-493. Washington, DC: United States Government Accountability Office. http://www.gao.gov/products/GAO-12-493.

GAO (2015). *Defense Inventory: Services Generally have Reduced Excess Inventory, but Additional Actions are Needed*, GAO-15-350. Washington, DC: United States Government Accountability Office. http://www.gao.gov/products/GAO-15-350.

GAO (2019). *Substantial Efforts Needed to Achieve Greater Progress on High-Risk Areas*, GAO-19-157SP. Washington, DC: United States Government Accountability Office. http://www.gao.gov/assets/700/697245.pdf.

Gardner, E.S. (1980). Inventory theory and the Gods of Olympus. *Interfaces* 10: 42–45.

Gardner, E.S. and Koehler, A.B. (2005). Comments on a patented bootstrapping method for forecasting intermittent demand. *International Journal of Forecasting* 21: 617–618.

Ghobbar, A.A. and Friend, C.H. (2002). Sources of intermittent demand for aircraft spare parts within airline operations. *Journal of Air Transport Management* 8: 221–231.

Ghobbar, A.A. and Friend, C.H. (2003). Evaluation of forecasting methods for intermittent parts demand in the field of aviation: a predictive model. *Computers and Operations Research* 30: 2097–2114.

Gilliland, M. (2002). Is forecasting a waste of time? *Supply Chain Management Review* 6: 16–23.

Gilliland, M. (2010). *The Business Forecasting Deal*. Hoboken, NJ: Wiley.

Glueck, J.J., Koudal, P., and Vaessen, W. (2007). *The Service Revolution: Manufacturing's Missing Crown Jewel*. Research Report. Deloitte Development LLC. https://www.researchgate.net/publication/259216993_The_service_revolution_manufacturing's_missing_crown_jewel.

Gneiting, T., Balabdaoui, F., and Raftery, A.E. (2007). Probabilistic forecasts, calibration and sharpness. *Journal of the Royal Statistical Society: Series B (Statistical Methodology)* 68: 243–268.

Goodwin, P. (1998). Enhancing judgmental sales forecasting: the role of laboratory research. In: *Forecasting with Judgment* (ed. G. Wright and P. Goodwin). Chichester: Wiley. 91–111.

Goodwin, P. and Lawton, R. (1999). On the asymmetry of the symmetric MAPE. *International Journal of Forecasting* 15: 405–408.

Green, K. and Tashman, L. (2008). Should we define forecast error as e = F − A or e = A − F?. *Foresight: The International Journal of Applied Forecasting* 10: 38–40.

Green, K. and Tashman, L. (2009). Percentage error: what denominator? *Foresight: The International Journal of Applied Forecasting* 12: 36–40.

Guijarro, E., Cardós, M., and Babiloni, E. (2012). On the exact calculation of the fill rate in a periodic review inventory policy under discrete demand patterns. *European Journal of Operational Research* 218: 442–447.

Gupta, S. (1988). Impacts of sales promotions on when, what, and how much to buy. *Journal of Marketing Research* 25: 342–355.

Gutierrez, R.S., Solis, A.O., and Mukhopadhyay, S. (2008). Lumpy demand forecasting using neural networks. *International Journal of Production Economics* 111: 409–420.

Hadley, G. and Whitin, T.M. (1963). *Analysis of Inventory Systems*. Englewood Cliffs, NJ: Prentice-Hall.

Hamilton, J.D. (1994). *Time Series Analysis*. Princeton, NJ: Princeton University Press.

Hanley, J.A., Joseph, L., Platt, R.W. et al. (2001). Visualizing the median as the minimum-deviation location. *The American Statistician* 55: 150–152.

Harrison, P.J. and Davies, O.L. (1964). The use of cumulative sum (CUSUM) techniques for the control of routine forecasts of product demand. *Operations Research* 12: 325–333.

Hasni, M., Babai, M.Z., Aguir, M.S., and Jemai, Z. (2019). An investigation on bootstrapping forecasting methods for intermittent demands. *International Journal of Production Economics* 209: 20–29.

Hastie, T., Tibshirani, R., and Friedman, J. (2009). *The Elements of Statistical Learning*, 2e. New York, NY: Springer.

Heinecke, G., Syntetos, A.A., and Wang, W. (2013). Forecasting-based SKU classification. *International Journal of Production Economics* 143: 455–462.

Herniter, J. (1971). A probabilistic market model of purchase timing and brand selection. *Management Science* 18: 102–113.

Hoover, J. (2006). Measuring forecast accuracy: omissions in today's forecasting engines and demand-planning software. *Foresight: The International Journal of Applied Forecasting* 4: 32–35.

Hu, Q., Boylan, J.E., Chen, H., and Labib, A. (2018). OR in spare parts management: a review. *European Journal of Operational Research* 266: 395–414.

Hua, Z.S., Zhang, B., Yang, J., and Tan, D.S. (2007). A new approach of forecasting intermittent demand for spare parts inventories in the process industries. *Journal of the Operational Research Society* 58: 52–61.

Hurvich, C.M. and Tsai, C.L. (1989). Regression and time series model selection in small samples. *Biometrika* 76: 297–307.

Hyndman, R.J. (2006). Another look at forecast-accuracy measures for intermittent demand. *Foresight: The International Journal of Applied Forecasting* 4: 43–46.

Hyndman, R.J. (2014). *Errors on percentage errors.* https://robjhyndman.com/hyndsight/smape.

Hyndman, R.J. and Athanasopoulos, G. (2020). *Forecasting: Principles and Practice*, 3e. Melbourne: OTexts. https://OTexts.com/fpp3.

Hyndman, R.J. and Koehler, A.B. (2006). Another look at measures of forecast accuracy. *International Journal of Forecasting* 22: 679–688.

Hyndman, R.J. and Kourentzes, N. (2018). thief: Temporal HIErarchical Forecasting. R package. http://pkg.robjhyndman.com/thief/.

Hyndman, R.J., Ahmed, R.A., Athanasopoulos, G., and Shang, H.L. (2011). Optimal combination forecasts for hierarchical time series. *Computational Statistics and Data Analysis* 55: 2579–2589.

Hyndman, R.J., Koehler, A.B., Ord, J.K., and Snyder, R.D. (2008). *Forecasting with Exponential Smoothing: The State Space Approach*. Berlin: Springer-Verlag.

Inglot, T. and Ledwina, T. (2006). Towards data driven selection of a penalty function for data driven Neyman tests. *Linear Algebra and its Applications* 417: 124–133.

Jandhyala, R., Kusters, J., Mane, P., and Sinha, A. (2018). *Sales and Operations Planning with SAP IBP*. Boston, MA: Rheinwerk Publishing.

Janssen, E. (2010). *Inventory control in case of unknown demand and control parameters.* PhD thesis. Tilburg University, The Netherlands.

Janssen, E., Strijbosch, L., and Brekelmans, R. (2009). Assessing the effects of using demand parameters estimates in inventory control and improving the performance using a correction function. *International Journal of Production Economics* 118: 34–42.

Januschowski, T. and Kolassa, S. (2019). A classification of business forecasting problems. *Foresight: The International Journal of Applied Forecasting* 52: 36–43.

Jeuland, A.P., Bass, F.M., and Wright, G.P. (1980). A multibrand stochastic model compounding heterogeneous Erlang timing and multinomial choice processes. *Operations Research* 28: 255–277.

Johansen, S.G. and Thorstenson, A. (1993). Optimal and approximate (Q, r) inventory policies with lost sales and gamma-distributed lead time. *International Journal of Production Economics* 30–31: 179–194.

Johnson, M.E. and Davis, T. (1998). Improving supply chain performance by using order fulfillment metrics. *National Productivity Review*. 17 (3): 3–16.

Johnson, M.E., Lee, H.L., Davis, T., and Hall, R. (1995). Expressions for item fill rates in periodic inventory systems. *Naval Research Logistics* 42: 57–80.

Johnston, F.R. (1980). An interactive stock control system with a strategic management role. *Journal of the Operational Research Society* 31: 1069–1084.

Johnston, F.R. and Boylan, J.E. (1996). Forecasting for items with intermittent demand. *Journal of the Operational Research Society* 47: 113–121.

Johnston, F.R. and Harrison, P.J. (1986). The variance of lead-time demand. *Journal of the Operational Research Society* 37: 303–308.

Johnston, F.R., Boylan, J.E., Meadows, M., and Shale, E. (1999a). Some properties of a simple moving average when applied to forecasting a time series. *Journal of the Operational Research Society* 50: 1267–1271.

Johnston, F.R., Boylan, J.E., Shale, E., and Meadows, M. (1999b). A robust forecasting system, based on the combination of two simple moving averages. *Journal of the Operational Research Society* 50: 1199–1204.

Johnston, F.R., Boylan, J.E., and Shale, E. (2003). An examination of the size of orders from customers, their characterisation and the implications for inventory control of slow moving items. *Journal of the Operational Research Society* 54: 833–837.

Johnston, F.R., Shale, E.A., Kapoor, S. et al. (2011). Breadth of range and depth of stock: forecasting and inventory management at Euro Car Parts Ltd. *Journal of the Operational Research Society* 62: 433–441.

Johnston, F.R., Taylor, S.J., and Oliveria, R.M.M.C. (1988). Setting company stock levels. *Journal of the Operational Research Society* 39: 15–21.

Jung, R.C. and Tremayne, A.R. (2006). Coherent forecasting in integer time series models. *International Journal of Forecasting* 22: 223–238.

Kachour, M. (2014). On the rounded integer-valued autoregressive process. *Communications in Statistics - Theory and Methods* 43: 355–376.

Kachour, M. and Yao, J.F. (2009). First-order rounded integer-valued autoregressive (RINAR(1)) process. *Journal of Time Series Analysis* 30: 417–448.

Kahn, K.B. (1998). Benchmarking sales forecasting performance measures. *Journal of Business Forecasting* (Winter 1998-1999): 19–23.

Kahneman, D. (2011). *Thinking, Fast and Slow*. London: Allen Lane.

Kalchschmidt, M., Verganti, R., and Zotteri, G. (2006). Forecasting demand from heterogeneous customers. *International Journal of Operations and Production Management* 26: 619–638.

Katti, R. (2008). Some observations on the measurement of forecast error and accuracy. *Journal of Business Forecasting* (Summer 2008): 33–35.

KBV Research (2017). *Global Retail Analytics Market* (2017–2023). Available (for purchase) at: https://www.kbvresearch.com/news/retail-analytics-market/.

Kelle, P. and Silver, E.A. (1989). Forecasting the returns of reusable containers. *Journal of Operations Management* 8: 17–35.

Kennedy, W.J., Patterson, J.W., and Fredendall, L.D. (2002). An overview of recent literature on spare parts inventories. *International Journal of Production Economics* 76: 201–215.

Kim, S. and Kim, H. (2016). A new metric of absolute percentage error for intermittent demand forecasts. *International Journal of Forecasting* 32: 669–679.

Kim, S.-H., Cohen, M.A., and Netessine, S. (2007). Performance contracting in after-sales service supply chains. *Management Science* 53: 1843–1858.

Knod, E. and Schonberger, R. (2001). *Operations Management: Meeting Customer Demands*, 7e. New York: McGraw-Hill.

Kolassa, S. (2016). Evaluating predictive count distributions in retail sales forecasting. *International Journal of Forecasting* 32: 788–803.

Kolassa, S. (2020). Why the "best" point forecast depends on the error or accuracy measure. *International Journal of Forecasting* 36: 208–211.

Kolassa, S. and Hyndman, R.J. (2010). Free open-source forecasting using R. *Foresight: The International Journal of Applied Forecasting* 17: 19–24.

Kolassa, S. and Schütz, W. (2007). Advantages of the MAD/Mean ratio over the MAPE. *Foresight: The International Journal of Applied Forecasting* 6: 40–43.

Kostenko, A.V. and Hyndman, R.J. (2006). A note on the categorization of demand patterns. *Journal of the Operational Research Society* 57: 1256–1257.

Kourentzes, N. (2013). Intermittent demand forecasts with neural networks. *International Journal of Production Economics* 143: 198–206.

Kourentzes, N. (2014). On intermittent demand model optimisation and selection. *International Journal of Production Economics* 156: 180–190.

Kourentzes, N. and Athanasopoulos, G. (2019). Cross-temporal coherent forecasts for Australian tourism. *Annals of Tourism Research* 75: 393–409.

Kourentzes, N. and Athanasopoulos, G. (2020). Elucidate structure in intermittent demand series. *European Journal of Operational Research* 228: 141–152.

Kwan, H.W. (1991). *On the demand distributions of slow-moving items*. PhD thesis. University of Lancaster, UK.

Larsen, C. and Thorstenson, A. (2008). A comparison between the order and the volume fill rate for a base-stock inventory control system under a compound renewal demand process. *Journal of the Operational Research Society* 59: 798–804.

Latour, A. (1998). Existence and stochastic structure of a non-negative integer-valued autoregressive process. *Journal of Time Series Analysis* 19: 439–455.

Ledwina, T. (1994). Data-driven version of Neyman's smooth test of fit. *Journal of the American Statistical Association* 89: 1000–1005.

Lengu, D., Syntetos, A.A., and Babai, M.Z. (2014). Spare parts management: linking distributional assumptions to demand classification. *European Journal of Operational Research* 235: 624–635.

Lewis, C.D. (1981). *Scientific Inventory Control*, 2e. London: Butterworths.

Liang, L. and Atkins, D. (2013). Designing service level agreements for inventory management. *Production and Operations Management* 22: 1103–1117.

Liboschik, T., Fokianos, K., and Fried, R. (2017). tscount: An R package for analysis of count time series following generalized linear models. *Journal of Statistical Software* 82: 1–51.

Lolli, F., Gamberini, R., Regattieri, A. et al. (2017). Single-hidden layer neural networks for forecasting intermittent demand. *International Journal of Production Economics* 183: 116–128.

Makridakis, S. (1993). Accuracy measures: theoretical and practical concerns. *International Journal of Forecasting* 9: 527–529.

Makridakis, S. and Hibon, M. (2000). The M3-competition: results, conclusions and implications. *International Journal of Forecasting* 16: 451–476.

Makridakis, S., Spiliotis, E., and Assimakopoulos, V. (2018). The M4 competition: results, findings, conclusion and way forward. *International Journal of Forecasting* 34: 802–808.

Makridakis, S., Wheelwright, S.C., and Hyndman, R.J. (1998). *Forecasting: Methods and Applications*, 3e. New York, NY: Wiley.

Manufacturing Management (G. Devine) (2018). *After-sales service is the key profit-lever for 2018*. https://www.manufacturingmanagement.co.uk/features/after-sales-service-is-the-key-profit-lever-for-2018.

Mathews, B.P. and Diamantopoulos, A. (1986). Managerial intervention in forecasting. An empirical investigation of forecast manipulation. *International Journal of Research in Marketing* 3: 3–10.

Mathews, B.P. and Diamantopoulos, A. (1989). Factors affecting subjective revision in forecasting. A multi-period analysis. *International Journal of Research in Marketing* 6: 283–293, 296–297.

Mathews, B.P. and Diamantopoulos, A. (1992). Judgemental revision of sales forecasts: the relative performance of judgementally revised versus non-revised forecasts. *Journal of Forecasting* 11: 569–576.

McKenzie, E. (1985). Some simple models for discrete variate time series. *Water Resources Bulletin* 21: 645–650.

McKenzie, E. (1988). Some ARMA models for dependent sequences of Poisson counts. *Advances in Applied Probability* 20: 822–835.

Mohammadipour, M. (2009). *Intermittent demand forecasting with integer autoregressive moving average models*. PhD thesis. Buckinghamshire New University, Brunel University, UK.

Mohammadipour, M. and Boylan, J.E. (2012). Forecast horizon aggregation in integer autoregressive moving average (INARMA) models. *Omega* 40: 703–712.

Molenaers, A., Baets, H., Pintelon, L., and Waeyenbergh, G. (2012). Criticality classification of spare parts: a case study. *International Journal of Production Economics* 140: 570–578.

Morlidge, S. (2015). Measuring the quality of intermittent–demand forecasts: it's worse than we've thought! *Foresight: The International Journal of Applied Forecasting* 37: 37–42.

Morlidge, S. (2018). *The Little (Illustrated) Book of Operational Forecasting*. Kibworth Beauchamp: Matador.

Motiwalla, L. and Thompson, J. (2014). *Enterprise Systems for Management*, 2e. Harlow: Pearson Education.

Mukhopadhyay, S., Solis, A., and Guttierez, R.S. (2012). The accuracy of non-traditional versus traditional methods of forecasting lumpy demand. *Journal of Forecasting* 31: 721–735.

Muller, M. (2019). *Essentials of Inventory Management*, 3e. Nashville, TN: Harpercollins Focus.

Naddor, E. (1975). Optimal and heuristic decisions in single- and multi-item inventory systems. *Management Science* 21: 1234–1249.

Nahmias, S. and Demmy, W.S. (1982). The logarithmic Poisson gamma distribution: a model for leadtime demand. *Naval Research Logistics Quarterly* 29: 667–677.

Neal, P. and Rao, T.S. (2007). MCMC for integer-valued ARMA processes. *Journal of Time Series Analysis* 28: 92–110.

Nikolopoulos, K. (2021). We need to talk about intermittent demand forecasting. *European Journal of Operational Research*. 291: 549–559.

Nikolopoulos, K., Babai, M.Z., and Bozos, K. (2016). Forecasting supply chain sporadic demand with nearest neighbor approaches. *International Journal of Production Economics* 177: 139–148.

Nikolopoulos, K., Syntetos, A.A., Boylan, J.E. et al. (2011). An aggregate–disaggregate intermittent demand approach (ADIDA) to forecasting: an empirical proposition and analysis. *Journal of the Operational Research Society* 62: 544–554.

Nuel, G. (2008). Cumulative distribution function of a geometric Poisson distribution. *Journal of Statistical Computation and Simulation* 78: 385–394.

Ord, J.K. and Bagchi, U. (1983). The truncated normal-gamma mixture as a distribution for lead time demand. *Naval Research Logistics Quarterly* 30: 359–365.

Ord, K., Fildes, R., and Kourentzes, N. (2017). *Principles of Business Forecasting*, 2e. New York, NY: Wessex Press.

Ord, J.K., Koehler, A.B., and Snyder, R.D. (1997). Estimation and prediction for a class of dynamic nonlinear models. *Journal of the American Statistical Association* 92: 1621–1629.

Ozaki, T. (1977). On the order determination of ARIMA models. *Journal of the Royal Statistical Society: Series C (Applied Statistics)* 26: 290–301.

Özel, G. and İnal, C. (2010). The probability function of a geometric Poisson distribution. *Journal of Statistical Computation and Simulation* 80: 479–487.

Park, C. (2007). An analysis of the lead time demand distribution derivation in stochastic inventory systems. *International Journal of Production Economics* 105: 263–272.

Pearson, R.L. and Wallace, W.A. (1999). *Appropriate measures of forecast error for business decision making*. Presented at the 19th International Symposium on Forecasting, Washington DC, USA. https://www.researchgate.net/publication/342479669_Appropriate_measures_of_forecast_error_for_business_decision_making.

Petropoulos, F. and Kourentzes, N. (2015). Forecast combinations for intermittent demand. *Journal of the Operational Research Society* 66: 914–924.

Petropoulos, F., Fildes, R., and Goodwin, P. (2016). Do 'big losses' in judgmental adjustments to statistical forecasts affect experts' behaviour? *European Journal of Operational Research* 249: 842–852.

Petropoulos, F., Kourentzes, N., Nikolopoulos, K., and Siemsen, E. (2018). Judgmental selection of forecasting models. *Journal of Operations Management* 60: 34–46.

Petropoulos, F., Nikolopoulos, K., Spithourakis, G.P., and Assimakopoulos, V. (2013). Empirical heuristics for improving intermittent demand forecasting. *Industrial Management and Data Systems* 113: 683–696.

Popper, K.R. (1959). *The Logic of Scientific Discovery*. New York, NY: Basic Books.

Popovic, J.B. (1987). Decision making on stock levels in cases of uncertain demand rate. *European Journal of Operational Research* 32: 276–290.

Porras, E. and Dekker, R. (2008). An inventory control system for spare parts at a refinery: an empirical comparison of different re-order point methods. *European Journal of Operational Research* 184: 101–132.

Porteus, E.L. (1985). Numerical comparisons of inventory policies for periodic review systems. *Operations Research* 33: 134–152.

Prak, D.R.J. (2019). *Practice-inspired contributions to inventory theory*. PhD thesis. The Netherlands: University of Groningen.

Prak, D., Teunter, R., and Syntetos, A. (2017). On the calculation of safety stocks when demand is forecasted. *European Journal of Operational Research* 256: 454–461.

Prestwich, S.D., Rossi, R., Tarim, S.A., and Hinch, B. (2014a). Mean-based error measures for intermittent demand forecasting. *International Journal of Production Research* 52: 6782–6791.

Prestwich, S.D., Tarim, S.A., Rossi, R., and Hinch, B. (2014b). Forecasting intermittent demand using hyperbolic–exponential smoothing. *International Journal of Forecasting* 30: 928–933.

Prichard, J.W. and Eagle, R.H. (1965). *Modern Inventory Management*. New York, NY: Wiley.

Ptak, C.A. and Smith, C.J. (2011). *Orlicky's Material Requirements Planning*, 3e. New York, NY: McGraw Hill.

Rao, A.V. (1973). A comment on: Forecasting and stock control for intermittent demands. *Operational Research Quarterly* 24: 639–640.

Regattieri, A., Gamberi, M., Gamberini, R., and Manzini, R. (2005). Managing lumpy demand for aircraft spare parts. *Journal of Air Transport Management* 11: 426–431.

Rego, J.R. and Mesquita, M.A. (2015). Demand forecasting and inventory control: a simulation study on automotive spare parts. *International Journal of Production Economics* 161: 1–16.

Rekik, Y., Syntetos, A.A., and Glock, C.H. (2019). *Inventory inaccuracy in retailing: does it matter? Efficient Consumer Response (ECR) report*. https://www.cardiff.ac.uk/parc-institute-manufacturing-logistics-inventory/research/publications/industry-insights.

Research Excellence Framework (REF) (2014). *Intermittent demand categorization and forecasting (Impact case study)*. http://impact.ref.ac.uk/CaseStudies/CaseStudy.aspx?Id=9144.

Ritchie, E. and Kingsman, B.G. (1985). Setting stock levels for wholesaling: performance measures and conflict of objectives between supplier and stockist. *European Journal of Operational Research* 20: 17–24.

Romeijnders, W., Teunter, R., and van Jaarsveld, W. (2012). A two-step method for forecasting spare parts demand using information on component repairs. *European Journal of Operational Research* 220: 386–393.

Rostami-Tabar, B., Babai, M.Z., Syntetos, A., and Ducq, Y. (2013). Demand forecasting by temporal aggregation. *Naval Research Logistics* 60: 479–498.

Rostami-Tabar, B., Babai, M.Z., Syntetos, A., and Ducq, Y. (2014). A note on the forecast performance of temporal aggregation. *Naval Research Logistics* 61: 489–500.

Sanders, N.R. and Manrodt, K.B. (2003). The efficacy of using judgmental versus quantitative forecasting methods in practice. *Omega* 31: 511–522.

Sani, B. (1995). *Periodic inventory control systems and demand forecasting methods for low demand items*. PhD thesis. Lancaster University, UK.

Sani, B. and Kingsman, B.G. (1997). Selecting the best periodic inventory control and demand forecasting methods for low demand items. *Journal of the Operational Research Society* 48: 700–713.

Schultz, C.R. (1987). Forecasting and inventory control for sporadic demand under periodic review. *Journal of the Operational Research Society* 38: 453–458.

Segerstedt, A. (1994). Inventory control with variation in lead times, especially when demand is intermittent. *International Journal of Production Economics* 35: 365–372.

Shale, E.A., Boylan, J.E., and Johnston, F.R. (2006). Forecasting for intermittent demand: the estimation of an unbiased average. *Journal of the Operational Research Society* 57: 588–592.

Shale, E.A., Boylan, J.E., and Johnston, F.R. (2008). Characterizing the frequency of orders received by a stockist. *IMA Journal of Management Mathematics* 19: 137–143.

Shenstone, L. and Hyndman, R.J. (2005). Stochastic models underlying Croston's method for intermittent demand forecasting. *Journal of Forecasting* 24: 389–402.

Sherbrooke, C.C. (1968). Discrete compound Poisson processes and tables of the geometric Poisson distribution. *Naval Research Logistics Quarterly* 15: 189–203.

Silver, E.A., Pyke, D.F., and Thomas, D.J. (2017). *Inventory and Production Management in Supply Chains*, 4e. Boca Raton, FL: CRC Press.

Smart, C.N. (2002). Accurate intermittent demand forecasting for inventory planning: new technologies and dramatic results. *Proceedings of APICS 2002 International Conference*, Nashville, TN. White paper version available at: http://www.scribd.com/document/230239300/Intermittent-Demand-Forecasting-White-Paper.

Smart, C.N. and Willemain, T.R. (2000). Get real - a new way to forecast intermittent demand. *APICS - the Performance Advantage*: June 2000, 64–68.

Smith, M. and Babai, M.Z. (2011). A review of bootstrapping for spare parts forecasting. In: *Service Parts Management: Demand Forecasting and Inventory Control* (ed. N. Altay and L.A. Litteral). London: Springer-Verlag. 125–141.

Smith, M.A.J. and Dekker, R. (1997). On the (*S-1,S*) stock model for renewal demand processes: Poisson's poison. *Probability in the Engineering and Informational Sciences* 11: 375–386.

Snapp, S. (2018). How should a company set service levels? Perception vs. reality. *Foresight: The International Journal of Applied Forecasting* 49: 11–17.

Snook, B., Taylor, P.J., and Bennell, C. (2004). Cognitive profiling: the fast, frugal and accurate way. *Applied Cognitive Psychology* 18: 105–121.

Snyder, R.D. (1984). Inventory control with the gamma probability distribution. *European Journal of Operational Research* 17: 373–381.

Snyder, R.D. (1985). Recursive estimation of dynamic linear models. *Journal of the Royal Statistical Society: Series B (Methodological)* 47: 272–276.

Snyder, R.D. (2002). Forecasting sales of slow and fast moving inventories. *European Journal of Operational Research* 140: 684–699.

Snyder, R.D., Koehler, A.B., Hyndman, R.J., and Ord, J.K. (2004). Exponential smoothing models: means and variances for lead-time demand. *European Journal of Operational Research* 158: 444–455.

Snyder, R.D., Koehler, A.B., and Ord, J.K. (1999). Lead time demand for simple exponential smoothing: an adjustment factor for the standard deviation. *Journal of the Operational Research Society* 50: 1079–1082.

Snyder, R.D., Ord, J.K., and Beaumont, A. (2012). Forecasting the intermittent demand for slow-moving inventories: a modelling approach. *International Journal of Forecasting* 28: 485–496.

Sobel, M.J. (2004). Fill rates of single-stage and multistage supply systems. *Manufacturing and Service Operations Management* 6: 41–52.

Soll, J.B. and Klayman, J. (2004). Overconfidence in interval estimates. *Journal of Experimental Psychology: Learning, Memory, and Cognition* 30: 299–314.

Sterman, J.D. (1989). Modeling managerial behaviour: misperceptions of feedback in a dynamic decision making environment. *Management Science* 35: 321–339.

Steutel, F.W. and van Harn, K. (1979). Discrete analogues of self-decomposability and stability. *The Annals of Probability* 7: 893–899.

Stevens, C.F. (1974). On the variability of demand for families of items. *Operational Research Quarterly* 25: 411–419.

Strijbosch, L.W.G. and Moors, J.J.A. (2005). The impact of unknown demand parameters on (R,S)-inventory control performance. *European Journal of Operational Research* 162: 805–815.

Strijbosch, L.W.G., Heuts, R.M.J., and van der Schoot, E.H.M. (2000). A combined forecast-inventory control procedure for spare parts. *Journal of the Operational Research Society* 51: 1184–1192.

Strijbosch, L.W.G., Moors, J.J.A., and de Kok, A.G. (1997). On the Interaction between Forecasting and Inventory Control. *Research Memorandum FEW 742*. Faculty of Economics and Business Administration, Tilburg University, The Netherlands.

Sugiura, N. (1978). Further analysis of the data by Akaike's information criterion and the finite corrections. *Communications in Statistics - Theory and Methods* 7: 13–26.

Svetunkov, I. and Boylan, J.E. (2019). *Multiplicative state space models for intermittent time series*. Lancaster University Management School working paper. https://www.researchgate.net/publication/320910865_Multiplicative_State-Space_Models_for_Intermittent_Time_Series/link/5e2cb987299bf152167e1d61/download.

Svetunkov, I. and Petropoulos, F. (2018). Old dog, new tricks: a modelling view of simple moving averages. *International Journal of Production Research* 56: 6034–6047.

Svetunkov, I. and Sagaert, Y.R. (2020). *Greybox: Toolbox for model building and forecasting. R package*. https://cran.r-project.org/web/packages/greybox/index.html.

Syntetos, A.A. (2001). *Forecasting of intermittent demand*. PhD thesis. Buckinghamshire Chilterns University College, Brunel University, UK.

Syntetos, A.A. (2011). *Notes from After Sales Advanced Planning* (ASAP: www.asapsmf.org) CEO meeting, Florence, Italy, 21 September 2011.

Syntetos, A.A. and Boylan, J.E. (2001). On the bias of intermittent demand estimates. *International Journal of Production Economics* 71: 457–466.

Syntetos, A.A. and Boylan, J.E. (2005). The accuracy of intermittent demand estimates. *International Journal of Forecasting* 21: 303–314.

Syntetos, A.A. and Boylan, J.E. (2006). On the stock control performance of intermittent demand estimators. *International Journal of Production Economics* 103: 36–47.

Syntetos, A.A. and Boylan, J.E. (2008). Demand forecasting adjustments for service-level achievement. *IMA Journal of Management Mathematics* 19: 175–192.

Syntetos, A.A. and Boylan, J.E. (2010). On the variance of intermittent demand estimates. *International Journal of Production Economics* 128: 546–555.

Syntetos, A.A., Babai, M.Z., Boylan, J.E. et al. (2016a). Supply chain forecasting: theory, practice, their gap and the future. *European Journal of Operational Research* 252: 1–26.

Syntetos, A.A., Kholidasari, I., and Naim, M.M. (2016b). The effects of integrating management judgement into OUT levels: in or out of context? *European Journal of Operational Research* 249: 853–863.

Syntetos, A.A., Babai, M.Z., Dallery, Y., and Teunter, R. (2009a). Periodic control of intermittent demand items: theory and empirical analysis. *Journal of the Operational Research Society* 60: 611–618.

Syntetos, A.A., Keyes, M., and Babai, M.Z. (2009b). Demand categorisation in a European spare parts logistics network. *International Journal of Operations and Production Management* 29: 292–316.

Syntetos, A.A., Nikolopoulos, K., Boylan, J.E. et al. (2009c). The effects of integrating management judgement into intermittent demand forecasts. *International Journal of Production Economics* 118: 72–81.

Syntetos, A.A., Babai, M.Z., Davies, J., and Stephenson, D. (2010). Forecasting and stock control: a study in a wholesaling context. *International Journal of Production Economics* 127: 103–111.

Syntetos, A.A., Babai, M.Z., and Gardner, E.S. (2015a). Forecasting intermittent inventory demands: simple parametric methods vs. bootstrapping. *Journal of Business Research* 68: 1746–1752.

Syntetos, A.A., Babai, M.Z., and Luo, S. (2015b). Forecasting of compound Erlang demand. *Journal of the Operational Research Society* 66: 2061–2074.

Syntetos, A.A., Boylan, J.E., and Croston, J.D. (2005). On the categorization of demand patterns. *Journal of the Operational Research Society* 56: 495–503.

Syntetos, A.A., Boylan, J.E., and Teunter, R. (2011a). Classification for forecasting and inventory. *Foresight: The International Journal of Applied Forecasting* 20: 12–17.

Syntetos, A.A., Georgantzas, N.C., Boylan, J.E., and Dangerfield, B.C. (2011b). Judgement and supply chain dynamics. *Journal of the Operational Research Society* 62: 1138–1158.

Syntetos, A.A., Lengu, D., and Babai, M.Z. (2013). A note on the demand distribution of spare parts. *International Journal of Production Research* 51: 6356–6358.

Taleb, N.N. (2007). *The Black Swan: The Impact of the Highly Improbable*. New York, NY: Random House.

Tashman, L.J. and Hoover, J. (2001). Diffusion of forecasting principles through software. In: *Principles of Forecasting* (ed. J.S. Armstrong). Dordrecht: Kluwer. 631–676.

Taylor, C.J. (1961). The application of the negative binomial distribution to stock control problems. *Operational Research Quarterly* 12: 81–88.

Teunter, R.H. (2009). Note on the fill rate of single-stage general periodic review inventory systems. *Operations Research Letters* 37: 67–68.

Teunter, R.H. and Duncan, L. (2009). Forecasting intermittent demand: a comparative study. *Journal of the Operational Research Society* 60: 321–329.

Teunter, R.H. and Sani, B. (2009a). Calculating order-up-to levels for products with intermittent demand. *International Journal of Production Economics* 118: 82–86.

Teunter, R.H. and Sani, B. (2009b). On the bias of Croston's forecasting method. *European Journal of Operational Research* 194: 177–183.

Teunter, R.H., Babai, M.Z., and Syntetos, A.A. (2010). ABC classification: service levels and inventory costs. *Production and Operations Management* 19: 343–352.

Teunter, R.H., Syntetos, A.A., and Babai, M.Z. (2011). Intermittent demand: linking forecasting to inventory obsolescence. *European Journal of Operational Research* 214: 606–615.

Teunter, R.H., Syntetos, A.A., and Babai, M.Z. (2017). Stock keeping unit fill rate specification. *European Journal of Operational Research* 259: 917–925.

Thomopoulos, N.T. (2015). *Demand Forecasting for Inventory Control*. Switzerland: Springer International.

Thonemann, U.W., Brown, A.O., and Hausman, W.H. (2002). Easy quantification of improved spare parts inventory policies. *Management Science* 48: 1213–1225.

Tokar, T., Aloysius, J., Williams, B., and Waller, M. (2014). Bracing for demand shocks: an experimental investigation. *Journal of Operations Management* 32: 205–216.

Trimp, M.E., Sinnema, S.M., Dekker, R., and Teunter, R.H. (2004). Optimise Initial Spare Parts Inventories: An Analysis and Improvement of an Electronic Decision Tool. *Econometric Institute Report 2004-52*. The Netherlands: Erasmus University. https://ideas.repec.org/p/ems/eureir/1830.html.

Turrini, L. and Meissner, J. (2019). Spare parts inventory management: new evidence from distribution fitting. *European Journal of Operational Research* 273: 118–130.

Tavares, L.V. and Almeida, L.T. (1983). A binary decision model for the stock control of very slow moving items. *Journal of the Operational Research Society* 34: 249–252.

Van der Auweraer, S., Boute, R.N., and Syntetos, A.A. (2019). Forecasting spare part demand with installed base information: a review. *International Journal of Forecasting* 35: 181–196.

Van Wingerden, E., Basten, R.J.I., Dekker, R., and Rustenburg, W.D. (2014). More grip on inventory control through improved forecasting: a comparative study at three companies. *International Journal of Production Economics* 157: 220–237.

Veinott, A.F. and Wagner, H.M. (1965). Computing optimal (s, S) inventory policies. *Management Science* 11: 525–552.

Verganti, R. (1997). Order overplanning with uncertain lumpy demand: a simplified theory. *International Journal of Production Research* 35: 3229–3248.

Viswanathan, S. and Zhou, C. (2008). *A new bootstrapping based method for forecasting and safety stock determination for intermittent demand items*. Working paper, Nanyang Business Schoool, Nanyang Technological University, Singapore. (Available from Prof. S. Viswanathan, on request.)

Wagner, H.M. (1975). *Principles of Management Science (with Applications to Executive Decisions)*, 2e. Englewood Cliffs, NJ: Prentice-Hall.

Waller, M.A., Williams, B.D., and Eroglu, C. (2008). Hidden effects of variable order review intervals in inventory control. *International Journal of Physical Distribution and Logistics Management* 38: 244–258.

Wallin, C., Rungtusanatham, M.J., and Rabinovich, E. (2006). What is the "right" inventory management approach for a purchased item? *International Journal of Operations and Production Management* 26: 50–68.

Wallström, P. and Segerstedt, A. (2010). Evaluation of forecasting error measurements and techniques for intermittent demand. *International Journal of Production Economics* 128: 625–636.

Weiß, C.H. (2007). Controlling correlated processes of Poisson counts. *Quality and Reliability Engineering International* 23: 741–754.

Weller, M. and Crone, S. (2012). *Supply Chain Forecasting: Best Practices and Benchmarking Study*. Lancaster University, Lancaster Centre for Forecasting. https://www.lancaster.ac.uk/media/lancaster-university/content-assets/documents/lums/forecasting/practitionerpapers/Weller_Crone_Techical_Report_Supply_Chain_Forecasting_Best_Practices_and_Benchmarking_Study.pdf.

Willemain, T.R. (2006). Forecast-accuracy metrics for intermittent demands: look at the entire distribution of demand. *Foresight: The International Journal of Applied Forecasting* 4: 36–38.

Willemain, T.R. (2018). Choosing and achieving a target service level. *Foresight: The International Journal of Applied Forecasting* 49: 6–10.

Willemain, T.R. and Hartunian, N.S. (2013). *Cluster based processing for forecasting intermittent demand*. US Patent, Patent No. US 2013/0166350 A1. https://patents.google.com/patent/US20130166350A1/en.

Willemain, T.R. and Smart, C.N. (2001). *System and method for forecasting intermittent demand*. US Patent, Patent No. US 6,205,431 B1. https://patents.google.com/patent/US6205431B1/en.

Willemain, T.R., Smart, C.N., and Schwarz, H.F. (2004). A new approach to forecasting intermittent demand for service parts inventories. *International Journal of Forecasting* 20: 375–387.

Willemain, T.R., Smart, C.N., Shockor, J.H., and DeSautels, P.A. (1994). Forecasting intermittent demand in manufacturing: a comparative evaluation of Croston's method. *International Journal of Forecasting* 10: 529–538.

Woodward, R.H. and Goldsmith, P.L. (1964). *Cumulative Sum Techniques*, I.C.I. Monograph No. 3 in the 'Mathematical and statistical techniques for industry' series. Edinburgh: Oliver and Boyd.

Wright, D.J. (1986). Forecasting data published at irregular time intervals using an extension of Holt's method. *Management Science* 32: 499–510.

Wübben, M. and Von Wangenheim, F. (2008). Instant customer base analysis: managerial heuristics often "get it right". *Journal of Marketing* 72: 82–93.

Zhang, J. and Zhang, J. (2007). Fill rate of single-stage general periodic review inventory systems. *Operations Research Letters* 35: 503–509.

Zhang, R.Q., Hopp, W.J., and Supatgiat, C. (2001). Spreadsheet implementable inventory control for a distribution center. *Journal of Heuristics* 7: 185–203.

Zhou, C. and Viswanathan, S. (2011). Comparison of a new bootstrapping method with parametric approaches for safety stock determination in service parts inventory systems. *International Journal of Production Economics* 133: 481–485.

Zhu, S., Dekker, R., van Jaarsveld, W. et al. (2017). An improved method for forecasting spare parts demand using extreme value theory. *European Journal of Operational Research* 261: 169–181.

Author Index

Intermittent Demand Forecasting: Context, Methods and Applications, First Edition.
John E. Boylan and Aris A. Syntetos.
© 2021 John Wiley & Sons Ltd. Published 2021 by John Wiley & Sons Ltd.
Companion Website: www.wiley.com/go/boylansyntetos/intermittentdemandforecasting

Subject Index

Intermittent Demand Forecasting: Context, Methods and Applications, First Edition.
John E. Boylan and Aris A. Syntetos.
© 2021 John Wiley & Sons Ltd. Published 2021 by John Wiley & Sons Ltd.
Companion Website: www.wiley.com/go/boylansyntetos/intermittentdemandforecasting